Review Manual for the

Certified Healthcare Simulation

Educator™ (CHSE™) Exam

Linda Wilson, PhD, RN, CPAN, CAPA, BC, CNE, CHSE, CHSE-A, ANEF, FAAN, is an assistant dean for Special Projects, Simulation, and Continuing Nursing Education Accreditation, and an associate clinical professor at Drexel University, College of Nursing and Health Professions in Philadelphia, Pennsylvania. Dr. Wilson completed her bachelor of science in nursing (BSN) at Misericordia University in Dallas, Pennsylvania, and completed her master of science in nursing (MSN) in critical care and trauma at Thomas Jefferson University in Philadelphia. She completed her PhD in nursing research at Rutgers, the State University of New Jersey in Newark. Dr. Wilson has also obtained a postgraduate Certificate in Epidemiology and Biostatistical Methods from Drexel University and a postgraduate Certificate in Pain Management from the University of California, San Francisco. Dr. Wilson has dual certification in simulation: Certified Healthcare Simulation Educator™ (CHSE™) and Certified Healthcare Simulation Educator Advanced (CHSE-A), along with several additional certifications. Dr. Wilson served as the president of the American Society of Perianesthesia Nurses (2002–2003) and has been serving as site appraiser for the ANCC (American Nurses Credentialing Center) Commission on Accreditation, American Nurses Association, from 2000 to the present. Dr. Wilson is the project director/primary investigator for SimTeam: The Joint Education of Health Professionals and Assistive Personnel Students in a Simulated Environment, a project funded by the Barra Foundation Inc. Dr. Wilson is also the project director/primary investigator for Faculty Development: Integrating Technology into Nursing Education and Practice, a nearly $1.5 million, 5-year project funded by the Health Resources and Services Administration (HRSA), Department of Health and Human Services (Grant # 1 U1KHP09542-01-00). Dr. Wilson is also the coeditor of *Human Simulation for Nursing and Health Professions* published by Springer Publishing Company.

Ruth A. Wittmann-Price, PhD, RN, CNS, CNE, CHSE, ANEF, is chairperson and professor at Francis Marion University, Department of Nursing, in South Carolina. Dr. Wittmann-Price has been an obstetrical/women's health nurse for 35 years. She received her associate of applied science (AAS) and BSN degrees from Felician College in Lodi, New Jersey (1978, 1981); and her master's in science as a perinatal clinical nurse specialist (CNS) from Columbia University, New York, New York (1983). Dr. Wittmann-Price completed her PhD at Widener University, Chester, Pennsylvania (2006), and was awarded the Dean's Award for Excellence. She developed a midrange nursing theory, Emancipated Decision-Making in Women's Health Care. She was the coordinator for the nurse educator track in the DrNP (Doctor of Nursing Practice) program at Drexel University in Philadelphia (2007–2010) and the director of Nursing Research for Hahnemann University Hospital (2007–2010), overseeing all evidence-based practice projects for nursing. The Hahnemann University Hospital was awarded initial Magnet status (American Nurses Credentialing Center) in December 2009. Dr. Wittmann-Price has taught all levels of nursing students over the past 15 years (AAS, BSN, MSN, DNP, PhD) and is a part of three dissertation committees on decisional science. At Francis Marion University, she developed the simulation program, the MSN program, an interprofessional rural health initiative, and is on the steering committee that is developing a physician assistant program. She has published over 20 articles and is coeditor and chapter contributor to 12 books and series editor of Nursing Test Success, a series of unfolding case studies, published by Springer Publishing Company. She has presented regionally, nationally, and internationally.

Review Manual for the Certified Healthcare Simulation Educator™ (CHSE™) Exam

Linda Wilson, PhD, RN, CPAN, CAPA, BC, CNE, CHSE, CHSE-A, ANEF, FAAN

Ruth A. Wittmann-Price, PhD, RN, CNS, CNE, CHSE, ANEF

Editors

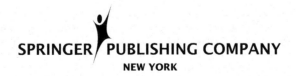

SPRINGER PUBLISHING COMPANY
NEW YORK

Springer Publishing Company, LLC
11 West 42nd Street
New York, NY 10036
www.springerpub.com

Acquisitions Editor: Margaret Zuccarini
Composition: Exeter Premedia Services Private Ltd.

ISBN: 978-0-8261-2011-3
e-book ISBN: 978-0-8261-2012-0

18 / 7

The Certified Healthcare Simulation Educator™ and CHSE™ marks are trademarks of the Society for Simulation in Healthcare. This manual is an independent publication and is not endorsed, sponsored, or otherwise approved by the Society. SSH is not liable or responsible for any errors, omissions or timeliness of the information or data available in this manual, any individual's negligence in connection with the manual, or any other liability resulting from the use or misuse of the manual.

The author and the publisher of this Work have made every effort to use sources believed to be reliable to provide information that is accurate and compatible with the standards generally accepted at the time of publication. Because medical science is continually advancing, our knowledge base continues to expand. Therefore, as new information becomes available, changes in procedures become necessary. We recommend that the reader always consult current research and specific institutional policies before performing any clinical procedure. The author and publisher shall not be liable for any special, consequential, or exemplary damages resulting, in whole or in part, from the readers' use of, or reliance on, the information contained in this book. The publisher has no responsibility for the persistence or accuracy of URLs for external or third-party Internet websites referred to in this publication and does not guarantee that any content on such websites is, or will remain, accurate or appropriate.

Library of Congress Cataloging-in-Publication Data
Review manual for the Certified Healthcare Simulation Educator™ (CHSE™) exam / Linda Wilson, Ruth A. Wittmann-Price, editors.
    p. ; cm.
  Includes bibliographical references.
  ISBN 978-0-8261-2011-3—ISBN 978-0-8261-2012-0 (e-book)
  I. Wilson, Linda, 1962– editor.   II. Wittmann-Price, Ruth A., editor.
  [DNLM: 1. Patient Simulation—Problems and Exercises.   2. Teaching—Problems and Exercises.   3. Certification—Problems and Exercises.   4. Health Occupations—education—Problems and Exercises.   W 18.2]
  R834.5
  610.76—dc23

                                                                                              2014023141

Special discounts on bulk quantities of our books are available to corporations, professional associations, pharmaceutical companies, health care organizations, and other qualifying groups. If you are interested in a custom book, including chapters from more than one of our titles, we can provide that service as well.

For details, please contact:
Special Sales Department, Springer Publishing Company, LLC
11 West 42nd Street, 15th Floor, New York, NY 10036-8002
Phone: 877-687-7476 or 212-431-4370; Fax: 212-941-7842
E-mail: sales@springerpub.com

Printed in the United States of America by Gasch Printing.

Contents

SECTION IV: USING SIMULATION TO EDUCATE AND ASSESS LEARNERS

SECTION V: MANAGING SIMULATION RESOURCES AND ENVIRONMENT

SECTION VI: ENGAGE IN SCHOLARLY ACTIVITY

Contributors

Deborah S. Arnold, MSN, RN, CMSRN, CHSE Manager of the Transform Patient and Safety Program, Sentara Healthcare, Chesapeake, Virginia

Anthony Battaglia, MS, BSN, RN Corporate Counsel, Pocket Nurse, Monaca, Pennsylvania

Melanie Leigh Cason, MSN, RN, CNE Simulation Nurse Educator, Collaborative Partner Coordinator, Health Care Simulation South Carolina (HCSSC), Medical University of South Carolina, Charleston, South Carolina

Brittny D. Chabalowski, RN, MSN, CEN, CNE, CHSE Instructor, Program Director, Upper Division/2nd Degree Nursing Sequence, Coordinator, Undergraduate Simulation, University of South Florida, Tampa, Florida

Deborah Coltrane, MBA, MSN, RN Director of Corporate Relations and Education, Pocket Nurse, Monaca, Pennsylvania

John T. Cornele, MSN, RN, CEN, EMT-P, CNE Director, Center for Interdisciplinary Clinical Simulation & Practice, Drexel University College of Nursing and Health Professions, Philadelphia, Pennsylvania

Mark C. Crider, PhD, MSN Assistant Professor and Chair of Undergraduate Programs, Duquesne University School of Nursing, Pittsburgh, Pennsylvania

Anthony Errichetti, PhD, CHSE Chief of Virtual Medicine, Director, MS in Medical/Health Care Simulation, New York Institute of Technology—College of Osteopathic Medicine, Old Westbury, New York

Rosemary Fliszar, PhD, RN, CNE Director, RN-BSN Program and Assistant Professor II, Rider University, Lawrenceville, New Jersey

Karen K. Gittings, DNP, RN, CNE, Alumnus CCRN Assistant Professor of Nursing, Francis Marion University, Florence, South Carolina

Mary Ellen Smith Glasgow, PhD, RN, CS, FAAN Dean and Professor, Duquesne University School of Nursing, Pittsburgh, Pennsylvania

Crystal Graham, MSN-Ed, RN, CHSE Instructor and Simulation Coordinator, Francis Marion University, Florence, South Carolina

Sharon Griswold, MD, MPH   Associate Professor of Emergency Medicine, Director, Simulation Division, Department of Emergency Medicine, Director, Master's Degree in Medical/Healthcare Simulation, Drexel University College of Medicine, Philadelphia, Pennsylvania

Bonnie A. Haupt, DNP(c), MSN, RN, CNL, CHSE   Clinical Nurse Leader, VA Connecticut Healthcare System; Acute Care Clinical Nurse Leader, Providence Veterans Administration Medical Center, Providence, Rhode Island

Terry Kirk, EdD, RN, NEA-BC   Associate Clinical Professor, School of Nursing, University of Houston–Victoria, Houston, Texas

Frances Wickham Lee, DBA, CHSE   Professor, College of Health Professions, Director of Instructional Operations, HCSSC, Medical University of South Carolina, Charleston, South Carolina

Colleen H. Meakim, MSN, RN, CHSE   Director of Simulation and Learning Resources, Villanova University College of Nursing, Villanova, Pennsylvania

Kymberlee Montgomery, DrNP, WHNP-BC, CNE   Nurse Faculty Leadership Fellow, Department Chair, Nurse Practitioner Program, Assistant Clinical Professor, Drexel University College of Nursing and Health Professions, Philadelphia, Pennsylvania

Kate Morse, PhD, CRNP-BC, CNE, CCRN   Jonas Scholar Alumni, Director, Graduate Interprofessional Simulation, Assistant Clinical Professor, Drexel University College of Nursing and Health Professions, Philadelphia, Pennsylvania

Nina Multak, MPAS, PA-C   Associate Clinical Professor, Physician Assistant Department, Drexel University College of Nursing and Health Professions, Philadelphia, Pennsylvania

Judy I. Murphy, PhD, RN, CNE, CHSE   VA Nursing Academic Partner Faculty and Simulation Coordinator, Providence Veterans Administration Medical Center and Rhode Island College, Providence, Rhode Island

Carol Okupniak, DNP, RN-BC Nursing Informatics   Assistant Clinical Professor, Drexel University College of Nursing and Health Professions, Philadelphia, Pennsylvania

Gregory J. Owsik, MD   Department of Emergency Medicine, Drexel University College of Medicine, Philadelphia, Pennsylvania

Fabien Pampaloni, BSN, RN   International Business Affairs Specialist, Pocket Nurse, Monaca, Pennsylvania

Samuel W. Price, MFA   Research, Technology, and Events Assistant, Drexel University College of Nursing and Health Professions, Philadelphia, Pennsylvania

Leland J. (Rocky) Rockstraw, PhD, RN   Assistant Dean, Simulation, Clinical and Technology Academic Operations, Associate Clinical Professor, Drexel University College of Nursing and Health Professions, Philadelphia, Pennsylvania

Carolyn H. Scheese, MS, RN, CHSE   Assistant Professor, Director, RN to BS in Nursing Program, College of Nursing, University of Utah, Salt Lake City, Utah

Beth A. Telesz, MSN, RN   SimEMR, Customer Service and Education Manager, Pocket Nurse, Monaca, Pennsylvania

Brenda Reap Thompson, MSN, RN, CNE   Assistant Clinical Professor, Drexel University College of Nursing and Health Professions, Philadelphia, Pennsylvania

Linda Wilson, PhD, RN, CPAN, CAPA, BC, CNE, CHSE, CHSE-A, ANEF, FAAN   Assistant Dean for Special Projects, Simulation and Continuing Nursing Education Accreditation; Associate Clinical Professor, Drexel University College of Nursing and Health Professions, Philadelphia, Pennsylvania

Ruth A. Wittmann-Price, PhD, RN, CNS, CNE, CHSE, ANEF   Professor and Chairperson, Department of Nursing, Francis Marion University, Florence, South Carolina

Foreword

I've been a teacher for a very long time and have used many teaching tools and techniques to impart knowledge to students. I have mastered the art of the lecture and can hold most classes captive, although every now and then I need to work extra hard to maintain the students' attention. The seminar, whether in person or online, is one of my favorite teaching methods—10 to 12 students, cogent questions prepared in advance, in-depth discussion of multifaceted issues, wrap-up, and a cataloguing of student "takeaways." *And then there is simulation—the most powerful pedagogy of all.* Whether learning and practicing psychomotor skills on high-fidelity mannequins or engaging with patient actors in complex healthcare scenarios—simulation takes teaching and learning to the next level, the iterative level, where both student and teacher learn; the former about the complex world of practice in a safe learning environment and the latter about how students perceive, think, and respond to the complexity of practice situations.

I know that had I experienced simulation in my own education, I would have been a more effective nurse in a shorter period of time. My teachers would have designed the most common, yet compelling, scenarios in which I could practice and reflect on my knowledge and skill application and my thought and decision-making processes. Simulation is about the deconstruction of complexity in healthcare and nursing education. It is a pedagogy through which both teachers and students can explore the rationale for clinical action, gain insights, and make corrections and updates to the knowledge and skill base. Simulation is a pedagogy that enriches both teacher and student; it fires the imagination and heightens awareness of the complexity of attentional, interpersonal, and cognitive processes in clinical care.

The authors of this review manual have captured all of the elements of simulation, from establishing the objectives of simulated learning experiences, to constructing scenarios, to debriefing students and the simulation team, to assessing and evaluating the learning that has accrued. They have also described the range of simulation options and the contexts for their most effective use. Learning everything that you can about simulation and applying that knowledge in your role as a teacher ensures that you are contributing ultimately to promoting positive patient outcomes in the future.

Gloria F. Donnelly, PhD, RN, FAAN, FCPP
Dean and Professor
Drexel University
College of Nursing and Health Professions

Preface

This book was created as an interprofessional, international project to assist healthcare simulation educators become certified for the very important work that is being accomplished during every simulation experience around the world. Simulation is one of the mechanisms needed to improve patient safety because it teaches healthcare providers interprofessional collaboration, communication, and cooperation like never before in the history of healthcare. Becoming certified in simulation is a wonderful step to promoting excellence in healthcare education, and we applaud your efforts.

This book will be an invaluable resource in the certification process. The contributing authors have analyzed the certification test plan (Society for Simulation in Healthcare [SSH], 2014) in order to bring you all the important information that may be presented on the examination and placed it in a user-friendly format. The information is divided into short chapters. The authors are simulation and education experts who have added features that will assist in critically analyzing the content.

Teaching Tips are provided for those educators who would like further explanation and exploration of topics, many of which provide practical hints to incorporate into simulation experiences. *Evidence-Based Simulation Practice (EBSP)* boxes assist you in focusing on the current simulation research. *Case Studies* and *Practice Questions* at the end of each chapter promote critical thinking and situational decision making.

Section I includes Chapter 1, which covers the specifics of the examination, the activities needed to reach advanced certification, and recertification. Chapter 2 concentrates on the current certification test plan. Chapter 3 provides you with test-taking strategies, which are always beneficial for "the student in all of us."

Section II discusses professional values and capabilities in relation to teaching with simulation. Chapter 4 covers leadership in educational simulation. Chapter 5 includes special considerations about simulation experiences with learners and describes learning styles.

Section III reviews foundational knowledge about simulation and includes a chapter on the theoretical background of learning using simulation (Chapter 6). Integrating simulation education into a professional healthcare curriculum is discussed in Chapter 7, and the legal and ethical issues that are sometimes encountered with simulation experiences are fully explored in Chapter 8.

Other foundational issues include principles, practice, and methodologies related to the human patient simulator (Chapter 9), along with the art of moulage (Chapter 10). Standardized patient simulation is the topic of Chapter 11, and Chapter 12 talks about using hybrid simulation. A separate chapter reviews using task trainers as a valuable learning experience (Chapter 13). Chapter 14 addresses interprofessional simulation experiences, and two chapters (Chapter 15 and Chapter 16) are devoted to the very important postsimulation experiences of debriefing and providing learners with feedback. Chapter 17 provides important information about the ever-increasing use of virtual reality as a teaching/learning tool.

Section IV focuses on the practicalities of simulation laboratories (Chapter 18). Chapter 19 discusses planning, implementing, and evaluating the learners using simulation activities.

Section V reviews simulation laboratory resource management and the environment considerations (Chapter 20). Chapter 21 reviews accreditation and standards of simulation laboratories.

Section VI addresses academic considerations of simulation educators, including professional development and career advancement (Chapter 22) and the role and current status of simulation research (Chapter 23). A simulated practice test begins the back matter of the book, which also contains answers and rationales to end-of-chapter tests and the practice test. Good luck!

Our hope in developing this review manual is that it will be another valuable tool to assist you in reaching your career goal of recognized excellence. We applaud your efforts as colleagues in the quest to educate the next generation of healthcare workers. We thank you for your efforts to recognize excellence in the simulation field and the very important role simulation plays in patient safety.

Linda Wilson
Ruth A. Wittmann-Price

Acknowledgments

To H. Lynn Kane, Helen "Momma" Kane, and Linda Webb, thank you for your amazing friendship and for being my family. To Lou Smith, Evan Babcock, and Steve Johnson, thank you for your friendship and support. To Sam Price, thank you for your endless help and support.

—*Linda Wilson*

Thank you to all my colleagues and friends who so graciously contributed to this awesome project and, of course, thank you to Margaret Zuccarini, whose publishing assistance and support is invaluable.

—*Ruth A. Wittmann-Price*

Overview of the Certification Examination, Advanced Certification, and Recertification

BRITTNY D. CHABALOWSKI

Do not go where the path may lead,
go instead where there is no path and leave a trail.
—Ralph Waldo Emerson

LEARNING OUTCOMES

- Describe the benefits of certification
- Review the requirements for initial certification
- Review the recertification process
- Describe the requirements for advanced certification

Obtaining specialty certification is a well-recognized way to demonstrate expertise, both in the clinical and academic setting. In both of these settings, healthcare educators have used simulation for many years. Simulation can range from simple task trainers to high-fidelity simulated patient care experiences. The goal of the complex patient-simulated experiences is to provide learners the opportunity to deliver care in high-risk, low-volume scenarios. These are situations that are seen infrequently in the clinical setting, but require swift and accurate intervention.

Unlike direct clinical instruction, simulation education requires a specialized skillset. Skilled healthcare simulation educators must be able to develop scenarios that are appropriate for the learners, administer the scenarios in a supportive atmosphere, and debrief the learners to complete an effective learning experience. It becomes clear that there is an "unmet need for a uniform mechanism to educate, evaluate, and certify simulation instructors for the health care profession" (McGaghie, Issenberg, Petrusa, & Scalese, 2010, p. 59).

Recognizing this need, the Society for Simulation in Healthcare (SSH) developed the basic certification examination and the advanced certification standards (SSH, 2014). The benefits of these certifications go beyond the individual or the individual's organization. One of the goals is to identify, recognize, and pool the knowledge of best practices. This will serve to standardize the unique body of knowledge that belongs to healthcare simulation educators.

INITIAL CERTIFICATION

- Eligibility
  - Bachelor's degree or equivalent (any candidate who does not have a bachelor's degree may petition the committee for consideration of equivalency based on experience)
  - Minimum of 2 years' experience in healthcare simulation setting
  - Demonstrate their simulation experience is focused on learners in healthcare at any level
  - Continued use of simulation in healthcare education, research, or administration in the past 2 years (SSH, 2014)
- Application
  - Can be completed online at https://ssih.org/certification
  - Includes information about simulation experience, education, and employment
  - Narrative descriptions required include
    - Relevant simulation-based educational activity that demonstrates evidence of your capabilities as a simulation-based educator
    - Relevant activities that demonstrate your advocacy for simulation-based education (this would include your activities at your place of employment, on the local level, as well as in professional societies)
    - Scholarly activities relevant to simulation-based education (such as participation in research, abstract preparation, publications, posters, workshops, curriculum development, and course construction)
  - Contact information for at least three references to complete the Confidential Structured Report of Performance (CSRP) online
  - Application processing takes approximately 3 weeks (SSH, 2014)
- Fees as of 2014
  - $395 for members of the SSH, the Association of Standardized Patient Educators (ASPE), and the International Nursing Association for Clinical Simulation & Learning (INACSL)
  - $495 for all others (SSH, 2014)
- Taking the test
  - Computer-based testing sites can be located on the ISO-Quality Testing, Inc., site: www.isoqualitytesting.com
  - Scheduled on a space-available basis
  - Must be taken within 90 days of application approval
  - Candidates are notified of results at the time of exam completion (SSH, 2014)

- Certification
  - Valid for 3 years from the successful completion of the exam
  - The initials of certification may be used as a credential after the candidate's name (SSH, 2014)

RECERTIFICATION/RENEWAL OF CERTIFICATION

- Retake the examination at or near the expiration date *or*
- Demonstrate ongoing professional development
  - Over the 3-year period, not just activity in a narrow time frame
  - In education or simulation-focused activities
  - Including, but not limited to:
    - Participation in continuing education (CE) activity such as attending conferences, webinars, or other education events
    - Publication of research, such as journal articles, chapters, books, or similar items
    - Presenting at educational events, such as conferences
- If the certification expires, candidates must reapply to take the exam and must meet the eligibility requirements in place at that time (SSH, 2014)

ADVANCED CERTIFICATION

- Eligibility
  - A basic certification
  - Participation in healthcare simulation in an educational role
  - Focused simulation expertise with learners in undergraduate, graduate, allied health, or healthcare courses
  - Master's degree or equivalent experience (any candidate who does not have a master's degree may petition the committee for consideration of equivalency based on experience)
  - Five years of continued use of simulation in healthcare education, research, or administration
- Application
  - Submission of an extensive portfolio, including a media submission and reflective statements
  - Portfolio is peer-reviewed and evaluated against the standards (SSH, 2014)

SUMMARY

The decision to prepare and take a certification examination is a personal and professional goal that will enhance your knowledge and ability. Both certifications promote the facilitation of the learning of future healthcare providers, and becoming certified will ultimately benefit patients receiving care. Congratulations on choosing to study and become a Certified Healthcare Simulation Educator™ to promote quality education that will benefit your students and all their patients.

REFERENCES

McGaghie, W. C., Issenberg, S. B., Petrusa, E. R., & Scalese, R. J. (2010). A critical review of simulation-based medical education research: 2003–2009. *Medical Education, 44,* 50–63.

Society for Simulation in Healthcare (SSH). (2014). *Certified healthcare simulation educator handbook.* Retrieved from http://ssih.org/certification/CHSE/handbook

The Certification Examination Test Plan

RUTH A. WITTMANN-PRICE

*We learn by example and by direct experience because there
are real limits to the adequacy of verbal instruction.*
—Malcolm Gladwell

LEARNING OUTCOMES

- Discuss the importance of certification in simulation for healthcare educators
- Discuss the specifics of the test plan
- Discuss case studies and practice questions as learning tools

For many reasons, simulation in healthcare education is here to stay. Simulation experiences provide a wealth of benefits for learners of educational organizations. The Society for Simulation in Healthcare (SSH) has developed the preliminary and advanced certifications to recognize healthcare educators who are experts in this important and growing field of using simulation to teach all aspects of healthcare delivery to improve patient safety.

The test plan for the examination was developed in 2011 and can be found in the SSH *Handbook* (2014) at http://ssih.org/certification/handbook. There are five broad areas covered by the exam, which include professional values and capabilities; knowledge of simulation principles, practice, and methodologies; educating and assessing learners; managing simulation resources; and engaging in scholarly activities as they pertain to simulation education. The largest number of questions on the test (52%) concentrate on the education and assessment of learners. Two test areas, professional values and scholarly activity, each comprise only 4% of the questions. Test questions regarding knowledge of simulation principles, practice, and methodologies comprise the second largest part of the test questions at 34%, and managing resources accounts for the final 6% (SSH, 2014).

The five major test areas listed above are broken down into criteria that are less general and therefore easier to dissect and understand. Each of those areas is discussed. It is understood that not all healthcare educators who teach in simulation laboratories are expert in all five areas, but for the test, each educator needs a working knowledge of every area. For example, a healthcare educator working in a large simulation laboratory may not be responsible for the stocking, ordering, or maintenance of the laboratory, but will need to have a working knowledge of the resources needed and used for simulation education.

CONTENT AREA 1: PROFESSIONAL VALUES AND CAPABILITIES

The first area of the test is the display of professional values and capabilities (SSH, 2014). This area includes

- Demonstrating leadership in the role of simulation education
- Acting as a role model and mentor to novice simulation educators
- Advocating for simulation within the educational unit and in the community
- Understanding diversity issues in the simulation environment just as an educator would in the clinical or classroom setting

Professional values and capabilities comprise only 4% of the test. So there may only be four or five questions pertaining to this area. Section II of this book (Chapters 4 and 5) discusses these content areas in depth. Below is a quick synopsis of each area.

Leadership

Leadership in simulation is thoroughly addressed in Chapter 4.

Transformational leadership, first described by Burns (1978), is the current leadership theory discussed in organizations and education. Transformational leaders are described as exhibiting positive attributes, which include

- Vision for future development
- The ability to engage others in the vision
- Developing values surrounding the vision
- Moving people toward the vision
- Effecting positive change (Bass, 1985)

Transformational leadership is different from *transactional leadership*. Transactional leadership is equated with more authoritarian management that directs people without motivating them. Some of the attributes associated with transactional leadership are

- Hierarchical decisions
- Institution of a reward-and-punishment system
- Micromanaging from the top of the organization (Motacki & Burke, 2011)

Role Modeling and Mentorship

The principles of role modeling and mentorship are based on Patricia Benner's (1982) novice-to-expert theory. Benner described five levels of expertise patterned on studies of how nurses grow in their role, and they include

A *novice* is a beginner with no experience who relies on

- General rules to help perform tasks
- Rules that are context-free, independent of specific cases, and applied universally
- Behavior that is limited and inflexible

An *advanced beginner* is at the point of demonstrating acceptable performance and

- Has gained prior experience in actual situations to recognize some patterns
- Uses principles, based on experiences, which begin to be formulated to guide actions

A *competent nurse* is typically a nurse with 2 to 3 years' experience in the same role and

- Is aware of long-term goals
- Has a perspective about planning care with conscious, abstract, and analytical thinking
- Has greater efficiency and organization

Proficient is a nurse who perceives and understands situations as a whole and

- Understands patients holistically and has improved decision making
- Learns from experiences what to expect in certain situations
- Is flexible and can modify plans of care

Expert is a nurse who no longer relies on principles, rules, or guidelines to understand patient needs and determine actions and

- Has an intuitive grasp of practice situations
- Is flexible and highly proficient

Although Benner's theory studied nurses, it has been applied to many healthcare professionals and learning situations. Mentorship programs are built on the understanding that a person can be an expert in one area, such as practice, while being a novice in another, such as healthcare education. Chapter 4 applies the theory directly to the development of simulation educators.

Advocating for Simulation

It is generally understood that the use of simulation was developed for two major purposes: to improve healthcare safety and increase educational experiences for learners. Even with positive educational student learning outcomes (SLOs) contributing to simulation's success, there is still resistance for its use from some educators. Part of the controversy hinges on how much simulation is appropriate in a curriculum. Currently, organizations are researching SLOs related to different percentages of clinical and simulation experiences for groups of learners (National Council State Boards of Nursing [NCSBN], 2013). Until investigational results are disseminated and the body of knowledge increases, simulation educators will need to use the positive studies already completed to increase the understanding of the benefits of simulation.

Additionally, simulation experiences can be expanded to community activities, for both the healthcare communities and the laity. Simulation can be an experience used in acute care, outpatient, and community settings. Disaster planning with simulation has made many groups aware of its educational ability. Whenever possible, all simulation educators should explain and demonstrate the positive learning experiences that can be attained through simulation.

Diversity

Simulation experiences provide a unique opportunity of a "safe space" for diversity issues as well as a platform to cultivate cultural awareness and humility among learners. Scenarios can easily contain culturally diverse characteristics with high-fidelity mannequins, standardized (simulated) patients (SPs), or healthcare professionals. Additionally, scenarios can be developed to assist learners to communicate with patients of diverse backgrounds, sexual orientation, and cultures to improve healthcare outcomes. Some current simulation scenarios include

- An adolescent telling his parents he is homosexual, which was a scenario demonstrated at the Drexel Simulation Conference in 2012
- A low-income immigrant family trying to obtain public resources
- A healthcare scene in which the patient does not speak English
- Eliciting complementary healthcare practices for patients of different cultures
- End-of-life issues from other cultures

The list of scenarios that can be created to develop learners' cultural sensitivity and understanding is endless.

CONTENT AREA 2: DEMONSTRATE KNOWLEDGE OF SIMULATION PRINCIPLES, PRACTICE, AND METHODOLOGY

The second content area covered in the examination makes up 34% of the examination or approximately 34 to 40 questions (SSH, 2014). It is divided into 18 criteria and 13 subcriteria, which are listed in the *Certified Healthcare Simulation Educator Handbook* (SSH, 2014). The chapters in this book address all areas, and before the introduction to each chapter, the criteria being addressed are stated.

CONTENT AREA 3: EDUCATE AND ASSESS LEARNERS USING SIMULATION

Content area 3 is the largest part of the test and comprises 52 to 60 questions (SSH, 2014). This section contains 5 major criteria and 18 subcriteria. The content in this section of the test comprises questions regarding the actual use of simulation with learners. Questions contain education scenarios, and you have to choose the correct assessment, plan, intervention, or

Simulation Teaching Tip 2.1
Introducing simulation experiences in the first semester of healthcare education may increase the learners' comfort level with the methodology as it is repeated semester after semester.

evaluation of the situation by the correct combination of educator and learner, learner and learner, learner and SP, or educator and SP. Expect application questions in which the knowledge from this area is applied to situations. Each of the criteria is also addressed in the upcoming, labeled chapters.

CONTENT AREA 4: MANAGE OVERALL SIMULATION RESOURCES AND ENVIRONMENTS

Content area 4 of the examination is made up of four criteria and comprises 6%—or six to seven questions—of the examination (SSH, 2014). This content area is addressed in depth in Chapters 20 and 21. The criteria under this content area are as follows

- Understand the basic operational principles associated with delivering simulation activities
- Assess and modify the physical environment to maximize simulation-based learning
- Follow policies, procedures, and practices of the simulation program
- Understand and respond to technical and material issues (e.g., video capture, simulator failures, material supplies)

Chapter 18 discusses how a simulation coordinator or educator sets up activities for the learners by

- Securing the administrative buy-in
- Arranging schedules
- Securing equipment
- Developing lesson plans
- Communicating with learners, simulation team members, and other educators
- Establishing policies for consistency and fairness

Chapter 19 addresses accreditation of simulation laboratories and provides information on stimulation standards, best practices, and benchmarking.

CONTENT AREA 5: ENGAGE IN SCHOLARLY ACTIVITIES

Content area 5 is 4%, or encompasses four to six questions of the exam. This area has three criteria, all related to professional development of the simulation educator. The criteria are

- Participation in professional development (e.g., conferences, courses)
- Identification and use of credible resources in simulation education (e.g., websites, listservs, literature)
- Understanding of the role of qualitative and quantitative research (SSH, 2014)

The importance of professional development cannot be underestimated, not only for examination purposes but also for self-development and the dissemination of simulation knowledge. Additionally, participating in simulation conferences as a participant or presenter will assist you in developing your professional "simulation education portfolio." Simulation educators will be in demand for years to come, and a portfolio will showcase your expertise; so begin collecting all your activities related to simulation education (Wittmann-Price, 2012). They will also be used for your certification renewal in 3 years and for supporting evidence for advanced certification; therefore, it is important to keep your documentation up to date and safe in a simulation education portfolio.

This last content area on the test also addresses two very important simulation elements: interdisciplinary education and research or *evidence-based simulation practice* (EBSP). Simulation activities that can be related to learning outcomes and patient safety increase knowledge for all healthcare professionals. Dissemination of project results is a professional obligation for all healthcare simulation educators.

EVIDENCE-BASED SIMULATION PRACTICE (EBSP) 2.1

Ammenwerth and colleagues (2012) used simulation to pilot a new computerized medication system in a safe environment. Fifty simulation attempts, using the new technology, were completed using physicians ($n = 5$) and SPs ($n = 10$). Simulation was used successfully to field-test technology in a more comprehensive manner than previously able with just laboratory testing but without the safety issues of testing technology in the clinical field.

CASE STUDY 2.1

Linda is an expert clinician hired as one of three educational coordinators for the simulation laboratory for undergraduate healthcare students. Linda is expert in the critical care units at the local acute care hospital. She is assisting in setting up a simulation experience for first-semester healthcare learners. During the experience, using a high-fidelity mannequin, Linda uses the computer controls to cause the patient to "code," and then in the debriefing, acknowledges that she thought the learners would know how to handle it better. How would you address this with Linda using Benner's theory?

PRACTICE QUESTIONS

1. A new simulation educator is hired in the simulation laboratory. The simulation educator who has been working at the laboratory for 5 years should be aware that when orientating the novice educator, the best method would be to

   A. Describe the purpose of simulation globally and then locally
   B. Have the novice educators observe first
   C. Teach the novice educator to evaluate learners
   D. Discuss step-by-step procedures for the activity

2. A healthcare educator is interviewing for a job as a simulation coordinator at a small, private institution. The educator asks about the simulation laboratory budget, and the administrative interviewer tells the educator that the budget has been set and that all the supplies needed have been purchased. The educator understands this type of leadership is

   A. Transactional
   B. Situational
   C. Laissez-faire
   D. Transformational

3. An administrator discusses the development of a simulation laboratory with a healthcare educator and states that the needs of the community must also be considered. What aspect of leadership is this demonstrating?

   A. Negotiation
   B. Resources management
   C. Strategic planning
   D. Governance

4. An expert simulation educator is hired and states that at his previous place of employment, they used highly effective high-fidelity simulation and that this institution would benefit from purchasing a better equipped mannequin. You know that the current budget will not allow the purchase; therefore, your best answer is

   A. "We can put it on our wish list."
   B. "There are many methods to do effective simulation."
   C. "Can you think of a way to raise funds?"
   D. "We don't have the money for that."

5. Which of the following activities by a simulation educator would not be considered as professional development?

   A. Taking the role of the SP in a culturally sensitive situation
   B. Presenting a poster about simulation at a general education conference
   C. Developing a simulation education portfolio to demonstrate to other educators the depth and breadth of simulation learning
   D. Surveying learners about their anxiety pre- and postsimulation experience

6. During a scenario debriefing, a learner is questioning the simulation educator about his simulation evaluation grade. The educator describes the learner's behavior and tells him, calmly and professionally, that the behavior is inappropriate. The simulation educator asks the learner to dialogue with her about appropriate ways to address the issue. This situation best describes

   A. Mentoring
   B. Leadership
   C. Educating
   D. Role modeling

7. An educator is asked to play a belligerent family member during a scenario and states the he is uncomfortable playing that role in front of learners because it may cause them to disrespect him. As a seasoned simulation educator your best response would be

    A. "I understand your concern but it is important that you participate."
    B. "You should not worry about such things; we are pretending."
    C. "The simulation laboratory is safe space, so do not worry."
    D. "All learners have been instructed on the nature of the simulation environment."

8. A learner tells the novice simulation educator who is demonstrating on a task trainer that he is doing the procedure wrong. The best response to the learner would be

    A. "This is the way we do it in practice."
    B. "I think I have more experience than you."
    C. "Please do not interrupt during the procedure; we can discuss it afterward."
    D. "Please show me the procedural steps in your textbook."

9. The education department's leader tells the simulation team that he can envision the simulation program growing and eventually making money for the institution by doing simulated team-building exercises for local organizations. The simulation team members regard the leader as

    A. Transactional
    B. Transformational
    C. Hierarchical
    D. Inspirational

10. The simulation educator has been in her role for several years, but needs a better understanding when she states that simulation resources involve

    A. "Administrative support"
    B. "Current financial concerns of the institution"
    C. "Legal and ethical concerns"
    D. "Laboratory personnel"

REFERENCES

Ammenwerth, E., Hackl, W. O., Binzer, K., Christoffersen, T. E. H., Jensen, S., Lawton, K., . . . Nohr, C. (2012). Simulation studies for the evaluation of health information technologies: Experiences and results. *Health Information Management Journal, 41*(2), 14–21.

Bass, B. M. (1985). *Leadership and performance beyond expectation*. New York, NY: Free Press.

Benner, P. (1982). From novice to expert. *American Journal of Nursing, 82*(3), 402–407.

Burns, J. M. (1978). *Leadership*. New York, NY: Harper & Row.

Gladwell, M. (2005). *Blink: The power of thinking without thinking*. New York, NY: Little, Brown.

Motacki, K., & Burke, K. (2011). *Nursing delegation and management of patient care*. St. Louis, MO: Mosby.

National Council State Boards of Nursing (NCSBN). (2013). *National simulation study.* Retrieved from https://www.ncsbn.org/2094.htm

Society for Simulation in Healthcare (SSH). (2014). *Certified healthcare simulation educator handbook.* Retrieved from http://ssih.org/certification/handbook

Wittmann-Price, R. A. (2012). *Fast facts for developing a nursing academic portfolio.* New York, NY: Springer Publishing.

Test-Taking Strategies

BRENDA REAP THOMPSON

Education is not preparation for life; education is life itself.
—John Dewey

LEARNING OUTCOMES

- Identify the process to best prepare for the certification examination
- Discuss tips for success to promote understanding of key concepts
- Describe how to integrate standards from practice into information that is outlined in the examination blueprint
- Discuss how to improve comprehension by eliminating anxiety related to test taking

WHY BECOME CERTIFIED IN SIMULATION?

Simulation allows the student or healthcare professional the ability to become involved in a valuable learning experience, which may not have been present in clinical practice. A former student told me that she was hired to work in a step-down unit. The first day on the job, her patient coded. Students may receive the theory and possibly a case study about the appropriate response during a specific healthcare emergency, but may not observe this situation until they are licensed and are responsible for the patient. Practicing in a simulation can better prepare the student for these types of situations and ultimately improve patient outcomes. Simulation allows the student to "think on her feet" in a controlled clinical environment instead of relying on learning theory while sitting in the classroom. Faculty may be surprised when students who score well on written exams are unable to provide an accurate assessment, react appropriately when a patient has a deteriorating medical condition, or communicate effectively with other members of the healthcare team. As educators and clinicians, it is our responsibility to provide simulations that develop individual and team skills as well as promote clinical reasoning to improve the competency of healthcare providers.

Educators and clinicians with years of experience in simulation can now validate their expertise and knowledge by certification. Obtaining a certification is an invaluable resource for the current system for the progression of future role models, mentors, and visionaries. The following list outlines a few of the ways in which those who are certified can affect the healthcare environment.

- Support patient safety guidelines
- Close the gap between theory and practice
- Provide standardization of practice within healthcare
- Impact patient outcomes and quality improvement
- Develop evidence-based practice and research

ARE YOU A QUALIFIED CANDIDATE TO TAKE THE EXAMINATION?

Ask yourself the following questions.

1. Have I participated in simulation within a healthcare arena?
2. Have I assumed an educational role during the experience?
3. Was the simulation developed to concentrate on learners in allied health programs or healthcare practitioners?
4. Do I have a baccalaureate degree or an equivalent experience?
5. Have I used simulation in healthcare education, research, or administration continuously over the past 2 years?

The certification committee can be contacted if there is a question regarding requirements (SSH, 2014).

HOW TO PREPARE FOR SUCCESS

- Set up a study schedule. Everyone studies differently, but it is best to set up a study calendar so you don't become overwhelmed. Make sure you have enough time to study before securing an examination date. Print the information that is available from the *SSH Certified Healthcare Simulation Educator Handbook* (2014) at http://ssih.org/chse/handbook.
- Use charts and diagrams to organize information so you can review at a glance. These visual aids also allow the learner to compare and contrast content.
- Practice questions on a routine basis. This will provide the learner with the ability to recognize gaps in knowledge. Schedule time to research the content that was incorrect on the practice exams.
- Look at the list of examination preparation references, most of which are journal publications. It is to your advantage to read multiple articles related to the categories, which carry the highest percentage of the examination.
- Group information that is related. Focusing on one topic at a time will help you to remember information by comparing and contrasting content. Use the concept of the deep learning approach by critically examining new facts and making links between ideas. It is also helpful to relate new knowledge to previous

knowledge. Adequate time management will allow you to understand content thoroughly and have confidence. If you are overworked and do not have enough time to study, there is a tendency to use the surface approach to learning, which is good for short-term memory only. This entails storing new facts as isolated information and may result in high anxiety (Biggs, 1999; Wittmann & Fasolka, 2010).

- Organize a study group with your colleagues. Reviewing information while in a group may be worthwhile if all members of the group are committed and prepared for the study sessions. It is essential for the group to stay focused. Studying with representatives of various healthcare disciplines can be a valuable learning experience. Discussion and debate are critical for those who are auditory learners.

- Develop mnemonics or checklists. In order to promote patient safety and standardization of care, mnemonics and checklists have been developed to promote a quick memory aid in specific situations. Mnemonics are used in Advanced Cardiac Life Support (ACLS) certification to recall algorithms. Healthcare professionals also use the SBAR mnemonic to promote optimal communication during patient handoff.

S = Situation

B = Background

A = Assessment

R = Recommendations

There is a tremendous amount of information to remember, so you may want to develop your own mnemonics while you study.

- Healthcare professionals always care for others; now it is time to take care of yourself. Even though you feel that you deserve a sweet high-calorie dessert for all your hard work—think energy and brain power. Blueberries, strawberries, red beets, broccoli, tomatoes, pomegranate juice, vegetable juice, and nuts can enhance your brain power. Whole-grain foods, nuts, and legumes have a low glycemic index and release glucose into the bloodstream slowly, which provides energy, for hours. Keep your body hydrated by drinking at least eight glasses of water daily (Table 3.1).

> **Simulation Teaching Tip 3.1**
> When designing a simulation experience, think about activities to enhance different types of learning styles. Students can access the VARK website (http://www.vark-learn.com /english/index.aspquestionnaire) to determine how they learn best (Fleming, 2001).

KNOW YOUR EQUIPMENT/TECHNOLOGY

- **Task trainers**—used to practice procedures, such as wound care and intravenous (IV) insertion.
- **Human patient simulators**—mannequin-based equipment in human form.

TABLE 3.1 Key Topics for Discussion in Your Review	
The designing stage	Determine a needs assessment by deciding whether cognitive, behavioral, and technical issues will be incorporated into the scenario. Determine the participants—individual, team, systems. Define the goals for the activity. Develop measurable learning objectives. Write the scenario and integrate complications, distractions, and roles. Select the tool that will be used to evaluate the participants.
The planning stage	Organize the simulation team. Schedule the simulation laboratory with time allocated for setup, scenario, and reorganization of the environment. Determine whether the simulation will be videotaped. Reserve the capital equipment needed for the scenario. Schedule standardized (simulated) patients (SPs) if needed. Plan the scene setting. Determine the type of moulage needed. Make a list of supplies and drugs to be used in the scenario. Prepare written information for the simulation team.
The implementation stage	Provide an overview of the goals and objectives. Orient the participants to the environment and the equipment. Brief the participants about the scenario. Assess the participants related to the objectives. Determine how to respond to unforeseen issues during simulation, such as equipment failure, drugs or equipment missing, unprofessional behavior, and knowledge gaps.
The postsimulation stage	Debriefing can include evaluation by self, peers, or faculty. Provide time, and schedule the room to view the video (if indicated). Know the debriefing models. Understand the responsibility of the facilitator.

- **Virtual reality simulation**—used to provide a computer-based simulation experience sometimes with the use of an avatar.
- **Standardized (simulated) patients (SPs)**—the use of actors to simulate patients in a standardized manner.
- **Hybrid simulation methodology**—a simulation that incorporates multiple types of simulation, with one being used to enhance the other. A task trainer can be used with an SP to provide a hybrid simulation experience.
- **Mixed simulation**—a simulation that incorporates multiple types of simulation, with each being a tool for educational purposes.

BECOME FAMILIAR WITH COMPUTERIZED TESTING

- Read directions for answering questions carefully. There is usually a tutorial for you to familiarize yourself with the process. Make sure you understand the directions that explain how to pause the test if you need to take a break.
- Pay attention to information such as how to change answers.
- If you are unsure of the answer, you can bookmark the question and return to it when you have completed the remainder of the test. Do not waste time on a question if you are unsure of the answer.
- Check the clock intermittently so you have time to answer all questions.

INCORPORATE STRATEGIES TO EASE THE FEAR OF TEST ANXIETY

It is normal to have some test anxiety about taking a certification examination.

- Anxiety is a natural response to new challenges in our lives.
- Some anxiety will cause heightened awareness and may improve test taking, whereas anxiety that is uncontrolled will impede the ability to think critically.
- Everyone who takes tests experiences some anxiety; however, recognizing and controlling anxiety is an important factor.

Some strategies that can be used to ease test anxiety include

1. Reduce anxiety related to time constraints.
   - Schedule the examination when you have a work schedule that is less stressful.
   - Start a study group and plan to meet once a week for 2 hours.
     - Use a detailed test plan to divide assignments.
     - Each member of the study group can complete an assignment and share notes with the group.
     - Each member of the group can also share the sources of information.

2. Reduce anxiety related to having limited experience in taking tests.
   - Develop a checklist by writing a list of content that concerns you, and cross each one off when you have mastered it.
   - Practice the questions in the book and review the rationales.
   - Self-evaluation will assist you in refocusing on specific content.
   - Practice will increase your confidence.

3. Reduce anxiety related to previous unfavorable testing experience.
   - Stop negative thoughts that begin with "what if."
   - Use positive affirmations about your goal, such as "I can answer more questions correctly" or "I understand that information now."
   - Take time each day to exercise; practice yoga or meditate.

Practice these strategies on a regular basis so that reducing anxiety becomes easy to achieve. Engage in activities that you find relaxing on the evening prior to the examination, such as watching a movie or going out to dinner with friends.

> **Simulation Teaching Tip 3.2**
> Anxious learners should write about their test-related concerns for approximately 8 to 10 minutes prior to testing. This will result in scoring closer to their potential (Beilock, 2010).

USE STRATEGIES TO BE A SAVVY TEST TAKER

Read or Misread

Read each question carefully, and determine the key words that provide details for answering the question. Misreading the question can dramatically change the objective of the question.

Visualization

If a simulation is described and you are unsure of the answer, close your eyes. Picture the scenario in your mind prior to answering the question.

Changing Answers

If you are sure you need to change an answer—do it. However, if you usually change answers from correct to incorrect—don't do it.

Understand the Types of Questions Developed From Cognitive Levels of Learning

Bloom's taxonomy of learning is used to determine whether the candidate has mastered definitive skills or competencies. The easiest or lower level questions would be within the knowledge or comprehension category. These questions include recalling or demonstrating an understanding of concepts. Chances are that you will not be responsible for answering many of these types of questions because of their uncomplicated nature.

When you study—think application. Application questions expect the candidate to provide an intervention to the problem. There is usually a large percentage of these questions. In such questions it would be important to apply ideas, concepts, principles, or theories to solve a problem. Exhibit 3.1 demonstrates an application question.

Analysis questions will also be evident. These questions expect a logical response to the detailed cause and effect after examining information or reports. This provides an opportunity to break down the relationship between the parts and decide how the whole functions. Ask yourself why a solution worked or

EXHIBIT 3.1

Example: During a simulation, the learners fail to recognize a negative response after a medication is administered. What action by the simulation facilitator would be most appropriate?

A. Decrease the other distractions in the environment.
B. Instruct the confederate to provide some information.
C. Continue the simulation as originally planned.
D. Stop the simulation.

The answer is: (C) Continue the simulation because this situation occurs in healthcare frequently.

It is important for the scenario to play out because it is a learning experience. The issue would be addressed and discussed during debriefing.

didn't work. Your conclusion should always be supported by facts or results. Keep this in mind while you study for the certification exam. Exhibit 3.2 is an example of an analysis question.

EXHIBIT 3.2

Example: A human simulation experience was designed as a formative assessment for learners who were midway through the nursing program. The learners stated that the experience was too difficult. Which information about the simulation experience should the educator examine first?

A. Course grades of the learners involved in the simulation
B. Training of the standardized (simulated) patients
C. Planning details of the encounter
D. Feedback from the standardized (simulated) patients (SPs)

The answer is: (D) Feedback from the SPs.

Learners are usually very anxious about simulation, which may alter their evaluation of the experience. Verbal feedback from the SPs as well as the information from the checklists will provide accurate information.

Another category within the high-level questions is synthesis (Exhibit 3.3). These types of questions are not used frequently in testing situations, but could be used in simulation because they require creating plans or constructing solutions to problems. All elements are combined into a unified whole to develop a tool or design a plan.

EXHIBIT 3.3

Example: Data has determined that the patient wait time in the emergency department has increased by 20% within the last quarter. The patient visits and patient acuity have remained the same. Three extra full-time RNs and one clerk have been hired within the past 11 months. Six months ago, a boarding area was constructed to accommodate patients waiting for inpatient beds to open. The manager decides to design a simulation experience for the team to promote best practice. What should be the focus of the simulation?

A. Perfecting skills
B. Team building
C. Effective communication
D. Use of ancillary staff

The answer is: (B) Team building.

The data that was collected does not reflect the fact that the nursing staff has increased and the boarding area is operational. Staff must communicate effectively, perfect their skills, and use ancillary staff appropriately. These issues would all be encompassed in team building.

Evaluation will also be tested to provide the candidate with the opportunity to make value judgments based on effectiveness of a simulation design, scenario progression, patient outcomes, or equipment. Exhibit 3.4 provides an evaluation question.

EXHIBIT 3.4

Example: The RN to BSN (bachelor of science in nursing) nursing program has 375 learners at present. This is an increase of 20% in 1 year. Approximately 60% of the class attends online. After evaluating the program, determine what equipment/technology should be discussed during the upcoming budget meeting.

A. Nasogastric (NG) and tracheostomy care trainer
B. Harvey, the cardiopulmonary patient simulator
C. Wound care trainer
D. Virtual reality simulation

The answer is: (D) Virtual reality simulation.

Learners attending online classes continue to increase. This technology would be accessible to those attending the classes live as well as those attending online. If the learners are already RNs, they should have skills to care for patients with NG tubes and tracheostomies. Skills as well as heart and lung sounds are available in most virtual simulation programs.

Keep in mind that the simulation certification is available to all healthcare professionals who have met the eligibility requirements. Therefore, the global approach to reviewing information for this examination is critical. Positive patient outcomes rely on the multidisciplinary approach to quality care. Think about concepts in relation to the types of questions (application, analysis, synthesis, evaluation) that will be tested. Examine your own activities as an educator and in practice and relate them to the content in the questions.

CASE STUDY 3.1

A course chair requested that faculty teaching the course use a simulation the last week of the term. There were five sections of the course. The goal was to provide a safe environment for learners to use assessment techniques and fundamental nursing skills with the use of a high-fidelity mannequin. The educators were provided with a choice of four different scenarios, objectives, lists of equipment, and medications needed for each simulation. A self-evaluation tool was also available for learners to complete after the simulation.

After the completion of the term, the course chair received multiple e-mails from learners stating that their section never had an opportunity to experience a simulation. The two sections involved were taught by the same educator. How would you approach this issue if you were the course chair?

RECERTIFICATION

The credential gained by passing the certification examination is valid for a total of 3 years from the date it was awarded. In order to recertify, you must submit an application for renewal. There are two options to meet the recertification standards.

1. Retake the certification examination by the expiration date from the original date of certification.
2. Demonstrate ongoing continued professional development that focuses on education or simulation activities.

Professional development includes
- Continued activity in simulation within the past 3 years
- Attendance at conferences, webinars, or other educational programs
- Presentations at educational conferences
- Publishing of journals articles, book chapters, or books (SSH, 2014)

Simplify the recertification process.
- Keep a record of specific activities, the dates, and continuing education (CE) credits accrued.
- Keep the original hard copies of certificates of attendance in a folder. Scan the certificates into a folder to maintain an electronic copy. Additional copies are important because original copies can become lost or damaged within the time period.
- Submit an application for renewal and other specified information outlined by the SSH approximately 8 weeks before the due date.

PRACTICE QUESTIONS

1. At a faculty meeting, a healthcare educator states that simulation cannot take the place of "real" clinical practice. The best response would be that simulation

   A. "Is not meant to take the place of clinical practice"
   B. "Is more productive than clinical practice"
   C. "Has advantages and disadvantages like all learning activities"
   D. "Is an adjunct to clinical practice"

2. A goal that high-fidelity simulation education does not usually support is

   A. Providing standardization for evaluation of learners
   B. Self-learning strategies
   C. Improved quality patient care
   D. Effective patient safety initiatives

3. Candidates eligible to sit for the Certified Healthcare Simulation Educator™ (CHSE™) exam may

   A. Be a healthcare administrator who has a simulation lab in the organizational structure
   B. Have a master's degree in a healthcare education discipline
   C. Understand the importance of simulation
   D. Develop simulation scenarios for healthcare learners

4. An important goal of simulation is

   A. Learner assessment
   B. Managing simulation resources
   C. Understanding simulation principles
   D. Developing professional values

5. An effective method of studying for many examination candidates would be

   A. Independent studying
   B. Using mnemonics
   C. Memorizing details
   D. Elevating anxiety to a point for action

6. A candidate taking a computerized test is anxious because the questions appear to be progressing in difficulty, and the candidate can narrow the answers down to two distracters for each question. The candidate is probably experiencing questions written at which level of Bloom's taxonomy?

   A. Application
   B. Comprehension
   C. Knowledge
   D. Understanding

7. A reason to become certified as a simulation healthcare educator is to

   A. Better understand teaching with simulation
   B. Develop scenarios that can be widely used by others
   C. Publish about simulation techniques
   D. Validate expertise in an area

8. The ultimate goal for having an interdisciplinary certification for healthcare simulation educators rather than discipline-specific certification is to

   A. Promote interdisciplinary conferences
   B. Clarify roles in patient care
   C. Promote quality patient care
   D. Develop collaboration

9. Clinical learning differs from simulated clinical experiences for healthcare in the concepts of

   A. Patient safety
   B. Procedural accuracy
   C. Interprofessional communication
   D. Deliberate practice

10. During a simulation experience, the learner is asked to review the patient's complete laboratory data, x-rays, and health history, and come up with a diagnosis. This type of scenario develops clinical decision making and uses a skillset on which level of Bloom's taxonomy?

    A. Evaluation
    B. Application
    C. Comprehension
    D. Knowledge

REFERENCES

Beilock, S. (2010). *Choke: What the secrets of your brain reveal about getting it right when you have to.* New York, NY: Free Press Simon & Schuster.

Biggs, J. (1999). What the student does: Teaching for enhanced learning. *Higher Education Research & Development, 18*(1), 57–75.

Fleming, N. (2001). *VARK a guide to learning styles.* Retrieved from http://www.vark-learn .com/english/page.asp?p=categories

Society for Simulation in Healthcare (SSH). (2014). *Certified healthcare simulation educator handbook.* Retrieved from http://ssih.org/certification/handbook

Wittmann-Price, R. A., & Fasolka, B. (2010). Objectives and outcomes: The fundamental difference. *Nursing Education Perspective, 31*(4), 233–236. doi:10.1043/1536-5026-31.4.233

Leadership in Simulation

BRITTNY D. CHABALOWSKI

The task of the leader is to get people from where they are to
where they have not been.
—Henry A. Kissinger

This chapter addresses Content Area 1: Display Professional Values
and Capabilities (Society for Simulation in Healthcare [SSH], 2014).

LEARNING OUTCOMES

- Discuss the role of certification in simulation leadership
- Discuss activities that contribute to leadership in simulation
- Review resources available for faculty development in simulation instruction

Simulation in healthcare requires experienced, confident, and well-trained educators. However, without any formal simulation education training available, experienced educators are responsible for passing along the bulk of this knowledge to novice educators. Demonstration of leadership in the field includes development of future simulation educators.

In addition to building the unique body of simulation knowledge, educators are responsible for understanding and disseminating best practices. Leadership in the field of simulation education includes innovation and collaboration. Activities that demonstrate leadership include publication, presentation, and continued training. Sharing experiences in simulation and novel ideas builds the specialty and improves the delivery of simulation education on a large scale.

As a leader in the field of simulation education, being a champion of this pedagogy is a principal responsibility. The use of simulation as a teaching strategy can be intimidating for experienced educators because many did not use high-fidelity simulation in their own educational process. Being an enthusiastic mentor to novice simulation educators will have a monumental impact on the specialty of simulation education.

KNOWLEDGE ACQUISITION

Without a formal training program in place, how did we get to specialty certification? One study surveyed users at a simulation conference to determine how they acquired their simulation expertise. The responses included

- Attending workshops
- Working with an experienced individual or observing an experienced individual
- Reading about simulation
- Working alone using trial and error

Additionally, the majority of these educators reported that their facility did not have a faculty development plan for simulation education. This study recommends faculty practice with feedback from an experienced simulation educator as an appropriate method for developing novice simulation educators (Anderson, Bond, Holmes, & Cason, 2012).

FACULTY TRAINING

As stated in Chapter 2, the use of Patricia Benner's novice-to-expert theory (1982) has been proposed as a framework for faculty development in simulation education. Using those stages, the Bay Area Simulation Collaborative Model describes the steps for instructor training (Waxman & Telles, 2009).

- Novice
  - Technical training
  - May include training through simulator manufacturer
- Advanced beginner
  - Foundations of simulation methodology
  - May include written or online resources
- Competent
  - Begins observation with experienced simulation educator
  - Collaborates on scenario development
  - Practices facilitating simulation with feedback from experienced simulation educator
  - Leads debriefing sessions with feedback
  - Receives advanced technical training
  - Receives discipline-specific training
- Proficient
  - Facilitates simulations independently
  - Gains experience in simulation
  - Develops scenarios independently
- Expert
  - Acts as experienced simulation educator and mentor for novice simulation educators
  - Demonstrates innovation in simulation

FACULTY MENTORSHIP

In a fashion very similar to designing learning outcomes, mentorship for simulation educators begins with an assessment of learning style and current knowledge. There are a number of resources available, both in print and online, that are useful in the *advanced beginner* stage of training. When the educator moves into the *competent stage*, the mentor provides a comfortable learning environment for the educator.

Simulation should be a safe and supportive environment for the learners and the new educator. As with any new experience, learners can become frustrated if they feel they do not have the tools or support necessary to be successful. Some things to consider:

- Begin with observation of one or more experienced simulation educators
- Start new simulation educators in their content area "comfort zone"
- Provide the new educator with a clear and concise template for the scenario
- Allow new educators to engage at their own pace (initial interaction may be as minimal as controlling the technical aspect of a high-fidelity simulator)
- Model positive behaviors with the learners
- Promote a supportive environment for the learners
- Demonstrate effective debriefing techniques

Once the new educator has reached the *proficient level* and is functioning independently, continue to serve as a resource for questions and support the development of innovation. As the new simulation educator designs and implements new scenarios, be sure to provide continuous guidance. As faculty grow into this role, there is a tendency to try to incorporate too much information into an experience. Emphasis on clear and concise learning objectives is imperative. There should be between three and five objectives for each scenario. Having more than five objectives diminishes the experience for the learners and they may become easily overwhelmed.

While transitioning to independence as a new simulation educator, it is easy to fall back onto teaching methods that are more familiar. Experienced clinical faculty who transition to the role of simulation educators may tend to interact with the learners during the scenario. This is the method that they might find the most comfortable and they may have difficulty allowing the learners to work independently without "real-time" guidance from the educator. As a mentor in simulation, it is important to continue to provide support to new educators. This includes the reassurance that the best learning experience develops by allowing the learners to work with minimal intervention from the educator.

That being said, one of the greatest challenges new simulation educators face when they begin to function independently is making modifications on the fly. What if the scenario does not go as planned? Anticipating and planning for complications during simulation will improve the confidence of the new simulation educator.

What if the learners

- Do not perform the required behaviors to progress to the next phase of the simulation?
- Make an error that would cause great harm to the patient?
- "Kill" the patient?

As a mentor, it is important to discuss the what ifs with the new simulation educator. Although the goal is to provide all learners with a similar simulation experience, that is not always the case. Oftentimes, the learners' behaviors will drive the scenario down an unexpected path. After facilitating a scenario multiple times, the educator can begin to identify the most common errors. Those errors can be anticipated, and cues to refocus the learners can be developed.

There is evidence to suggest that unexpected death in simulation can negatively impact the learning experience. Some studies suggest that unless death is one of the learning objectives, the facilitator should not allow the simulator to "die" (Corvetto & Taekman, 2013; Fraser et al., 2014). Mentoring a new simulation educator should include the development of an escape plan for each scenario. These can include transfer to a higher level of care or intervention by a critical care team.

Mentorship for new simulation faculty is a continuous process. As a certified educator, the expectation regarding leadership and mentorship extends to all levels of simulation. This includes continuing to ensure best practices and serving as a resource for the simulation educators.

RESOURCES FOR FACULTY DEVELOPMENT

As a leader in simulation, development of a formal training program may not be a feasible short-term goal. However, there are a number of training resources available for faculty development.

- SSH
  - Annual conference—International Meeting on Simulation in Healthcare (IMSH)
- CAE Healthcare
  - Annual conference—Human Patient Simulation Network (HPSN)
- National League for Nursing (NLN) Simulation Innovation Resource Center (SIRC)
  - Online training modules
  - Content continuously updated
  - Appropriate for novice-to-expert simulation educators
  - http://sirc.nln.org
- Drexel University's Certificate in Simulation
  - One week-long training program
  - Offered throughout the year
  - On-site at Drexel University in Philadelphia, Pennsylvania
  - www.drexel.edu/cne/conferencesCourses/conferences/Certificate_in_Simulation
- *Simulation in Nursing Education: From Conceptualization to Evaluation*
  - Edited by Pamela Jefferies, PhD, RN, FAAN, ANEF
  - Published by the NLN, Washington, DC
- *Developing Successful Health Care Education Simulation Centers: The Consortium Model*
  - Written by Pamela Jeffries, PhD, RN, FAAN, ANEF, and Jim Battin, BS
  - Published by Springer Publishing Company, New York, New York

- *Human Simulation for Nursing and Health Professions*
  - Edited by Linda Wilson, PhD, RN, CPAN, CAPA, BC, CNE, CHSE, CHSE-A, ANEF, FAAN, and Leland Rockstraw, PhD, RN
  - Published by Springer Publishing Company, New York, New York

ADVOCATING FOR SIMULATION

Many healthcare training facilities have incorporated simulation into their program on some level. However, advocating for simulation means increasing the use of simulation in a curriculum and cultivating new simulation educators. Acceptance of increasing simulation activities may initially be met with some resistance. Some anticipated challenges include

- Time to prepare for simulation activities
- Lack of training
- Belief that it is not a useful teaching method
- Lack of space or equipment
- Complicated scheduling
- Lack of funding
- Lack of staffing
- Concerns about student engagement (Adamson, 2010; Jansen, Johnson, Larson, Berry, & Brenner, 2009)

As a champion for simulation integration, acknowledging and addressing these challenges will be imperative. Some strategies include

- Identifying educators who are interested in being trained in simulation
- Meeting with content or course leaders to explore opportunities for simulation
- Suggesting simulation activities that do not require elaborate equipment or space (i.e., Second Life simulations or use of standardized [simulated] patients [SPs])
- Reviewing course or training objectives and identifying ways to incorporate simulation to meet those objectives
- Advocating for simulation as a tool to increase learner experience with diversity and high-risk, low-volume patient experiences

SUMMARY

The responsibilities of being a certified educator in the discipline of simulation include continuous knowledge development and acquisition of the best practices of simulation. Furthermore, the dissemination of this knowledge serves to develop new simulation faculty and the field of simulation. Serving as a champion for simulation means

- Mentoring new faculty
- Promoting innovation in simulation
- Participating in building the specialty

CASE STUDY 4.1

A new simulation educator has been training with an experienced simulation educator and feels ready to start designing and implementing her own simulation scenarios. After reviewing the simulation design, the experienced educator finds there are 15 objectives for the 30-minute activity. What is the best approach to use to mentor the new educator?

PRACTICE QUESTIONS

1. An experienced simulation educator wants to include simulation in a community-based course that does not currently use simulation as a teaching strategy. The course leader states that it is not feasible to include simulation because it is too difficult to schedule another course activity in the simulation lab. What is the best response?

    A. "There may be too many activities in your course already."
    B. "The simulation lab personnel will need to cancel another course to accommodate this activity."
    C. "There are many kinds of simulated activities that would not require time in the simulation lab."
    D. "Simulation might not be the right fit for your course."

2. A course leader is looking for a way to supplement a clinical experience. There is concern that the current experience is observational and not interactive for the learners. The course leader has had some experience with simulation in the past, but has never designed a scenario. What is the best way to mentor this educator?

    A. Refer the educator to some training resources and offer to help design a scenario that has clear objectives and addresses low-volume, high-risk clinical situations.
    B. Design the new scenario based on a conversation with the manager of the clinical site.
    C. Decline to assist because independent learning through trial and error is the best way to gain experience.
    D. Show the educator how to use the high-fidelity simulator.

3. An administrator wants to increase the amount of clinical time in an educational program. This will require additional simulation educators. Which of the following statements by the administrator demonstrates an understanding of simulation educator development?

    A. "I can ask the clinical educators to help out because they already have the experience."
    B. "I will need to replace my current educators and hire experienced simulation educators."
    C. "I will identify educators who are interested in the role and have them work with the more experienced simulation educators."
    D. "Anyone interested in becoming a simulation educator will need time off from work to go back to school."

4. A new simulation educator has been working with experienced educators and is now running simulation scenarios independently. According to Benner's stages, how would you describe the level of this educator?

   A. Novice
   B. Competent
   C. Advanced beginner
   D. Proficient

5. A new simulation educator is facilitating a scenario involving a diabetic patient in a medical–surgical area. The learner administers a potentially lethal dose of medication after committing a medication calculation error. The best response by the educator is to

   A. Intervene when the learner is calculating the incorrect dose.
   B. Stop the learner from administering the medication.
   C. Intervene as the critical care response team and administer the reversal agent.
   D. Program the simulator to go into cardiac arrest.

6. A simulation educator is running a scenario about diabetic ketoacidosis, and the students interpret the glucose sliding scale wrong and give too much insulin. The students realize the mistake and adjust the glucose intravenous (IV) drip. The simulation educator uses this as a teaching scenario during the debriefing and understands that this type of situation, when it arises in simulation, is referred to as

   A. An "as-is situation"
   B. A "critical incident"
   C. A "what if"
   D. An "escape plan"

7. A simulation educator is running the same scenario about diabetic ketoacidosis, and the students interpret the glucose sliding scale wrong and give too much insulin. The students do not realize the mistake. The simulation educator uses this as a teaching scenario during the simulation by sending in an experienced SP to question the dose. This type of situation, when it arises in simulation, is referred to as

   A. An "as-is situation"
   B. A "critical incident"
   C. A "what if"
   D. An "escape plan"

8. The simulation educator is providing first-year medical students and freshman nursing students with a scenario about a geriatric patient who has pneumonia. The patient's condition is declining, and the students discuss types of appropriate oxygenation. The appropriate progression of the scenario for this level of healthcare students would be to

   A. Discuss the scenario after it is done and let it progress.
   B. Let the scenario progress uninterrupted.
   C. Intervene and prompt them to the appropriate treatment.
   D. Allow the patient to deteriorate and observe the students' behavior.

9. A novice simulation educator has developed a scenario about a critically ill patient, and the students have not received the didactic content for overwhelming sepsis. As the mentor, you should

   A. Ask the novice simulation educator to redo the entire scenario.
   B. Teach all the variables that the students will need to know.
   C. Simplify the scenario for the novice simulation educator.
   D. Direct the novice simulation educator to re-examine the learning objectives.

10. A novice simulation educator develops a scenario for interprofessional learners. The scenario is well developed and at the appropriate level. As the mentor, you review the scenario for the novice simulation educator. In which part of the scenario would you provide guidance to the novice simulation educator?

    A. The "what if" that is worked into the scenario
    B. The 10 objectives that the scenario should facilitate
    C. The environmental description of the resources needed for the scenario
    D. The role of the learners participating in the scenario

REFERENCES

Adamson, K. (2010). Integrating human patient simulation into associate degree nursing curricula: Faculty experiences, barriers, and facilitators. *Clinical Simulation in Nursing, 6*(3), e75–e81. doi:http://dx.doi.org/10.1016/j.ecns.2009.06.002

Anderson, M., Bond, M. L., Holmes, T. L., & Cason, C. L. (2012). Acquisition of simulation skills: Survey of users. *Clinical Simulation in Nursing, 8*(2), e59–e65. doi:http://dx.doi.org/10.1016/j.ecns.2010.07.002

Benner, P. (1982). From novice to expert. *American Journal of Nursing, 82*(3), 402–407.

Corvetto, M. A., & Taekman, J. M. (2013). To die or not to die? A review of simulated death. *Simulation in Healthcare, 8*(1), 8–12. doi:10.1097/SIH.0b013e3182689aff

Dieckmann, P., Gaba, D., & Rall, M. (2007). Deeping the theoretical foundations of patient simulation as social practice. *Simulation in Healthcare, 2*(3), 183–193.

Fraser, K., Huffman, J., Ma, I., Sobczak, M., McIlwrick, J., Wright, B., & McLaughlin, K. (2014). The emotional and cognitive impact of unexpected simulated patient death: A randomized controlled trial. *Chest, 145*(5), 958–963. doi:10.1378/chest.13-0987

Jansen, D. A., Johnson, N., Larson, G., Berry, C., & Brenner, G. H. (2009). Nursing faculty perceptions of obstacles to utilizing manikin-based simulations and proposed solutions. *Clinical Simulation in Nursing, 5*(1), e9–e16. doi:http://dx.doi.org/10.1016/j.ecns.2008.09.004

Society for Simulation in Healthcare (SSH). (2014). *Certified healthcare simulation educator handbook.* Retrieved from http://ssih.org/certification/handbook

Waxman, K. T., & Telles, C. L. (2009). The use of Benner's framework in high-fidelity simulation faculty development: The Bay Area Simulation Collaborative model. *Clinical Simulation in Nursing, 5*(6), e231–e235. doi:http://dx.doi.org/10.1016/j.ecns.2009.06.001

Special Learning Considerations in Simulation

RUTH A. WITTMANN-PRICE AND CRYSTAL GRAHAM

It is time for parents to teach young people early on that in diversity there is beauty and there is strength.
—Maya Angelou

This chapter addresses Content Area 1: Display Professional Values and Capabilities (Society for Simulation in Healthcare [SSH], 2014).

LEARNING OUTCOMES

- Discuss the importance of recognizing diversity in learning styles, teaching styles, and in generational differences
- Discuss cultural diversity in the simulation learning experience
- Discuss the enactment of the Americans with Disabilities Act (ADA, 2014) in the simulation laboratory
- Describe diversity through a case study and practice questions

Diversity can be defined as "the condition of having or being composed of different elements" (Merriam-Webster, 2013). Diversity related to simulation experiences can include any or all of the following human attributes in any combination listed in Exhibit 5.1.

Simulation experiences used for learning and evaluation must consider the diversity inherent in all the participants of the experience. Personal characteristics and past experiences are "brought to the table" within any learning environment. The *realism* created within a simulation environment or scenario can easily trigger personal reactions that are guided by the participants' diversity. Simulation is a *social practice*. Dieckmann, Gaba, and Rall (2007) define it as a contextual event in space and time, conducted for one or more purposes, in which people interact in a goal-oriented fashion with each other, with technical artifacts (the simulator), and with the environment (including relevant devices). This chapter briefly outlines several elements of human diversity and relates them to the simulation environment. The outcome of understanding diversity and gaining tolerance for human

---

EXHIBIT 5.1

Diversity Attributes

Diversity attributes can be exhibited by any of the humans or simulated humans, such as the patient (including family or community), learner, or educator. The attributes can include any of the following elements.

- Demographic
  - Age
  - Gender
  - Ethnicity
  - Disabilities
- Experiential
  - Work–life experiences (e.g., adult learners)
- Informational
  - Educational background
  - Learning–teaching styles
- Fundamental
  - Different beliefs and values
  - Relationships with others

---

differences can be reached through learning and reflection, which are hallmarks of simulation.

DIVERSITY IN LEARNING STYLES

All learners come to the simulation, skills laboratory, or the virtual environment with their own unique learning styles. A learning style refers to the ways and conditions under which learners most efficiently perceive, process, store, and recall what they are attempting to learn (James & Gardner, 1995).

- Cassidy (2004) adds that the approach learners take to different tasks is also important.
- A learning style is an approach to learning that works for the individual learner.
- Learners may have more than one learning style.
- Educators must first assist learners in identifying their learning style(s) if they do not already know it, and then present information in a manner consistent with the students' learning styles.

The four most common learning styles are defined by the acronym VARK, as described by Fleming and Mills (1992).

- V = Visual
- A = Auditory
- R = Read/write
- K = Kinesthetic

Visual (V) or Spatial Learners

- Learn best through what they *see*
- Like pictures, diagrams, flow charts, timelines, maps, and demonstrations
- A good learning assignment for a visual learner might involve concept mapping
- Like using computers and graphics
- May also be called graphic (G) learners
- Important to note that visual learners do not usually care to learn by viewing movies, videos, or PowerPoint presentations (Fleming, 2001)

Aural or Auditory (A) Learners

- Prefer to learn through what is *heard or spoken*
- Learn best from lectures, tapes, tutorials, group discussions, speaking, web chats, e-mails, mobile phones, and talking things through out loud
- By talking about a topic, these learners are able to process the given information (Fleming, 2001)

Reading (R) or Writing Learners

- Prefer to have the information to be learned displayed as *written words*
- Prefer text-based input and output in all of its forms
- Many academics have a preference for this style of learning
- Are often fond of PowerPoint presentations, the Internet, lists, dictionaries, thesauri, quotations, or anything else featuring words (Fleming, 2001)

Kinesthetic (K) or Active Learners

- Use their bodies and sense of touch to enhance learning while engaged in physical activity
- Like to think about issues while working out or exercising
- Like to participate, play games, role-play, act, and model experiences
- Appreciate demonstrations, simulations, videos, and movies of "real things," as well as case studies, practice sessions, and applications (Fleming, 2001)
- Felder and Solomon (1998) refer to these learners as active learners

Multimodal/Mixture (M) Learners

- Prefer to learn via two or more styles of learning or using a variety of modes
- Like information to be context specific or might choose a single mode to suit a certain occasion or situation
- Like to gather information from each mode and often have a deeper and broader understanding of topics (Fleming, 2001)

In addition to the above, there are labels given to other learning styles by various authors, which include

- Verbal (linguistic) learners
- Tactile learners

- Global learners
- Intuitive learners
- Sequential learners
- Reflective learners
- Analytical learners
- Accommodative learners

Table 5.1 displays the characteristics of these alternative types of learning styles identified by various learning specialists.

Kolb's Learning Styles

Kolb describes *experiential learning* (Chapter 6) as a type of learning in which the student is actively engaged. Kolb also discusses learning styles in relation to experiential learning. Kolb's four learning styles are

1. **Diverging:** This style of learner likes to work in groups and generate ideas. Students are fine with feedback and reflecting on activities learned. This style of learner uses concrete experiences and reflective observation.

2. **Assimilating:** This style of learner prefers to read information, be presented with lectures, and then analyze topics. This type of learning style, according to Kolb, is generated by learners who prefer abstract conceptualization and reflective observation.

3. **Converging:** This style of learner likes to put ideas to practical application. This style of learning is generated from those who abstract, conceptualize, and actively experiment.

4. **Accommodating:** This style of learner enjoys hands-on work in teams to complete projects. This style of learning is derived from those people who use concrete experience and active experimentation (Kolb, 1984).

Generational Learners

In addition to learning styles, the era or context in which learners were born and reared will affect how they view receiving and retaining information. Just as homogeneous groups of healthcare learners are obsolete, having learners that all fall within one generation in higher education is also not a reality. Characteristic learning attributes have been noted in different generational learners, but of course, like any other categorization, individual differences and preferences may override any stereotypical attribute (Hills, Ryan, Smith, & Warren-Forward, 2012; Kgongwana, 2012). Table 5.2 shows attributes of generational learners.

DIVERSITY IN TEACHING STYLES OF HEALTHCARE EDUCATORS

Jeffries (2007) emphasizes the importance of the teacher's role in simulation as well as the facilitator–learner relationship. The method by which the teacher

TABLE 5.1
Various Diverse Learning Styles

Verbal (linguistic) learners (similar to auditory learning style)	• Get value from spoken words • Enjoy talking through procedures • Use recordings of content for repetition • Frequently use mnemonics to retain information
Tactile learners	• Learn by touching or manipulating objects • Require movement • Trace words and use letter tiles to learn to spell words (Scrabble) • Often doodle, sketch, write, or conduct experiments (Mahoney, 2007)
Global learners	• Make decisions based on their emotions and intuition • Are spontaneous and focus on creativity • Do not consider tidiness important • Enjoy learning • Use humor, tell stories, and enjoy group work • Like to participate in activities • Tend to absorb material randomly • Frequently do not see connections at first, but then suddenly "get it" • Are able to solve complex problems quickly or put things together in unique ways once they have grasped the big picture, but they may have difficulty explaining how they did it • Lack good sequential thinking abilities (Felder & Solomon, 1998; Mahoney, 2007)
Intuitive learners	• Like to discover the possibilities in relationships • Like solving problems using well-established methods • Do not like complications or surprises • Do not like repetition • Work fast • Are innovative • Do not like courses that involve memorization or routine calculations • Easily become bored • Are prone to careless mistakes on tests because they are impatient with details, such as checking math calculations (Felder & Solomon, 1998)
Reflective learners	• Prefer to think about new material by reflecting quietly • Prefer to work alone, rather than with groups • Do not like classes that cover large amounts of material quickly • Do not like to be asked simply to read and memorize • Like to stop periodically to review what they have read • Find it helpful to write short summaries of readings or class notes in their own words to help them retain the material better (Felder & Solomon, 1998)

(continued)

TABLE 5.1	
Various Diverse Learning Styles (*continued*)	
Analytical learners	• Base all of their decisions on logic • Plan and organize well • Focus on details and facts • Like a tidy, well-organized environment • Enjoy learning, take sequential steps, and follow "the rules" • Like examples and clear goals (Mahoney, 2007)
Accommodative learners	• Like a combination of concrete experiences and active experimentation • Complete tasks and are less concerned about the theories • Are risk-takers • Solve problems by trial and error • Are concerned with abstract concepts and assimilate abstract conceptualizations with reflective observations (Mahoney, 2007)

designs the simulation experience and the educational practices used to organize and deliver the experience will affect the quality of the learning (Elfrink, Nininger, Rohig, & Lee, 2009). The teaching style during the experience is another affecting variable.

Teaching styles permeate the development and orchestration of the experience, and teaching styles have been classified by many different methods. Educators rarely ascribe to just one teaching style. Most educators use a variety of styles, even within a single learning session. This mixed approach can appeal to the variety of learning styles and improve learning outcomes. Reflecting on the type of style used encourages self-understanding the most and may serve to improve effectiveness. Individual teaching styles involve teaching behaviors and are noteworthy because behaviors have a direct effect on the simulation teaching–learning environment. The next section describes some of the ways teaching styles are categorized and what experts say are good teaching behaviors and personality traits for educators.

Walton, Chute, and Ball (2011) identified teaching characteristics as well as strategies in a qualitative grounded study with nursing learners that promoted learning in simulation. Table 5.3 shows the identified teaching strategies and teacher characteristics that the learners deemed helpful for understanding simulation.

Grasha's Classification of Teaching Styles

Grasha's (1996) classification defines teaching styles as expert, formal authority, demonstrator, facilitator, and delegator. The characteristics of each teaching style are unique and are listed in Table 5.4.

TABLE 5.2
Generational Learners

GENERATIONAL LABEL	LEARNER ATTRIBUTES	WHAT MAY FACILITATE LEARNING
Baby boomers (born between 1946 and 1964)	• Most healthcare educators fall into this category	• Respond to competition due to large peer groups (80 million strong) • Are taught mainly by lecture • May think technology is nice but not essential
Generation X (born between 1965 and 1979)	• Challenge authority • Are independent problem solvers • Are multitaskers	• Respond to self-learning modules • Find demonstration useful • Are pragmatic and focus on the outcomes of learning • Want real-world skills
Generation Yers **Millennials** **Nexters** **MTV generation** (born after 1975 or between 1981 and 1999) **This generation is:** • More culturally diverse • One third raised in single-parent homes • 81 million strong	• Need constant stimulation • Respond to multimedia and instant information • Are critical consumers • Expect entertainment • Are active, hands-on learners • Prefer fast-paced experiences • Seek instant gratification • Respond to positive reinforcement • Are resourceful • Like the challenge of problem solving • Prefer group activities • May have poor reading and math skills • Display poor work habits • Are multitaskers • Have no time for school • Are visual learners due to computers	• Use critical reading • Use intertextuality—reading from multiple electronic sources to critically appraise the overlap for meaning • Display self-preferentiality—better critiquing if it is a topic they are passionate about or can relate to in their own lives • Consider different viewpoints or cultural interpretations • Journal to foster reflection and critical thinking • Like using technology • Use concept mapping • Respond to simulation in teams

TABLE 5.3
Helpful Teaching Strategies and Teacher Characteristics

TEACHING STRATEGIES	TEACHER CHARACTERISTICS
Uses repeat demonstrations	Knows learners
Role models good communication	Welcoming voice and demeanor
Is flexible about debriefing method	Dresses the part
Repeats instructions	Calm
Explains steps	Welcomes learners' questions
Does not rush	Experienced and current in practice
Discusses worst case scenarios to alleviate fear	Willing to learn with and from students
Provides feedback to learners	Uses teachable moments and errors to learn
Maintains civil environment	Communicates well
Provides learners with opportunity to think through a situation	Enthusiastic and passionate
Role-plays thinking in action	Empathizes with learners' feelings

TABLE 5.4
Grasha's Teaching Styles

STYLE	CHARACTERISTICS
Expert	Uses vast knowledge base to inform learners Challenges them to be well prepared Can be intimidating to the learner
Formal Authority	Educator is in control of the learners' knowledge acquisition Educator is not concerned with student–teacher relationships Focuses on the content to be delivered
Demonstrator	Educator coaches, demonstrates, and encourages active learning
Facilitator	Learner-centered, active learning strategies are encouraged Accountability for learning is placed on the learner
Delegator	Educator's role is that of a consultant Learners are encouraged to direct the entire learning process

Adapted from Grasha (1996).

Quirk's Classification of Teaching Styles

Another useful classification of teaching styles was devised by Quirk in 1994.

- **Assertive**—Educator is usually content specific and drives home information.
- **Suggestive**—Educator uses experiences to describe a concept and then requests that the learners research more information on the subject.
- **Collaborative**—Educator uses skills to promote problem solving and a higher level of thinking in the learners.
- **Facilitative**—Educator challenges the learners to reflect and use affective learning, ask ethical questions, and demonstrate skill in interpersonal relationships and professional behavior.

Kelly's Teaching Effectiveness

Kelly (2008) also studied learners' perceptions of teaching effectiveness and found that there were three main important attributes for teaching effectiveness. The first of these, educator knowledge, was rated the most important and consists of four separate domains, as shown in Figure 5.1.

FIGURE 5.1 Kelly's attributes of teaching effectiveness.

Feedback

Communication

Educator knowledge:
1. Clinical knowledge
2. Curriculum knowledge
3. Knowing the learner
4. Knowing teaching–learning theory

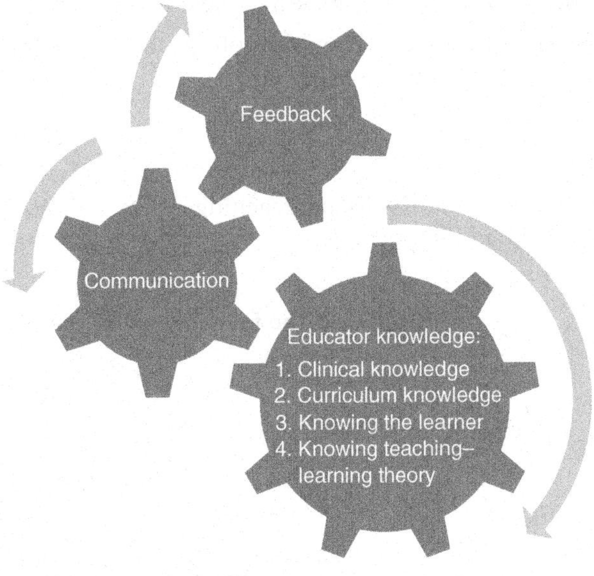

Adapted from Kelly (2008).

House, Chassie, and Spohn's Teaching Behaviors

House, Chassie, and Spohn (1999) provide examples of the following behaviors and their effect on learners.

- Making eye contact can encourage learner participation.
- Positive facial expressions that elicit a positive learner response, such as head nodding, can assist learners in feeling comfortable, whereas negative gestures, such as frowning, can discourage learners' class participation.
- Vocal tone is very important and can easily portray underlying feelings and encourage or discourage learner participation.

Choo's Positive Characteristics for Educators

Choo (1996) researched teachers and identified characteristics that students rated positive.

- Values learning
- Exhibits a caring relationship
- Provides learner independence
- Facilitates questioning
- Tries different approaches
- Accepts the differences among learners

Hicks and Burkus

Hicks and Burkus (2011) describe attributes of "master teachers," which include

- Clear communication
- Positive role modeling
- Professionalism demonstrated in lifelong learning and scholarship
- Reflective practice and making adjustments for improvement
- Use of philosophical, epistemological, and ontological influences in their practice of education

Story and Butts

Story and Butts (2010) discuss teaching delivery in the frame of the important four "Cs" shown in Figure 5.2.

FIGURE 5.2 The four "Cs" of teaching methods.

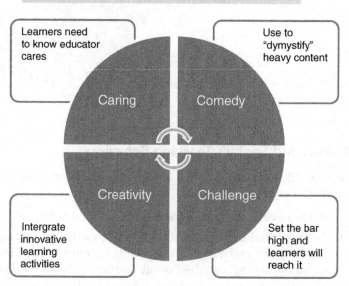

Adapted from Story and Butts (2010).

The Myers-Briggs Type Indicator

The Myers-Briggs Type Indicator (MBTI) measures Jung's 16 personality types by classifying them into four bipolar dimensions; the educator's personality also affects instruction.

- Extroversion–introversion
- Sensing–intuition
- Thinking–feeling
- Judgment–perception (Carifio & Everritt, 2007)

Silver, Hanson, and Strong

Silver, Hanson, and Strong (1996) developed a Teaching Style Inventory (TSI) based on Jung's theory of psychological types or personality types. It tests educators' propensity for one of four types.

- Sensing–thinking
- Sensing–feeling
- Intuitive–thinking
- Intuitive–feeling

Knowing your teaching style and understanding your personality style and how those two personal aspects mix in the simulation or skills environment can be very enlightening. Reflecting on these attributes can assist healthcare educators to provide learners with excellent environments for facilitating their knowledge acquisition.

CULTURALLY DIVERSE LEARNERS

The culture of the individual encompasses an individual's values, attitudes, perceptions, interpersonal needs, roles, and cognitive styles (Tomey, 2008). It is important for simulation educators to recognize that cultural diversity can influence learning ability and needs and may influence how learning is perceived by individuals. Perceptions of individuals must be considered during any educational session.

Despite the growing diversity of the nation, the healthcare workforce continues to be underrepresented by minorities (Burruss & Popkess, 2012). Moreover, culturally diverse learners face certain barriers that may impinge on their ability to achieve success in college. The most common of these barriers are

- The lack of ethnically diverse faculty
- Finances
- Academic preparation (Burruss & Popkess, 2012)
- Available role models
- Academic support
- Family support
- Peer support

The culture or customs of an individual learner may, at times, come into conflict with the values of a simulated clinical environment, and the individual's value system may be disrupted.

- A value represents a basic conviction about what is right, wrong, desirable, or just, and may support an individual's decision about how to act or perform in relation to what is perceived as preferable or valuable within the individual's culture.
- This can contribute to forming attitudes, which are similar to values that are learned from the individual's parents, caregivers, and family.
- Educators and peers may have a significant impact on one's actions.
- Some learners may experience a situation that differs from the values of their cultural tradition and usual behavior, thus causing them to experience cognitive dissonance.
- The inconsistencies revealed by cognitive dissonance are both uncomfortable and ambiguous for learners (Tomey, 2008).
- It is important for educators to offer clear directions and rationales for decision making to help alleviate any sense of dissonance a minority learner might experience.

A study by Amaro, Abriam-Yago, and Yoder (2006) interviewed ethnically diverse learners who had recently completed a college program and identified the major themes related to educational barriers. These include

- Personal needs (lack of finances, time issues, family responsibilities and obligations, and difficulties related to language and communication)
- Academic needs (large or heavy workload)
- Language needs (difficulty reading and understanding assignments, a prejudice due to their accents, verbal communication barriers)
- Cultural needs (expectations related to assertiveness and cultural norms, lack of diverse role models, and difficulty with communication)

An important issue among culturally diverse learners is their level of knowledge of the English language, which, if inadequate, can be problematic. Barriers may also exist for the English-as-a-second-language (ESL) learner in progressing in healthcare programs, once accepted.

Suggestions for accommodating learners from culturally and linguistically diverse backgrounds include

- Using nonstandardized and standardized methods of testing
- Dynamic assessments
- Nonverbal measures of ability
- Multiple methods of testing
- Testing in both the learner's native and second language
- The use of the TOEFL® test (Overton, Fielding, & Simonsson, 2004)

Hansen and Beaver (2012) discuss test development for ESL learners and provide the following tips.

- Use short simple sentences
- Be direct when stating information
- Use common vocabulary

EFFECT OF DIVERSITY ON SIMULATION SCENARIOS

Dieckmann, Lippert, Glavin, and Rall (2010) discuss simulation *lifesavers* (p. 219), that is, manipulations of a scenario when unexpected situations occur. Unexpected situations are listed below as identified by Dieckmann, Lippert, Glavin, and Rall and are pre-empted many times by the diversity of the simulation learners. Causes for unexpected situations are

- Comprehensiveness of the scenario is unclear to participants due to poor instructions or ambiguous clues during the scenario
- Inability to accept the scenario due to inexperience or distractibility of participants
- Unrealistic difficulty level of the scenario, which does not match the competency of the participants
- Participants in the scenario do not follow the procedural steps and produce unexpected actions
- Participants change the intended scenario to a familiar scenario that is also plausible

When unexpected occurrences take place during a scenario, debriefing (which will be discussed in depth in Chapter 15) may be affected. The lifesavers are the anticipated actions that may be needed during a scenario. Scenario lifesavers can be used to adapt to the situation or restore the scenario to its original form. These scenario-lifesaving actions are identified before the scenario and can come from "within" the scenario or simulation room itself by altering the patient or providing hints, or it can come from "outside" the scenario by using the director's voice to clarify, stop, or explain the scenario. Some lifesaving techniques are commonly used in many scenarios either to provide the participants with time or to emphasize missed clues, such as the patient asking learners to repeat information. Other lifesavers must be specific to the scenario, such as altering vital signs more drastically to gain the learners' attention.

LEARNER AND LEARNING DISABILITIES

Learning disabilities are the most common type of disability found on college campuses. Although increasing numbers of individuals with physical or affective disabilities are attending higher educational institutions and many disabilities are known and accommodated for before the learner enters college, other learners with learning disabilities begin college without their disability having been detected.

- In healthcare education, these disabilities are often noted when significant differences are noticed between a learner's classroom and simulation or clinical performance. Often, a learner may perform well in the simulation or clinical environment, but may be unable to demonstrate the same ability, skills, and competency in the classroom.

- Healthcare educators should always refer learners they suspect as having a learning disability to the appropriate counselors or office for accommodations for assistance (Frank, 2012).

Learners with documented disabilities are entitled to the same access to education as traditional learners. An office of academic services must be available to provide learners with *reasonable accommodations* and support services.

- Accommodations must be made for students with learning disabilities in accordance with the ADA (National Council of States Boards of Nursing, 2014).

- It is important for educators to be aware of learners with physical disabilities, such as learners with a documented or apparent physical limitation, substance abuse, chemical or alcohol impairments, and/or mental health problems (Frank, 2012).

BELONGINGNESS

Another important concept in learning is belongingness. Levett-Jones, Lathlean, Higgins, and McMilan (2009) studied the concept of belongingness in healthcare students related to clinical learning and the relationship learners have with their faculty. Learners who are marginalized are less likely to succeed; so, simulation and virtual experiences must be inclusive, providing a valued role for each learner. Belongingness is conceptually related to motivation, and the authors previously (Levett-Jones & Lathlean, 2008) identified themes about learning that assist learners to either succeed or disengage, which are listed in Exhibit 5.2.

EXHIBIT 5.2
Themes About Learning Motivation
Theme A = Motivation to learn or being accepted and valued as a learner Theme B = Self-directed learning (SDL) assists in building confidence Theme C = Anxiety is a barrier to learning Theme D = Confidence to ask questions

Adapted from Levett-Jones and Lathlean (2008).

SIMULATION LEARNING AS A SOCIAL PRACTICE

Goffman (1974) describes social meaning in terms of "frames" that are perceived by the individual about the reality that he or she is experiencing. It helps individuals understand what is happening at the moment and to make sense of the situation. Goffman breaks experiences down to two types of frames.

1. **Primary frames:** Assist the individual to make sense out of the current situation.

2. **Modulation frames:** Bring in the individual's perception of the world and therefore will include individual differences (all diversity issues previously discussed). These frames must be addressed to ensure positive learning experiences (Dieckmann, Manswer, Wehner, & Rall, 2007).

> **Simulation Teaching Tip 5.1**
> Elfrink, Nininger, Rohig, and Lee (2009) remind us that the exact learning mechanism by which simulation works is not fully understood because of its complexity, but it is understood that simulation is a social learning experience due to its interactivity.

SOCIALIZATION DURING SIMULATION

Walton, Chute, and Ball (2011) provide results of a grounded study with nursing learners that discusses socialization during simulation. Five phases of the process of "negotiating the role of the professional nurses" (p. 301) were identified and are as follows.

Phase I	Feeling like an imposter (includes anticipation, wanting further instructions, not knowing where to start, and anxiety)
Phase II	Trial and error (includes practice, replaying and reviewing, self-reflection, and mentoring)
Phase III	Taking the role seriously (includes having the scenario be realistic, dedication to learn, using nursing language, developing team leadership, analyzing, and better understanding of the situation)
Phase IV	Transference (includes gaining confidence, socializing into the healthcare role, feeling devastated after failing, then repracticing and rebuilding)
Phase V	Professionalism (includes growth in role as nurse and patient advocate, interprofessional collaboration, and career goal building)

The socialization aspects of simulation cannot be overlooked. Simulation is a powerful mechanism to provide learning environments in all three domains: cognitive, psychomotor, and affective.

CASE STUDY 5.1

A healthcare student tells the simulation educator that she needs time and a half to take tests, and she should have extra time to read and understand the patient history on the simulation scenario that is being used for evaluative purposes in a capstone course. As the simulation educator, how would you respond, and what (if any) provisions would you make and under what circumstances?

PRACTICE QUESTIONS

1. During a role-play simulation about poverty, a healthcare learner excuses himself and leaves the simulation laboratory. On the evaluation form he states that the scenario was humiliating, and people don't really understand what poverty is like. As the simulation educator, how would you first address this with the learner?

   A. Discuss with him that his reality contract was signed and that he needs to abide by it.
   B. Ask him why he felt the scenario was insensitive.
   C. Discuss his lack of achieving the learning outcomes.
   D. Develop a plan to achieve the outcomes in a different format.

2. A simulation educator is approached by an ESL learner who asks whether she can have the full written evaluative scenario in her hands because it is difficult for her to understand the patient's voice over the microphone. The simulation educator would best reply by

   A. Providing the entire script to the learner
   B. Explaining to the learner that it is copyrighted and would be giving her an unfair advantage
   C. Reviewing the scenario with her beforehand
   D. Asking another learner in the scenario to repeat the patient's responses

3. During a scenario, a group of four interdisciplinary learners arrives at the wrong conclusion for the patient's manifestations. As the patient is reporting postsurgical pain of 10 on a scale of 1 to 10, the group discusses the possibility of an infection when, in fact, a hematoma is developing in the surgical site. The simulation educator overseeing the scenario decreases the body temperature and increases the pulse above 120 bpm. This technique is referred to as

   A. Adjusting the primary frame
   B. Adjusting the secondary frame
   C. Adjusting from within
   D. Adjusting from outside

4. During a scenario, a learner stands in the background but does participate in the role assigned. When assessing the video replay of the scenario, the simulation educator discusses the actions of this learner as those that could possibly exemplify which learning style?

   A. Verbal (linguistic)
   B. Tactile
   C. Global
   D. Reflective

5. During an interdisciplinary scenario, a learner who is in the role of the nurse tells the learner in the role of a physician that the procedure being considered is not the best choice for the patient's condition. In reviewing the scenario, the simulation educators discuss the possible learning style of the learner in the role of the nurse as

A. Sequential
B. Tactile
C. Global
D. Reflective

6. During a hybrid simulation scenario, the learner tells a family member that she needs to give the healthcare professional team "a minute to think" when the family member keeps asking what is wrong with her son. The simulation educator decides that the best debriefing method for this learner would be to

A. Have him review the video and write a reflection
B. Individually counsel him on professionalism
C. Have a group review of all aspects of the scenario
D. Send him to student services for counseling

7. An interdisciplinary healthcare team of learners is experiencing its first scenario together, and one learner giggles frequently during the simulation scenario. The simulation educator understands that this may be a symptom of which of the following phases of learner development?

A. Transference
B. Trial and error
C. Professionalism
D. Feeling like an imposter

8. During a high-fidelity simulation scenario, a beginning learner is reluctant to place the monitor leads on the mannequin, turn on the cardiopulmonary monitor, and adjust the computer screen so the recording is visible. The simulation educator understands that this learner is most likely from which of the following generational groups?

A. Millennials
B. Generation X
C. Generation Y
D. Baby boomers

9. During a high-fidelity simulation, the interdisciplinary learners are drawing the wrong conclusion as the case is unfolding, and the simulation educator stops the case and provides some educational information. The educational technique is referred to as

A. Modulation framing
B. Lifesaving from outside
C. Preventing cognitive dissonance
D. Demonstrating authority in the educator role

10. A learner requests to use an amplified stethoscope during the scenario. The simulation educator allows her to use it because

A. Many learners are able to hear better with one.
B. It is an American with Disabilities Act mandate.
C. It demonstrates cultural sensitivity.
D. It is a reasonable accommodation.

REFERENCES

Amaro, D., Abriam-Yago, K., & Yoder, M. (2006). Perceived barriers for ethnically diverse students in nursing programs. *Journal of Nursing Education, 45*(7), 247–254.

Americans with Disabilities Act (ADA). (2013). Retrieved from http://www.ada.gov

Burruss, N., & Popkess, A. (2012). The diverse learning needs of students. In D. Billings & J. Halstead (Eds.), *Teaching in nursing: A guide for faculty* (4th ed., pp. 15–32). St. Louis, MO: Elsevier.

Carifio, J., & Everritt, A. (2007). Further validation of Hanson's learning profile indicator and Silver, Hanson, and Strong's teaching style inventory. *Work, 29*(2), 165–174.

Cassidy, S. (2004). Learning styles: An overview of theories, models, and measures. *Educational Psychology, 24*(4), 419–444.

Choo, L. A. (1996). Reflections: Learning at work. *Professional Nurse (Singapore), 23*(3), 8–11.

Dieckmann, P., Gaba, D., & Rall, M. (2007). Deepening the theoretical foundations of simulation as social practice. *Simulation in Healthcare, 2,* 183–193.

Dieckmann, P., Lippert, A., Glavin, R., & Rall, M. (2010). When things do not go as expected: Scenario life savers. *Simulation in Healthcare, 5*(4), 219–225.

Dieckmann, P., Manswer, T., Wehner, T., & Rall, M. (2007). Reality and fiction cues in medical patient simulation: An interview study with anesthesiologists. *Journal of Cognitive Engineering Decision Making, 1*(2), 148–168.

Elfrink, V. L., Nininger, J., Rohig, L., & Lee, J. (2009). The case for group planning in human patient simulation, *Nursing Education Perspectives, 30*(2), 83–86.

Felder, R. M., & Solomon, B. A. (1998). *Learning styles and strategies.* Retrieved November 28, 2008, from http://www4.ncsu.edu/unity/lockers/users/f/felder/public/ILSdir/styles

Fleming, N. (2001). *VARK: A guide to learning styles.* Retrieved from http://www.vark-learn.com/english/page.asp?p=categories

Fleming, N., & Mills, C. (1992). Not another inventory, rather a catalyst for change. In D. Wulff & J. Nygist (Eds.), *To improve the academy: Resources for faculty, instructional, and organizational development* (Vol. 11, pp. 137–155). Stillwater, OK: New Forums.

Frank, B. (2012). Teaching students with disabilities. In D. M. Billings & J. A. Halstead (Eds.), *Teaching in nursing: A guide for faculty* (pp. 18–31). St. Louis, MO: Mosby/Elsevier.

Goffman, E. (1974). *Frame analysis: An essay on the organization of experience.* New York, NY: Harper & Row.

Grasha, A. (1996). *Teaching with style.* Pittsburgh, PA: Alliance.

Hansen, E., & Beaver, S. (2012). Faculty support for ESL nursing students: Action plan for success. *Nursing Education Perspectives, 33*(4), 246–250.

Hicks, N. A., & Burkus, E. (2011). Knowledge development for master teachers. *Journal of Theory Construction and Testing, 15*(2), 32–35.

Hills, C., Ryan, S., Smith, D. R., & Warren-Forward, H. (2012). The impact of "Generation Y" occupational therapy students on practice education. *Australian Occupational Therapy Journal, 59*(2), 156–163.

House, B. M., Chassie, M. B., & Spohn, B. B. (1999). Questioning: An essential ingredient in effective teaching. *Journal of Continuing Education in Nursing, 21*(5), 196–201.

James, W. B., & Gardner, D. L. (1995). Learning styles: Implications for distance learning. *New Directions for Adult and Continuing Education, 67*(1), 19–32.

Jeffries, P. (Ed.). (2007). *Simulation in nursing: From conceptualization to evaluation.* New York, NY: National League for Nursing.

Kelly, C. (2008). Students' perceptions of effective clinical teaching revisited. *Nurse Education Today, 27*(8), 885–892.

Kgongwana, T. (2012). Mind the generation gap. *Nursing Update, 37*(11), 60–63.

Kolb, D. A. (1984). *Experiential learning: Experiences as the source of learning and development.* Englewood Cliffs, NJ: Prentice Hall.

Levett-Jones, T., & Lathlean, J. (2008). Belongingness: A prerequisite for nursing students' clinical learning. *Nurse Education in Practice, 8*(2), 103–111.

Levett-Jones, T., Lathlean, J., Higgins, J., & McMillan, M. (2009). Staff-student relationships and their impact on nursing students' belongingness and learning. *Journal of Advanced Nursing, 65*(2), 316–324. doi:10.1111/j.1365-2648.2008.04865.x

Mahoney, P. (2007). *Certified nurse educator preparation course.* Philadelphia, PA: Villanova University.

Merriam-Webster. (2013). *Merriam-Webster online.* Retrieved from http://www.merriam_webster.com/dictionary/diversity

Overton, T., Fielding, C., & Simonsson, M. (2004). Decision making in determining eligibility of culturally and linguistically diverse learners. *Journal of Learning Disabilities, 37*(4), 319–330.

Silver, H., Hanson, J. R., & Strong, R. W. (1996). *Teaching styles and strategies (Unity in Diversity Series, Manual No. 2).* Alexandria, VA: Silver and Strong.

Society for Simulation in Healthcare (SSH). (2014). *Certified healthcare simulation educator handbook.* Retrieved from http://ssih.org/certification/handbook

Story, L., & Butts, J. B. (2010). Compelling teaching with the four Cs: Caring, comedy, creativity, and challenging. *Journal of Nursing Education, 49*(5), 291–294. doi:10.3928/01484834-20100115-08

Tomey, A. M. (2008). *Nursing management and leadership* (8th ed.). St. Louis, MO: Mosby/Elsevier.

Quirk, M. E. (1994). *How to learn and teach in medical school: A learner-centered approach.* New York, NY: Charles C Thomas.

Walton, J., Chute, E., & Ball, L. (2011). Professional nurse: The pedagogy of simulation: A grounded study. *Journal of Professional Nursing, 27*, 299–310.

Educational Theories, Learning Theories,

and Special Concepts

RUTH A. WITTMANN-PRICE AND SAMUEL W. PRICE

The teacher who is indeed wise does not bid you to enter the house of his wisdom but rather leads you to the threshold of your mind.
—Khalil Gibran

This chapter addresses Content Area 2: Demonstrate Knowledge of Simulation Principles, Practice, and Methodology (Society for Simulation in Healthcare [SSH], 2014).

LEARNING OUTCOMES

- Discuss educational philosophies and theories and how they relate to simulation education
- Discuss learning and motivational theories
- Discuss concepts related to simulation education

Understanding educational and learning theories increases awareness of what and how educators do things and how learners assimilate knowledge presented to them or facilitated by educators. A simulation environment is an excellent milieu in which to synthesize cognitive, psychomotor, and affective learning. Development of competence in all three learning realms is important for healthcare providers. The goal of using a simulation environment for teaching and assessment is to promote patient safety, protect patients from harm, and provide healthcare learners with the best possible safe learning environment (Cleland, Abe, & Rethans, 2009).

Educational theories are contextual and change as societal values change. Educational theories spurn learning theories or how learners grasp, understand, and apply knowledge. This chapter provides an overview of educational theories including those used specifically for simulation.

EDUCATIONAL PHILOSOPHIES AND THEORIES

To facilitate learning in a simulation environment, a simulation educator must build experiences on sound theoretical foundations, which include understanding that educational philosophies

- Date back to ancient times, are never stagnant, and change as the larger social system matures
- Provide the foundations on which learning theories and educational pedagogies are built
- Consider the branch of philosophy that addresses why we teach, how we teach, and what the goals of education are for learners and society (Wortham, 2011)

Traditional educational theories were teacher centered and based on what the educator could provide to the learner. Postmodern theories more often take into account the social meaning of learning, the relationship of knowledge and power, and are more likely to consider multiple and innovative ways of learning (Mann, 2011).

Educational philosophies guide educational theories, and there is some overlap in terms and ideas. Some common terms regarding philosophies are shown in Figure 6.1.

Worldviews about education categorize how an educational philosophy relates to the social context. Learning theories have more defined concepts that are more applicable to the teaching situation. In learning theories, "Teaching is what the educator provides the learner in terms of goals, methods, objectives, and outcomes. Learning refers to the processes by which the learner changes skills, knowledge, and dispositions through a planned experience" (Kaakinen & Arwood, 2009, p. 1).

How people learn and how they store, connect, discover, and retrieve skills and information has been well studied and formalized into many theoretical frameworks. These frameworks try to explain the connection between knowledge and the human brain, a truly interesting subject that affects learners every day in simulation experiences.

FIGURE 6.1 Philosophy terminology.

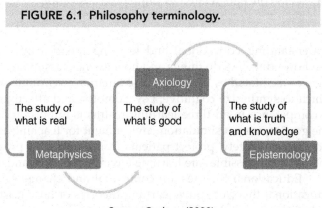

Source: Csokasy (2009).

The learning theories discussed today in education are mainly *behaviorism* and *constructivism*. Behaviorism is an ingrained theory in education and structures teaching plans. Constructivism is an ideal theory to encapsulate, ground, and expand what is done in the simulation laboratory because its major tenets promote active learning. Both behaviorism and constructivism are discussed further in this chapter. In Table 6.1, philosophical foundations are broken down into brief descriptions of general philosophies—sometimes referred to as "worldviews"—educational philosophies, and the corresponding teaching–learning theories.

> **Simulation Teaching Tip 6.1**
> Related to simulation, the cognitive theory is used to assess actual performance of learners compared to intended performance, whereas the behavioral theory would use the appraisal process to reinforce or change the behavior exhibited by the learner during simulation (Archer, 2010).

Behaviorism

Behaviorism is a learning theory that was developed in the 1940s. Some of the major tenets of behaviorism are

- Learning is observable through behavior.
- Learning is reinforced by response.
- Behavior modification leads to control.
- Token economies may be used for classroom management.
- Instructional objectives guide learning (Tyler, 1949).
- Learning is shaped by others.
- Learning is teacher centered.
- Behaviorists include Watson, Skinner, Pavlov, and Bandura.

Behaviorism posed a couple of difficult issues for education, including the following.

- Behaviorism does not explain the intrinsic motivation of the learner.
- All learning is not displayed in behavior.
- By predetermining objectives or outcomes, the depth and breadth of the learners' experiences may be squelched (Bevis & Watson, 1989; Diekelmann, 1997, 2005).

It is difficult, at best, to package the human intellect into a modifiable mold for convenience for grouping, evaluating, and justifying what is being taught or presented and what a learner carries forth from an experience. Behaviorism was made popular by Tyler's landmark book *Basic Principles of Curriculum and Instruction* (1949) in relation to writing instructional objectives or what the teacher expected the learner to learn by the end of a teaching session or course.

TABLE 6.1
Worldview Philosophies, Educational Philosophies, and Learning Theories

WORLDVIEW PHILOSOPHIES	EDUCATIONAL PHILOSOPHIES	LEARNING THEORIES
Traditional Philosophies and Theories		
Idealism (Plato, Socrates) • Ideas are important • People would like to live in a perfect world • Interactive immersion education, e.g., as designed experiences in serious gaming may participate in "ideal" worlds (Squire, 2006)	**Perennialism** (Thomas Aquinas) • Traditional education style • Teacher centered • Liberal education is valued • Includes great thinkers of the past • Prepares learners for adult life • Reading, writing, and arithmetic are important	**Information processing** (Gagne, 1970) • Describes how information is received, stored, and processed in the mind • Learning is a function of the brain (sometimes called brain-based learning) • Humans process information and store it in memory • Memory is achieved by sensory input that goes to short-term memory (working memory), which is stored, if significant, in long-term memory
Realism (Positivism) (Aristotle) • The world is orderly • Science can be viewed objectively and analyzed • Develops knowledge that is value and context free (Mann, 2011)	**Essentialism** (Bagley, Hirsh) • Traditional education approach • Develops learners' minds through knowledge passed from the educator to the learner • A core curriculum is valued, as are democracy and cultural heritage • Physical world is the true reality • Learners should appreciate the masterworks of art and literature • Learners need critical thinking skills to help society • Teacher-directed learning	**Behaviorism** (Pavlov, Watson, Skinner) • Stimulus–response is the basis for learning • An environment develops the person • Requires behavior modification and management • Positive reinforcement is used to encourage acceptable behavior • Generated the idea of "programmed learning" • Tyler (1949) introduced behavioral objectives • Faculty decides on the educational experience • Education is still steeped in behaviorism today with lockstep curricula **Social learning theory or social cognitive theory** (Bandura, 1997) • Role-modeling behavior for learners • Perception of confidence in oneself in the situation (self-efficacy) • Positive expectations are the incentives • Bandura's term, reciprocal determinism, means that the world and the person's behavior cause each other • Feedback to the learner is important

Poststructuralism or Modern Philosophies and Theories

Pragmatism (Dewey, Pierce)	Progressivism (Dewey)	Constructivism (Piaget, Vygotsky)
• Ideas can be tested scientifically • The human experience is important • Theory was influenced by social reform and the growth of citizenship in the early 19th century	• School mimics society • Real-life curriculum and problem-solving exercises are the most important • Attends to and optimizes inquisitive, active learning • Experiential learning to take place • Learners to have choices about what to learn • Learners are engaged in group and peer learning • Education experiences are learner centered	• "Active" learning theory • Learning is built by the learner, and it is built on previous knowledge in the reality of the learner • Learning is actively constructed through interaction with the environment, and it is marked by reflection • The learner tries to make sense out of his or her perceptions and experiences (Mann, 2011) • Doing is learning • Social negotiation is a part of learning • Multiple perspectives on subjects are supported • Taking ownership of learning is important • Being self-aware and reflective in the knowledge acquisition process is important to learning • The goal is problem solving, reasoning, critical thinking, and active and reflective use of knowledge • Most important, it is learner focused (Brandon & All, 2010) Piaget (1972) described cognitive learning as a process of: • Accommodation • Assimilation • Equilibration Knowles's (1980) adult learning theory (andragogy) • Supports constructivism because it also builds on the learner's previous experiences **Situated learning theory** • Closely linked with constructivism • Reality based • Learner is an active participant in learning • Especially helpful when applied to clinical practice (Mann, 2011)

Adapted from Chinn (2007).

Constructivism

Currently, constructivism is the theoretical paradigm that best fits educational processes and the social context of today, and it is described in Table 6.1. Constructivists view learning as an active process that builds new knowledge on knowledge already obtained, thereby connecting what is unknown to what is known. Adaptive behaviors are produced when learners take received stimuli and convert it or construct it into cognitive knowledge that makes sense to them. Constructivism is based in the reality of the learner and is therefore learner focused. The faculty role in constructivism includes coaching and facilitating (Brandon & All, 2010; Philpott & Batty, 2009).

Learning using simulation fits well into the constructivist theoretical framework because it is problem based and individually constructed knowledge though experiential learning (Dreifuerst, 2009).

LEARNING THEORIES

Experiential Learning Theory

A learning theory that fits within the constructivist framework is experiential learning. Experiential learning theory (ELT) is widely used in simulation experiences. It is defined as "the process whereby knowledge is created through the transformation of experience. Knowledge results from the combination of grasping and transforming an experience" (Kolb 1984, p. 41).

There are the four major concepts within Kolb's ELT theory.

1. **Concrete experience** or experiences built from reality
2. **Abstract conceptualization** (AC) or thinking about an experience
3. **Reflective observation** (RO) or taking in the experience
4. **Active experimentation** (AE) using hands-on experiences to learn (Kolb, Boyatzis, & Mainemelis, 1999)

ELT is learner centered because the learners are in control of the direction the simulation scenario takes. Although the student learning outcomes (SLOs) are formulated by the certified healthcare educator, the learners are in control of their actions and the consequences. As learners become more advanced in their healthcare studies, they are able to forsake a more passive role in scenarios and increase their active roles and participate in experiential learning (Alinier, 2011). The change from passive to active learning is depicted in Figure 6.2.

Gibbs (1988) also has a model for planning experiential learning, which includes

- Planning for action
- Carrying out the action
- Reflecting on the action
- Relating the action back to the theory

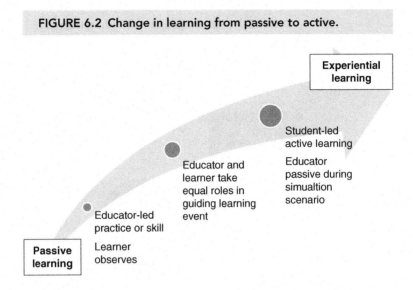

FIGURE 6.2 Change in learning from passive to active.

Grant and Marsden (1992) explain experiential learning as having the following components.

- Providing an experience
- Thinking about the experience
- Identifying improvements
- Planning the learning needed
- Putting the learning into practice

Simulation is well suited for experiential learning because it is a practiced experience in a controlled environment that allows for reflection (thinking) and ultimately changes in practice (doing) by adult professionals (Fanning & Gaba, 2007). Schaefer and colleagues (2011) reviewed 221 simulation studies; of those who based their research on an educational theory, 25% used Kolb's ELT.

Scaffolding Learning Theory

Congruent with ELT is cognitive scaffolding. This theory was introduced by Vygotsky (1978) to explain how a novice learns to be an expert. Just as a scaffold supports a building under construction, the novice learner needs resources and support from the expert or mentor to increase cognitive knowledge in a subject and build it progressively. The scaffolding sets the framework for learning and is intentionally established as a "stretch" for the learner. In order for the learner to reach higher levels of knowledge or understanding about a situation or process, supports must be in place, such as

- Constructive feedback
- Explanations
- Reflection
- Revision of knowledge building (Lax, Russell, Nelles, & Smith, 2009)

FIGURE 6.3 Outcomes of scaffolding learning.

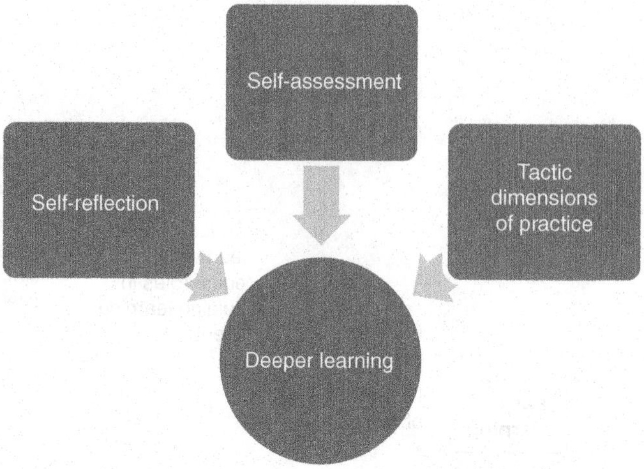

Source: Lax, Russell, Nelles, and Smith (2009).

Conceptually, scaffolding learning should promote deeper learning by assisting the learner in areas depicted in Figure 6.3.

Social Learning Theory

Social learning theory is also a proponent of reinforcement and modeling new behavior as learners observe it from certified healthcare educators (LeFlore & Anderson, 2009). Another popular concept that was attributed to social learning theory is self-efficacy coined by Bandura (1997). Self-efficacy is often measured in healthcare learners, and progressive or ongoing simulation experiences are an ideal environment for its measurement. Self-efficacy is the perception of confidence in one's self in a given situation. Self-efficacy is based on four principles

1. **Enactive mastery experiences**—the learner's own history of success
2. **Vicarious experiences**—the observed behaviors of a role model being successful at a task
3. **Verbal persuasion**—telling individuals they will be successful
4. **Physiological states**—the person's "gut feeling" that success can be achieved

PEDAGOGY VERSUS ANDRAGOGY AS EDUCATIONAL CONCEPTS

Pedagogy is generally defined as the art and science of teaching. It refers to the manner in which educators instruct. Its development was intended for children, and it is now used for all ages as well as for simulation (Walton, Chute, & Ball, 2011). *Andragogy* is the art and science of teaching adults and was coined by Malcolm Knowles in 1980 (Table 6.2).

TABLE 6.2
Andragogy and Pedagogy

EDUCATIONAL CONSIDERATIONS	ANDRAGOGY	PEDAGOGY
Demands of learning	Learners have life demands besides school.	Learners can devote more time to the demands of learning because responsibilities are minimal.
Role of instructor	Learners are autonomous and self-directed. Educators facilitate the learning, but do not supply all the facts.	Teacher centered because the educator directs the learning. Often uses surface learning.
Life experiences	Learners have a tremendous amount of life experience. Learners connect the learning to their knowledge base. Learners must recognize the value of the learning.	Learners do not have the knowledge base to make the connections of new knowledge to life experiences without facilitation.
Purpose of learning	Learners have a goal in sight for their learning.	Learners cannot always see the long-term necessity of information.
Permanence of learning	Learning is self-initiated and tends to last a long time.	Learning is compulsory and tends to disappear shortly after instruction.

Adult learners display a variety of learning characteristics.

- The most common reason an adult enters any learning experience is to create change in
  - Skills
  - Behavior
  - Knowledge level
  - Attitudes about things (Russell, 2006)

Adult learners sometimes experience unique barriers to learning, which include

- Lack of time
- Lack of confidence
- Lack of information about opportunities to learn
- Scheduling problems
- Red tape (Russell, 2006)

It is important to incorporate adult learning principles into simulated learning experiences to maximize learning potential for this population. Adult learners learn best when learning is

- Related to an immediate need, problem, or deficit
- Voluntary and self-initiated
- Person centered and problem centered
- Self-controlled and self-directed
- The role of the teacher is that of a facilitator
- Information and assignments are pertinent
- New material draws on past experiences and is related to information the learner already knows
- The learner's perception of threats to the self is reduced to a minimum in the educational situation
- Learners are able to participate actively in the learning process
- Learners are able to learn in a group
- The nature of the learning activity changes frequently
- Learning is reinforced by application and prompt feedback

Fanning and Gaba (2007) comment that much of simulation learning is done by adult learners who have undeniable previous life experiences, and frames and traditional teaching methods are not effective.

Wang (2011) describes adult learners as

- Needing to know why
- Leaning toward independence and self-direction
- Having a self-identity shaped by life experiences
- Valuing learning that can be applied
- Problem centered
- Internally motivated

SIMULATION LEARNING FRAMEWORKS

Several simulation learning frameworks describe how simulation specifically affects learning.

Kneebone

Kneebone (2005) describes simulation learning in the following stages.

1. Should allow for deliberate practice (DP) in a safe environment
2. Expert tutors should be available to the learners
3. Experiences should be similar to real life
4. Should be learner centered

Kirkpatrick

Kirkpatrick (1998) discusses four levels of learning with simulation as depicted in Figure 6.4.

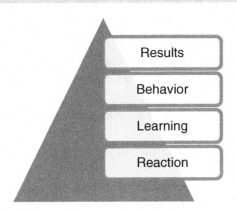

FIGURE 6.4 Kirkpatrick's levels of simulation learning.

Results

Behavior

Learning

Reaction

Doerr and Murray

Doerr and Murray (2008) describe the teaching–learning process of simulation by using the model of a four-step plan, which includes

1. The plan
   a. Developing learning outcomes
   b. Description of the scenario and certified healthcare educator responses to the learners
   c. Scripts for standardized (simulated) patients (SPs)
2. The situation
3. Debriefing
4. Transference

Meller

Meller (1997) described the elements of activity in relation to simulation.

- **Passive elements**—those things that try to stage the realism of the simulation experience, such as moulage (refer to Chapter 10)
- **Active elements**—those things that are programmed into the simulation experience that cause the learner to respond
- **Interactive elements**—those changes that the certified healthcare educator makes in reaction to the actions of the learner

REALISM IN SIMULATION

Although realism is a traditional worldview of education (refer to Table 6.1), it takes on a slightly different interpretation when applied to simulation. A certain amount of realism must be present during a scenario to meet SLOs. Some points about simulation scenario realism are as follows.

- The goal is to acquire experience in a safe environment
- The scenario must be real enough to suspend disbelief
- The scenario must mimic as closely as possible a real clinical scenario
- SPs, along with mannequins, increase the realism
- The environmental setup is also important in producing a realistic scenario (Alinier, 2011)
- SPs provide a transition from role-playing to real patients for healthcare professionals
- SPs can provide learners with "authentic" assessment or those assessment skills that are critical (Barrows, 1993)
- Boulet, Jeffries, Hatala, Korndorffer, Feinstein, and Roche (2011) discuss how the applicability of learning through simulation education is a link to real-life situations

Understanding the perspective of realism is also important for certified healthcare educators. Dieckmann, Gaba, and Rall (2007) state this when they profess that "it is not uniformly the case that more realism helps to achieve better educational goals" (p. 183). This emphasizes that there are many variables within any one scenario that can increase or decrease the realism of an experience.

Realism is sometimes referred to as the fidelity of the simulation experience. Issenberg, McGaghie, Issenberg, Petrusa, and Scalese (2010) describe fidelity as the exactness of duplication and remind us that simulation is never isomorphic with real life. The higher fidelity may be equated with increased realism. The goal of a simulated environment is to replicate a realistic situation. Fidelity in simulation includes

> **Simulation Teaching Tip 6.2**
> Dieckmann, Gaba, and Rall (2007) inform certified healthcare educators that learners experience simulation in two realities:
>
> 1. Real-time experience
> 2. Real-time educational event

- **Physical fidelity:** How real does the mannequin appear?
- **Psychological fidelity:** How mentally prepared are the learners?
- **Equipment fidelity:** What can the mannequin, task trainer, or virtual reality platform do?
- **Environmental fidelity:** How do the surroundings look? (Dieckmann, Gaba, & Rall, 2007)

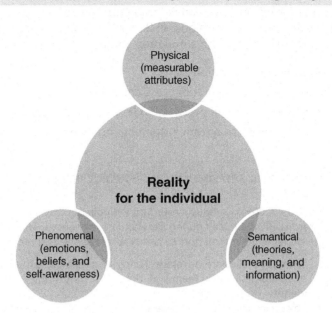

FIGURE 6.5 Laucken's theory of conceptualizing reality.

Dieckmann, Gaba, and Rall (2007) warn that high fidelity does not necessarily equate with better learning outcomes. Although realism of the simulation experience is the gold standard, it does not guarantee learner outcomes.

Laucken (2003) describes reality as three ways of thinking that are interactive with one another to create reality for the individual person in the experience. Figure 6.5 demonstrates the interconnectiveness of Laucken's theory of how reality is conceptualized.

Suspending Disbelief

Suspending disbelief or engaging in a fiction contract in a simulation experience encompasses the appropriate use of the "as-if" concept (Vaihinger, 1927). Certified healthcare educators running a scenario must integrate information that is believable and within the framework of the scenario, and learners must be open to changing information and understand that the scenario represents actual patient care (Dieckmann, Gaba, & Rall, 2007).

Deliberate Practice

One of the founding teaching principles of simulation is deliberate practice (DP). Ericsson, Krampe, and Tesch-Römer (1993) dicussed DP as a method of teaching and reinforcing skills for healthcare providers; it is a forerunner to simulation. Ericsson and colleagues understood the implications of translating practice on nonhuman materials to the clinical area as a means to promote expertise and safety.

Team Learning

Simulation encourages team learning through open communication in a safe space that protects the discussions while leveling the playing field. The safe space concept of learning through simulation contains the following features.

- Promotes collaboration
- Removes the actual patient care concerns
- Provides voice to all on an equal level
- Provides protection from judgment and incivility (Forsythe, 2009)

EVIDENCE-BASED SIMULATION PRACTICE (EBSP) 6.1

Forsythe (2009) qualitatively studied the collaboration of three interdisciplinary teams during simulation experiences. The following points were identified in the effort to create a safe space and teamwork.

- Team processes are developed and need reflection; the interactions of a team or its tactical teamwork become a part of the team's functioning identity
- Physicians verbalized the need to have their orders recognized
- Team members identified the importance of being named during the experience
- Team members identified that conversation "off topic" was not productive
- Equipment and supplies needed to be locatable

LEARNING DOMAINS

Learning is discussed as a process that takes place in three domains: cognitive, affective, and psychomotor. Learners in healthcare programs are evaluated for growth in all three domains due to the nature of the service work that they will provide to humanity. Bloom's taxonomy (Table 6.5) identifies learning mainly in the cognitive domain. Psychomotor domains are evident in the application of knowledge, such as demonstrating skills, and are not difficult to evaluate because they produce observable behavior. Psychomotor learning is often related to procedures, skills, and interventions, all of which can be evaluated in the simulation laboratory. The affective domain of learning is more difficult to assess because it is related to judgment and values (Partusch, 2007). Wong and Driscoll (2008) describe the learning development of the affective domain in five stages, which are

> **Simulation Teaching Tip 6.3**
> Facilitator-led group planning of learners' simulation experiences may be an ideal method to promote cooperation, collaboration, and teamwork (Elfrink, Nininger, Rohig, & Lee, 2009).

1. **Receiving:** Learners attend, listen, watch, and recognize.
2. **Responding:** Learners answer, discuss, respond, reply, and actively participate.
3. **Valuing:** Learners accept, adopt, initiate, or demonstrate a preference.

4. **Organizing:** Learners formulate, integrate, modify, and systematize.

5. **Internalizing:** Learners commit, exemplify, and incorporate professionalism into practice.

An example of an affective domain being evaluated in the simulation laboratory would include the learner's interactions with the simulation mannequin or the SPs or the learner's advocacy or professionalism during a situation. Often SLOs in the affective domain are the most difficult to write and evaluate.

Kardong-Edgen, Adamson, and Fitzgerald (2010) concur that simulation has the potential of effective learner evaluation in all three domains because it can evaluate learners using the same scenario under standard conditions. Simulation evaluation calls for effective instruments, which are still in developmental stages. Evaluation of simulation experiences is thoroughly addressed in Chapter 19.

MODES OF THINKING

Laucken (2003) describes three modes of *realistic* learner thinking during a simulation experience.

1. **Physical mode** of thinking includes the actual equipment and the fidelity of the equipment. Although mannequins simulate humans, there are many unrealistic attributes, and the same is true for other laboratory equipment.

2. **Semantical mode** of thinking includes the situation created in humans containing information that represents an event. For example, the situation of a patient having a myocardial infarction would include EKG and vital sign changes that would indicate to a learner that this was the event taking place.

3. **Phenomenal mode** of thinking includes the learners' perceptions, emotions, and thinking process during the simulation experience, as well as the participants' understanding of the relationship of the simulated experience to actual clinical practice (Dieckmann, Gaba, & Rall, 2007; Elfrink, Nininger, Rohig, & Lee, 2009).

Specifically in simulation experiences, the right fidelity in the experience needs to be used to emphasize the goal of the experience. The experience needs to be constructed with the goal in mind and framed within the learning outcomes. For example, if the goal is to have the learners practice effective chest compressions, then the primary frame of the scenario theoretically should be focused on the physical or the anatomical realism of a human chest, and modulations to the scenario may include understanding individual learners' previous experiences with a "code" situation (Dieckmann, Gaba, & Rall, 2007).

CRITICAL THINKING AND METACOGNITION

Critical thinking as an educational concept can be traced back to 1941, when Glaser defined composites of knowledge. Other historical developments in the concept of critical thinking are as follows.

- Miller and Malcolm (1990) adapted Glaser's definition into a model for critical thinking and advised educators to pay closer attention to learners' mental processes.

TABLE 6.3
Descriptions of Critical Thinking

AUTHOR	DESCRIPTION OF CRITICAL THINKING
Facione, Facione, and Sanchez (1994)	Critical thinking is the process of purposeful, self-regulating judgment.
Paul and Elder (2007)	Attitudes are central, rather than peripheral, to critical thinking as is independence, confidence, and responsibility, which are needed to arrive at one's own judgment.
Bandman and Bandman (1995)	Critical thinking as the rational examination of ideas, inferences, assumptions, principles, arguments, conclusions, issues, statements, beliefs, and actions. It covers scientific reasoning, decision making, and reasoning in controversial issues. It also includes deductive, inductive, informal, and practical reasoning.

- In the early days of concept development, educators were concerned with finding an appropriate definition for critical thinking in order to evaluate learners.
- A multitude of definitions arose, and some of the more prominent ones are listed in Table 6.3.

Scheffer and Rubenfield (2000) developed a consensus statement describing the attributes of critical thinking that is useful for healthcare education because it acknowledges its multifaceted characteristics (Table 6.4).

Walker (2003) reviewed some of the teaching strategies that enhance critical thinking; they work well with simulated experiences also. Walker suggests

- Questioning that promotes the evaluation and synthesis of facts
- Discussions and debates with open negotiation
- Short, focused assignments, such as the following.
  - Summarize five major points of the experience.
  - Discuss the essence of the experience using a metaphor.

TABLE 6.4
Attributes of Critical Thinking

PERSEVERANCE	CONTEXTUAL INSIGHT
• Open mindedness • Flexibility • Confidence • Creativity • Inquisitiveness • Reflection • Intellectual integrity • Intuition	• Perspective • Information seeking • Transformative knowledge • Applying standards • Logical reasoning • Discriminating • Analyzing

- Explain the experience to your neighbor, who has a high school education.
- How did the experience affect your life personally or professionally?

• Using case studies has also been reported as a learning strategy to increase critical thinking skills (Falco, 2009; Popil, 2011)

Assessment of learners' critical thinking skills has been completed by use of several different tools. Two of the most widely used tools are listed here.

• The California Critical Thinking Disposition Inventory. This tool evaluates seven "habits of the mind," which are

1. Truth seeking
2. Open mindedness
3. Analyticity
4. Systematicity
5. Self-confidence
6. Inquisitiveness
7. Cognitive maturity

• The Watson-Glaser Critical Thinking Appraisal (WGCTA, 1964) has three different forms of the instrument available, and the newest version has 16 scenarios and 40 items. There are five subcategories.

1. Inference
2. Recognition of assumptions
3. Deduction
4. Interpretation
5. Evaluation (Romeo, 2010)

Metacognition

Metacognition is a different concept from critical thinking. According to Hsu (2010, p. 2573), "Metacognition refers to an individual's knowledge, awareness and command of thinking and learning strategies." Metacognition is evaluating your own learning and ideas and being able to change them in order to understand and promote your own learning success (Hsu, 2010).

EVIDENCE-BASED SIMULATION PRACTICE

The foundations of evidence-based simulation practice (EBSP) are analogous to evidence-based practice (EBP). Healthcare educators use the same method of synthesizing and appraising evidence in the simulation environments in order to draw a conclusion or develop an opinion that is grounded and derived from logical, common ideas in the literature (Hicks & Butkus, 2011).

Overall, more research needs to be completed in order to produce evidence to support specific learning activities. Pearson, Wiechula, Court, and Lockwood (2007) opined that faculty members should use the acronym FAME when planning to make a change based on evidence.

F = Feasibility

A = Appropriateness

M = Meaningfulness

E = Effectiveness

GOFFMAN'S THEORY OF FRAME ANALYSIS

In order to make sense out of a situation, such as a simulated experience, Goffman (1974), who developed a theory about experience interpretation, discusses human perception in frames.

- **Primary frames** describe how the learner's mind or cognition makes sense out of a situation.
  - **Natural primary frames** are those that include natural law (physics, anatomy, and physiology).
  - **Social primary frames** include human factors such as decision making and communication.
- **Modulations** are learners' understanding that they are in a "what-if" situation that is predefined by the situation in the primary frame. Modulations should hold to learning rules, such as
  - Be within the primary frame and not be a surprise or deception
  - Have a time frame that is appropriate
  - Know the rules and roles within the modulation (Dieckmann, Gaba, & Rall, 2007; Elfrink, Nininger, Rohig, & Lee, 2009)

THEORIES OF KNOWING

Healthcare education also draws on theories about how learners come to understand concepts. There are two classic models that have been significant in healthcare education for the past several decades and are widely used as the theoretical foundations for many studies, curriculum, and learning activity development. They are Barbara Carper's (1978) Ways of Knowing, which is discussed briefly here and Patricia Benner's (1982) novice-to-expert theory, which was outlined in Chapter 2.

> **Simulation Teaching Tip 6.4**
> Using the new ISBARR (originally, S is for situation, B is for background, A is for assessment and R is for recommendation) communication tool during simulation, as in practice, may mitigate some of the study results that were identified, because the "I" is for introduction and the second "R" is for repeating the orders or results.

Carper (1978) described four ways that healthcare professionals understand practice situations.

1. **Empirical knowledge** or scientific knowledge (this includes EBP)
2. **Personal knowledge** or understanding how you would feel in the patient's position
3. **Ethical knowledge** or attitudes and understanding of moral decisions
4. **Esthetic knowledge** or understanding the situation of the patient at the moment

Munhall (1993) added a fifth way of knowing: *unknowing* or understanding that one cannot know everything about the patient and that one must place oneself in a position willing to learn from the patient's perspective.

DEEP, SURFACE, AND STRATEGIC LEARNING

Other ways to describe learning include Marton and Saljo's (1976) terms: deep surface and strategic learning. These terms describe student learning approaches and a method of knowledge acquisition. The approach a learner takes to comprehend information presented can fall into any one of the three classifications.

1. A deep learning approach is accomplished when a learner addresses material with the intent to understand both the concepts and meaning of the information.
   - The learner relates new ideas to existing experiences (constructs knowledge).
   - Formulates links in long-term memory.
   - The motivation for a deep learning approach is primarily intrinsic, created from the learner's interest and desire to understand the relevance of the information to applied practice.
2. A surface learning, or atomistic, approach facilitates learning by
   - Memorization of facts and details similar to rote learning
   - Learners assimilation of information presented at face value
   - Extrinsic motivation for surface learning is driven either by the learner's fear of failing or desire to complete the course successfully.
3. A third learning approach is called strategic learning.
   - The learner does what is needed to complete a course.
   - Strategic learning is a mixture of both deep and surface learning techniques (Wittmann-Price & Godshall, 2009).

All three approaches to learning can be measured by the Approaches to Student Inventory (ASSIST; Entwistle, 1999; Ramsden & Entwistle, 1981).

MOTIVATION TO LEARN

Not only do certified healthcare educators need to know how learners acquire information, they also need to know why they learn. What are their motivating factors? Motivation has been linked to learner retention and success. Many variables affect motivation; it can be influenced by the need for achievement or curiosity, or it can be a function of the situation at hand or a person's ability. A learner's locus of control can be motivated extrinsically or intrinsically.

- Extrinsic needs are those based on external variables, such as grades or earning money.
- Intrinsic motivation has to do with the feeling of accomplishment or learning for the sake of learning. Typically, intrinsic motivation is associated with better retention (Rose, 2011).
- Intrinsic motivation is correlated with the self-determination theory developed by Deci and Ryan (Deci, Eghrari, Patrick, & Leone, 1994). According to the theory, humans have three types of needs.

  1. To feel competent
  2. To feel related
  3. To feel autonomous

There are numerous models that conceptualize motivation in learning situations. Several of them are listed in the following text. All of them have an interactive component that includes the educator and the learner.

Designed Experiences Through "Serious Gaming"

Using the videogame simulation platform to build educational programs that enhance learning by *being* or becoming the character in the game and by *doing* to create and organize for a functional epistemology in which one learns through doing and through performance is a new frontier in education, but this mode of simulation also lacks research. Some of the concepts associated with serious gaming include

- **Interactivity:** Serious games can be played alone or as part of a community.
- **Agency:** The simulated world grants the player the right to create.
- **Parameters:** These are built-in barriers by the game designers (Squire, 2006).

Additional information about Second Life and gaming is provided in Chapter 17.

ARCS Model

Keller (1987) talks about the factors educators can implement to motivate learners in the ARCS model

A: Attention Keep the learner's attention through stimulus changes in the environment
R: Relevance Make the information relevant to the learner's goals
C: Confidence Make expectations clear so the learner will engage in learning
S: Satisfaction Have appropriate consequences for the learner's new skills

Brophy Model

Brophy (1986) listed the following methods by which motivation is formed.

- Modeling
- Communication of expectations
- Direct instruction
- Socialization by parents and educators

Vroom's Expectancy Model

Vroom's expectancy model (VEM; 1964) describes what people want and whether they are positioned to obtain it. The Vroom model describes three concepts, which are

1. **Force (F):** The amount of effort a person will place into reaching a goal
2. **Valence (V):** How attractive the goal is to the person
3. **Expectancy (E):** The possibility of the goal being achieved

The VEM model is $F = V \times E$ (Vroom, 1964).

DeYoung's Motivational Tips

DeYoung (2009) lists 10 principles to motivate learners (p. 62); they are applicable to a laboratory and virtual learning environment as well as to a traditional setting.

1. Use several senses
2. Actively involve the learner
3. Assess readiness
4. Determine whether the learner thinks the information is relevant
5. Repeat information
6. Generalize information
7. Make learning pleasant
8. Begin with what is known
9. Present information at an appropriate rate
10. Provide a learning-friendly environment

LEARNER SOCIALIZATION IN THE VIRTUAL, SIMULATION, AND SKILLS ENVIRONMENT

Simulation experiences are a social practice (Elfrink, Nininger, Rohig, & Lee, 2009) because they encompass a goal-oriented situation that calls for participant interaction in a setting (module) that influences behavior. The simulation setting includes

- Introduction
- Simulator briefing

- Scenario
- Debriefing—which can be done during the simulation or after the learning experience (Van Heukelom, Begaz, & Treat, 2010)
- Session ending (Dieckmann, Gaba, & Rall, 2007)

The social practice goal of simulation is to enhance positive learner socialization and extend it to healthcare practice. Socialization is defined as a process of internalizing the norms, beliefs, and values of a professional culture to which one hopes to gain admission (Philipin, 1999).

- New healthcare learners are instructed in ways and attitudes of the organization and gradually adopt the attitudes, values, and unspoken messages within the organization (Mooney, 2007).
- It is important to note that a lack of socialization has been associated with negative outcomes, such as turnover, attrition from the healthcare profession, and decreased productivity (Nesler, Hanner, Melburg, & McGowen, 2001).

The transition of a healthcare learner to the professional environment is challenging. Simulation environments are being used to decrease reality shock and familiarize learners using both social practice and social aspects within the social practice. Social aspects include interdisciplinary communication, teamwork, and role identification (Dieckmann, Gaba, & Rall, 2007).

Kramer (1974) describes reality shock that takes place when a neophyte realizes that what was learned in school does not match that which is experienced in actual clinical practice.

Kramer's four phases of reality shock are

1. Honeymoon
2. Shock or rejection
3. Recovery
4. Resolution

TEACHING SIMULATION

LeFlore and Anderson (2009) explain that most simulation scenarios begin with a "stem," or some information about the case, and then teaching during simulation experiences can take on one of three levels of facilitation by certified healthcare educators.

1. **Self-directed:** This approach allows experienced learners to proceed through scenarios without assistance from the certified healthcare educator.
2. **Cueing students:** In this approach, the certified healthcare educator provides hints or cues to the learners to ensure they progress through the scenario.
3. **Expert or instructor-model:** This is an approach in which the certified healthcare educator instructs during the scenario as the learners are experiencing the situation.

INSTRUCTIONAL OBJECTIVES AND LEARNING OUTCOMES

Objectives, which are still used today and are an expectation of most simulation learning sessions, are part of the behavioral paradigm. In order to standardize the format of objectives, educators have incorporated the action verbs outlined in Bloom's taxonomy, which has been revised. Bloom's *Taxonomy of Educational Objectives* (1956) describes an end behavior (see Table 6.5). The taxonomy uses "behavioral terms" to divide learning into leveled achievement, from knowledge acquisition to the synthesization or evaluation of new ideas (Novotny & Griffin, 2006).

Most sessions begin with objectives or learning outcomes in order to frame the content or experience. Objectives and learning outcomes are two terms used often in education; the differences between the terms may be slight on the surface, but they depict two approaches to evaluating learning that have emerged in recent years.

- An objective speaks to the process; therefore, it is teacher centric.
- An outcome, on the other hand, speaks to the product; thus, it is learner centric (Wittmann-Price & Fasolka, 2010).

TABLE 6.5
Bloom's Taxonomy

LEVEL	CONCEPT	VERBS USED WHEN WRITING LEARNING OUTCOMES
Evaluating (formerly called evaluation)	Judgment, selection	Appraise, argue, assess, attach, choose, compare, defend, estimate, judge, predict, rate, select, support, value, evaluate
Creating (formerly called synthesis and this step was formerly above evaluation)	Productive thinking, novelty	Arrange, assemble, collect, compose, construct, create, design, develop, formulate, manage, organize, plan, prepare, propose, set up
Analyzing (formerly called analysis)	Induction, deduction, logical order	Analyze, appraise, calculate, categorize, compare, contrast, criticize, differentiate, discriminate, distinguish, examine, experiment, question, test
Applying (formerly called application)	Solution, application	Apply, choose, demonstrate, dramatize, employ, illustrate, interpret, operate, practice, schedule, sketch, solve, use, write
Understanding (formerly called comprehension)	Explanation, comparison, illustration	Classify, describe, discuss, explain, express, identify, indicate, locate, recognize, report, restate, review, select, translate
Remembering (formerly called knowledge)	Memory, repetition, description	Arrange, define, duplicate, label, list, memorize, name, order, recognize, relate, recall, repeat, reproduce, state

Adapted from Bloom, Englehart, Furst, Hill, and Drathwohl (1956).

TABLE 6.6
Learning Outcomes

ANTECEDENT	LEARNER	VERB DESCRIBING BEHAVIOR	CONTENT	CONTEXT	CRITERIA
By the end of this session	the learner will	demonstrate	correct medication administration	in the simulated setting	100% of the time

Changing from objectives to outcomes is truly more of a conceptual change than an operational change. Some educators have simply switched words, but not thought processes. Others believe that neither objectives nor outcomes give us the freedom needed to encourage learners to think critically (Bevis & Watson, 1989; Diekelmann, 1997).

Depending on the length of the simulation scenario and the level of the practitioners, there are usually between one and four learning objectives (Alinier, 2011). Because most educational institutions still describe learning in terms of outcomes, the formula to write them is depicted in Table 6.6.

SLOs are tied to learner evaluation. Evaluating learning that takes place in simulation is addressed in Chapter 19. Simulation as an evaluation tool has become widespread because it is a controlled environment where all learners can be presented with testing in similar conditions; a leveled playing field. Traditional clinical experiences were not able to provide that, and education and evaluation were done by "random opportunity" (LeFlore & Anderson, 2009).

EVALUATING SLOs

Simulation experiences are used for either formative and summative learner assessment or evaluation. Evaluation is defined by Bourke and Ihrke (2012, p. 422) as "a means of appraising data or placing a value or data gathered through one or more measurements." Simulation-based evaluation is becoming increasingly popular, yet much research is needed on the two most important outcomes of simulation-based evaluation to understand if simulation.

1. Meets the SLOs and increases knowledge acquisition
2. Improves patient care and safety

An important consideration when using simulation-based evaluation is validity. Is the simulation experience measuring what it is intended to measure? Kane (2006) discusses the evaluation process of testing by breaking it down into four key areas.

1. **Scoring:** Was the test provided to learners under fair and consistent conditions?
2. **Generalization:** Are the results reliable and consistent when the evaluation technique is used with different groups?
3. **Extrapolation:** Is the assessment measuring the construct it is supposed to measure and not extraneous variables?
4. **Decision/interpretation:** Are the scores being used for their intended purpose and without manipulation?

Cant and Cooper (2010) searched the literature for studies that validated the learning results when simulation was used. They recovered 12 studies that supported simulation as a method used to increase learners' knowledge, critical thinking ability, confidence, and satisfaction by 7% to 11%. All the studies appraised used a control group and were qualitative.

Boulet and colleagues (2011) have identified multiple areas of research needed because simulation is increasingly being used as an assessment or evaluative mechanism of student learning. Some of the areas of research related to the development of sound assessment tools that are needed are studies related to

- Identifying measurement error in simulation-based assessment scores
- Developing scoring rubrics
- Supporting the theoretical basis for learning in the simulated environment
- Demonstrating the relationship between performance in the simulated environment and the actual patient care settings
- Understanding the impact simulation-based assessment has on the delivery of care

Jeffries (2007) emphasizes the need for increased research in simulation and relates it to the relationship of the learner and facilitator. As a pioneer in simulation learning, she states (p. 163) that more research is needed to "identify the hallmarks of a good simulation."

Research has been accomplished on learners' perception of simulation, which includes questions such as the following.

- What was helpful?
- What was not helpful?
- What would you change for the next experience? (Elfrink, Nininger, Rohig, & Lee, 2009)

Schaefer and colleagues (2011) reviewed simulation research studies for four distinct themes.

1. The validity and reliability of the simulator
2. The validity and reliability of the performance evaluation tool
3. The study design
4. The translational impact

The research team reviewed 221 articles that studied healthcare education simulation in one of the four themes above and rated the evidence of the studies. Out of 221 studies, only five were rated as unequivocal. Conclusions drawn by the review team were that more studies needed to be done on the validity and reliability of the simulator itself and on evaluation tools used to assess knowledge acquisition.

INNOVATIVE EDUCATIONAL RESEARCH

Innovation is a term often used in conjunction with simulation. When applying the term to simulation in healthcare education research, it takes on an added dimension. Research in simulation is only one area that needs additional effort; educational research is another area that is wrought with lack of evidence. Innovative educational research is using new technology to promote the synthesis of new methods of knowledge building for learners. This process is best described by Kanter (2008, p. 703): "Ideally, a report of an innovation will provide not just information but insight—the kind of insight that will sustain a cycle of progressive thinking that will lead to even newer and better ideas."

Historically, simulation is an innovative teaching and evaluation method for healthcare learning as known by the write-up about using SPs (called PIs [patient instructors]) in 1980 by Stillman, Ruggill, Rutala, and Sabers. Even early in the 1970s, it was recognized in medical education specifically that standard conditions needed to be sought for evaluation of learners, and SPs provided the standardization that clinical practice could not (Swanson & Stillman, 1990).

GAGNE'S CONDITIONS OF LEARNING

Gagne's (1970) steps for instruction are a classic list of tasks that is still referenced today and suited for learning in a simulated environment. Gagne's (1970) nine events of instruction are shown in Table 6.7.

Experienced educators "role model" learning. They convey concepts in an organized understandable manner, are learner oriented, and develop an appropriate relationship with learners (Hicks & Burkus, 2011).

LEARNING ACTIVITIES USED IN SIMULATION ENVIRONMENTS

Cooperative/Collaborative Learning Techniques

- These techniques support active learning using a peer-centered approach.
- This is an overall framework that supports many kinds of active learning techniques with a special focus on group engagement, such as learning circles and project-based learning.

Five attributes are needed to make cooperative learning successful.

1. Face-to-face interaction
2. Individual and group accountability
3. Interpersonal and small-group skills
4. Positive interdependence
5. Group processing (Johnson & Johnson, 2003)

Interprofessional Learning

Team-based education is needed for quality patient care and is the focus of many healthcare educational and simulation initiatives. The goal of interprofessional learning is to have all health professional learners "deliberately working

TABLE 6.7
Gagne's Conditions of Learning

INSTRUCTIONAL EVENT	ACTIVITIES OF TEACHING–LEARNING
1. Gain attention of the learner	Stimuli activates receptors
2. Inform learners of objectives	Sets expectations for the learner
3. Stimulate recall of prior learning	Activate short-term memory and the retrieval of information by asking questions
4. Present the content	Present content with features that can be remembered
5. Provide "learning guidance"	Assist the learner to organize the information for long-term memory
6. Elicit performance (practice)	Ask learners to perform to enhance encoding and verification
7. Provide appropriate feedback (feedback about simulation experiences is covered in Chapter 16)	Encourage performance
8. Assess performance	Evaluate
9. Enhance retention and transfer	Review periodically to decrease memory loss of information

together" as stated by the Interprofessional Educational Collaboration (IPEC) made up of six professional organizations (American Association of Colleges of Nursing, American Association of Colleges of Osteopathic Medicine, American Association of Colleges of Pharmacy, American Dental Education Association, Association of American Medical Colleges, and Association of Schools of Public Health, 2011). The IPEC outlined four core competencies needed for healthcare professionals to function effectively in interprofessional teams. The domains of the major four major competencies and related criteria are fully explained in Chapter 14.

Self-Directed Learning

Self-directed learning (SDL) is another term often heard in healthcare education and refers to a collection of learning activities that are truly learner focused. It originated with Knowles (1980) and is a process in which the learner decides his or her learning needs. The learner formulates the goals, develops the networking and resources, does the learning, and evaluates the learning. Learners must be ready to take on the task of SDL and they need to have the confidence, maturity, and tenacity to engage in SDL (Areewan, Nongkran, Acharaporn, & Sue, 2011). SDL activities can include virtual learning modules. To assess whether learners are ready for this type of knowledge acquisition, there is a self-directed learning readiness scale (SDLRS).

Reflection

Reflection is a method used to develop critical thinking and is used extensively in simulation experiences through debriefing (Chapter 15) and feedback (Chapter 16). Please refer to those chapters to better understand the essence of reflection, which is a critical component of simulation learning.

Environmental Management

The underpinning of positive learning environment management is respect for the learners. Once an atmosphere of trust and respect is established, there should be very few management issues. Chickering and Gamson's (1987) seven principles of good teaching practice are applicable to simulation learning environments and are listed here.

1. Encourage contact between learners and educators.
2. Develop reciprocity and cooperation among learners.
3. Encourage active learning.
4. Give prompt feedback.
5. Emphasize time on task.
6. Communicate high expectations.
7. Respect diverse talents and ways of learning.

According to Mulligan (2007), there are four pillars of classroom management; these are discussed here because they also fit the simulation learning environment very well.

Pillar 1: Educators should use instructional strategies (active learning strategies) that motivate and keep learners interested and engaged.

Pillar 2: Educators need to use instructional time wisely and take a proactive approach to teaching by charging the learners to be accountable for their learning.

Pillar 3: Social behaviors that need attention and correcting should be dealt with immediately, face to face, and privately.

Pillar 4: Educators need to create a flexible environment in order to adjust to the learners' needs.

SUMMARY

Simulation as a learning tool has a history of success in healthcare education. The theoretical foundations of experiential learning and realism are well represented in simulation. Successful simulation for healthcare education contains the following best-practice attributes as identified in a mega-analysis completed by McGaghie, Issenberg, Petrusa, and Scalese (2010).

- Feedback: formative or summative (discussed in Chapters 15 and 16)
- DP: encompasses nine educational goals:
  1. Occurs with motivated learners
  2. Define the learning outcomes
  3. Have the experience at the appropriate level for the learner
  4. Repeat the exercise or skill to gain proficiency
  5. Promote rigor in skill to ensure best practice
  6. Provide learner with feedback
  7. Promote self-regulation in learners
  8. Evaluate to reach a mastery standard
  9. Start process again with another task (McGaghie, Siddall, Mazmanian, & Myers, 2009)
- Curriculum integration
- Outcome measurement
- Simulation fidelity
- Skill acquisition and maintenance
- Mastery learning
- Transfer to practice
- Team training
- High-stake testing
- Instructor training
- Educational and professional context

CASE STUDY 6.1

Joseph is a new faculty member at a small baccalaureate school with a premed, nursing, and prepharmaceutical program. He is full time, tenure track, and working on his doctorate degree. Joseph is assigned a mentor and a 12-credit semester teaching load, which is normal for many institutions. He meets with his mentor, who goes over his syllabus with him. The mentor asks Joseph why he has so many assignments for the learners to do after they have completed their hybrid simulation experience. Joseph states that he believes that the learners' writing skills are lacking, and they need writing assignments and has them expand on the simulation day by describing the illness process of the simulated patient scenario in depth. If you were the mentor and saw a novice place 50% of the clinical course grade on writing assignments related to simulation, how would you handle it?

PRACTICE QUESTIONS

1. A novice nurse educator reports to the department chair that there are three learners in the back of the room who are chattering during class, and the nurse educator finds it very distracting. The nurse educator tells the department chair that the next step is to "call them out" and send them to the department chair's office to be "written up" for unprofessionalism. The best response by the department chair is

   A. "Calling them out in front of their peers should take care of the problem."
   B. "I will tell them that if they are unprofessional again, they will be excused from the program."
   C. "Before the next class, move their seats to separate areas."
   D. "After the next class, speak with them and explain how their behavior is affecting you."

2. A nurse educator is developing a test and formulating a test item at an application level on Bloom's taxonomy. Which type of test question would best evaluate the learner's cognitive level of understanding?

   A. A true/false question that has two different interventions
   B. A hot spot that asks the learner to place an X on an anatomical part
   C. A multiple-choice question that asks for the best nursing assessment for a patient with a complaint of costovertebral tenderness
   D. A select-all-that-applies question that asks for the appropriate nursing interventions for a postoperative abdominal hysterectomy

3. A nurse educator has submitted a syllabus with the following learning outcomes. Which learning outcome is written at the highest level of Bloom's taxonomy?

   A. Demonstrate caring to geriatric patients
   B. Discuss common healthcare concerns of geriatric patients
   C. Evaluate geriatric patients' understanding of home safety
   D. Formulate a plan of care for a geriatric patient

4. During a curriculum meeting, a nurse educator states, "I think we should coordinate the clinical skills checklists for all the classes to make sure they are appropriately leveled and each is measurable." The philosophical foundations for this analysis would be

   A. Narrative pedagogy
   B. Behaviorism
   C. Constructivism
   D. Feminism

5. During a faculty interview, a nurse educator candidate states that a preferred learning activity to facilitate learner understanding is storytelling. What nursing educational philosophy or theory is indicated by this learning activity?

   A. Narrative pedagogy
   B. Behaviorism
   C. Constructivism
   D. Feminism

6. A nurse educator would like learners to each become responsible for a section of a case study and to articulate how their work contributes to the patient care picture. An active learning activity that would best accomplish this outcome would be

    A. An unfolding case study approach
    B. Socratic questioning
    C. A learning circle
    D. A jigsaw activity

7. A nurse educator states at a faculty meeting that switching from traditional care planning to concept mapping will not teach the learners the nursing process. Which statement by the department director would address this concern?

    A. Ask the other faculty members what they think.
    B. Request the nurse educator making the comment to provide evidence.
    C. Ask the group to vote on one of the learning tools, care plans, or concept maps.
    D. Tell the faculty that the evidence shows that concept mapping increases critical thinking.

8. When interviewing for a job, a nurse educator is asked about her education philosophy, and she says that she is primarily concerned with equality in the classroom. This nurse educator most likely subscribes to the philosophy of

    A. Phenomenology
    B. Emancipatory education
    C. Narrative pedagogy
    D. Constructivism

9. At a faculty retreat, a nurse educator is telling the group about her philosophy and says, "I believe in rewarding learners for good behavior and doing well on tests." What philosophy is the educator a proponent of?

    A. Realism
    B. Essentialism
    C. Perennialism
    D. Behaviorism

10. Which statement by a learner should alert a nurse educator to consider using another learning activity to increase learner comprehension?

    A. "I have never been given such low grades before."
    B. "I read the book before class."
    C. "I do extra questions every night."
    D. "I understand the material in class, but cannot pick the right test answer."

REFERENCES

Alinier, G. (2011). Developing high-fidelity health care simulation scenarios: A guide for educators and professional. *Simulation & Gaming, 42*(1), 9–29. doi:10.1177/1046878109355683

Archer, J. C. (2010). State of the science in health professional education: Effective feedback, *Medical Education, 44,* 101–108. doi:10.1111/j.1365.2923.2009.03546.x

Areewan, K., Nongkran, V., Acharaporn, S., & Sue, T. (2011). Readiness for self-directed learning among nursing students in Thailand. *Nursing and Health Sciences, 12*, 177–181. doi:10.1111/j.1442-2018.2010.00515.x

Bandman, E. L., & Bandman, B. (1995). *Critical thinking in nursing* (2nd ed.). Norwalk, CT: Appleton & Lange.

Bandura, A. (1997). *Self-efficacy: The exercise of control.* New York, NY: W. H. Freeman.

Barrows, H. S. (1993). An overview of the uses of standardized (simulated) patients for teaching and evaluating clinical skills. *Academic Medicine, 68*(6), 443–451.

Benner, P. (1982). From novice to expert. *American Journal of Nursing, 82*(3), 402–407.

Bevis, E., & Watson, J. (1989). *Toward a caring curriculum: A new pedagogy for nursing.* New York, NY: National League for Nursing.

Bloom, B., Englehart, M., Furst, E., Hill, W., & Drathwohl, D. (Eds.). (1956). *Taxonomy of educational objectives.* New York, NY: Longmans, Green.

Boulet, J. R., Jeffries, P. R., Hatala, R. A., Korndorffer, J. R., Feinstein, D. M., & Roche, J. P. (2011). Research regarding methods of assessing learning outcomes. *Simulation in Healthcare, 6*(7), S48–S51.

Bourke, M., & Ihrke, B. (2012). The evaluation process: An overview. In D. Billings & J. Halstead (Eds.), *Teaching in nursing: A guide for faculty* (4th ed.). St. Louis, MO: Elsevier/Saunders.

Brandon, A. F., & All, A. C. (2010). Constructivism theory analysis and application to curricula. *Nursing Education Perspectives, 31*(2), 89–92.

Brophy, J. (1986). *On motivating students. Occasional Paper No. 101.* East Lansing, MI: Institute for Research on Teaching, Michigan State University.

Cant, R. P., & Cooper, S. J. (2010). Simulation-based learning in nurse education: Systematic review. *Journal of Advanced Nursing, 66*(1), 3–15. doi:10.1111/j.13652648.2009.05240.x

Carper, B. A. (1978). Fundamental patterns of knowing in nursing. *Advances in Nursing Science, 1*(1), 13–24.

Chickering, A. W., & Gamson, Z. F. (1987). Seven principles for good practice in undergraduate education. *Wingspread Journal, Volume 9, No. 2.* Retrieved from http://www.johnsonfdn.org/Publications/ConferenceReports/SevenPrinciples

Chinn, P. (2007). Philosophical foundations for excellence in nursing. In B. Moyer & R. A. Wittmann-Price (Eds.), *Nursing education: Foundations of practice excellence* (pp. 15–28). Philadelphia, PA: F. A. Davis.

Cleland, J. A., Abe, K., & Rethans, J. (2009). The use of simulated patients in medical education: AMEE Guide No. 42. *Medical Teacher, 31*, 477–486.

Csokasy, J. (2009). Philosophical foundations of the curriculum. In D. Billings & J. A. Halstead (Eds.), *Teaching in nursing: A guild for faculty* (pp. 125–144). St. Louis, MO: Elsevier Saunders.

Deci, E., Eghrari, H., Patrick, B. C., & Leone, D. R. (1994). Facilitating internalization: The self-determination theory perspective. *Journal of Personality, 62*(1), 119–142. doi:10.1111/j.1467-6494.1994.tb00797.x

DeYoung, S. (2009). *Teaching strategies for nurse educator* (2nd ed.). Upper Saddle River, NJ: Prentice Hall.

Dieckmann, P., Gaba, D., & Rall, M. (2007). Deepening the theoretical foundations of patient Simulation as social practice. *Simulation in Healthcare, 2*, 183–193.

Diekelmann, N. L. (1997). Creating a new pedagogy for nursing. *Journal of Nursing Education, 36*(4), 147–148.

Diekelmann, N. L. (2005). Engaging the students and the teacher: Co-creating substantive form with narrative pedagogy. *Journal of nursing Education, 44*(6), 249–252.

Doerr, H., & Murray, W. B. (2008). How to build a successful simulation scenario = obstacle course + treasure hunt. In R. R. Kyle & W. B. Murray (Eds.), *Clinical simulation: Operations, engineering and management* (pp. 745–749). London, UK: Elsevier/Academic Press.

Dreifuerst, K. T. (2009). The essentials of debriefing in simulation learning: A concept analysis. *Nursing Education Perspectives, 30*(2), 109–114.

Elfink, V. L., Nininger, J., Rohig, L., & Lee, J. (2009). The case for group planning in human patient simulation. *Nursing Education Perspectives, 30*(2), 83–86.

Entwistle, N. J. (1999). Approaches to studying and levels of understanding: The influences of teaching and assessment. In J. C. Smart (Ed.), *Higher education: Handbook of theory and research* (p. xv). New York, NY: Agathon Press.

Ericsson, K. A., Krampe, R. T., & Tesch-Römer, C. (1993). The role of deliberate practice in the acquisition of expert performance. *Psychology Review, 100*(3), 363–406.

Facione, N. C., Facione, P. A., & Sanchez, C. A. (1994). Critical thinking disposition as a measure of competent judgment: The development of the California Critical Disposition Inventory. *Journal of Nursing Education, 33*, 345–350.

Falco, P. A. (2009). Teaching nursing critical thinking strategies to nursing students. *Metas de Enfermería, 12*(9), 68–72.

Fanning, R. M., & Gaba, D. M. (2007). The role of debriefing in simulation-based learning. *Simulation in Healthcare, 2*(2), 115–125.

Forsythe, L. (2009). Research, simulation, team communication, and bringing the tacit into voice society for simulation in healthcare. *Simulation in Healthcare, 4*, 143–148.

Gagne, R. (1970). *The conditions of learning* (2nd ed.). New York, NY: Holt, Rinehart and Winston.

Gibbs, G. (1988). *Learning by doing: A guide to teaching and learning methods.* London, UK: Fell.

Glaser, E. M. (1941). *An experiment in the development of critical thinking.* New York, NY: Teacher's College, Columbia University.

Goffman, E. (1974). *Frame analysis. An essay on the organization of experience.* Boston, MA: Northeastern University Press.

Grant, J., & Marsden, P. (1992). *Training senior house officers by service based training.* London, UK: Joint Conference for Education in Medicine.

Hicks, N. A., & Burkus, E. (2011). Knowledge development for master teachers. *Journal of Theory Construction and Testing, 15*(2), 32–35.

Hsu, L. (2010). Metacognitive Inventory for nursing students in Taiwan: Instrument development and testing. *Journal of Advanced Nursing, 66*(11), 2573–2581. doi:10.1111/j.1365-2648.2010.05427.x

Issenberg, S. B., McGaghie, W. C., Issenberg, E. R., Petrusa, D. L., & Scalese, R. J. (2010). Features and uses of high-fidelity medical simulations that lead to effective learning: A BEME systematic review. *Medical Teacher, 27*(1), 10–28.

Jeffries, P. (Ed.). (2007). *Simulation in nursing: From conceptualization to evaluation.* New York, NY: National League for Nursing.

Johnson, D. W., & Johnson, F. P. (2003). *Joining together: Group theory and group skills* (8th ed.). Boston, MA: Pearson.

Kaakinen, J., & Arwood, E. (2009). Systematic review of nursing simulation literature for use of learning theory. *International Journal of Nursing Education Scholarship, 6*(1), 1–20. doi:10.2202/1548-923X.1688

Kane, M. (2006). Validation. In R. L. Brennan (Ed.), *Educational measurement* (4th ed, pp. 17–64). Westport, CT: American Council on Education/Praeger.

Kanter, S. L. (2008). Toward better descriptions of innovations. *Academic Medicine, 83*, 703–704.

Kardong-Edgen, S., Adamson, K. A., & Fitzgerald, C. (2010). A review of currently published evaluations for human patient simulation. *Clinical Simulation in Nursing, 6*, e25–e35.

Keller, J. M. (1987). Development and use of the ARCS model of motivational design. *Journal of Instructional Development, 10*(3), 2–10.

Kirkpatrick, D. L. (1998). *Evaluating training programs: The four levels* (2nd ed.). San Francisco, CA: Berrett-Koehler.

Kneebone, R. (2005). Evaluating clinical simulations for learning procedural skills: A theory-based approach. *Academic Medicine, 80*(6), 549–553.

Knowles, M. (1980). *The modern practice of adult education.* Chicago, IL: Follett.

Kolb, D. A. (1984). *Experiential learning: Experience as the source of learning and development.* New Jersey, NJ: Prentice-Hall.

Kolb, D. A., Boyatzis, R. E., & Mainemelis, C. (1999). *Experiential learning theory: Previous research and new directions.* Department of Organizational Behavior Weatherhead School of Management, Case Western Reserve University. Retrieved from http://www.d.umn.edu/~kgilbert/educ5165-731/Readings/experiential-learning-theory.pdf

Kramer, M. (1974). *Reality shock: Why nurses leave nursing.* St. Louis, MO: C.V. Mosby.

Laucken, U. (2003). *Theoretical psychology.* Oldenburg: Bibliotheks und Informationssystem der Universität Oldenburg.

Lax, L. R., Russell, M. L., Nelles, L. J., & Smith, C. M. (2009). Scaffolding knowledge building in a web-based communication and cultural competence program for international medical graduates. *Academic Medicine, 84*(10 Suppl.), S5–S8.

LeFlore, J. L., & Anderson, M. (2009). Alternative educational models for interdisciplinary student teams. *Simulation in Healthcare, 4,* 135–142.

Mann, K. V. (2011). Theoretical perspectives in medical education: Past experience and future possibilities. *Medical Education, 45,* 60–68. doi:10.1111/j.1365-2923.2010.03757.x

Marton, F., & Saljo, R. (1976). On qualitative differences in learning: I—Outcome and process. *British Journal of Educational Psychology, 46*(1), 4–11.

McGaghie, W. C., Issenberg, S. B., Petrusa, E. R., & Scalese, R. J. (2010). A critical review of simulation-based medical education research: 2003–2009. *Medical Education, 44,* 50–63. doi:10.1111/j.1365-2923.2009.03547.x

McGaghie, W. C., Siddall, V. J., Mazmanian, P. E., & Myers, J. (2009). Lessons for continuing medical education from simulation research in undergraduate and graduate medical education: Effectiveness of continuing medical education: American College of Chest Physicians evidence-based educational guidelines. *Chest, 135*(Suppl. 3), 62–68.

Meller, G. (1997) A typology of simulators for medical education. *Journal of Digital Imaging, 10*(3, Suppl. 1), 194–196.

Miller, M. A., & Malcolm, N. S. (1990). Critical thinking in the nursing curriculum. *Nursing & Healthcare, 11*(2), 66–73.

Mooney, M. (2007). Professional socialization: The key to survival as a newly qualified nurse. *International Journal of Nursing Practice, 13,* 75–80.

Mulligan. R. (2007). Management strategies in the educational setting. In B. Moyer & R. A. Wittmann-Price (Eds.), *Teaching nursing: Foundations of practice excellence* (pp. 109–125). Philadelphia, PA: F. A. Davis.

Munhall, P. L. (1993). Unknowing: Toward another pattern of knowing in nursing. *Nursing Outlook, 41*(3), 125–128.

Nesler, M. S., Hanner, M. B., Melburg, V., & McGowan, S. (2001). Professional socialization of baccalaureate nursing students: Can students in distance nursing programs become socialized? *Journal of Nursing Education, 40*(7), 293–302.

Novotny, J., & Griffin, M., T. (2006). *A nuts-and-bolts approach to teaching nursing.* New York, NY: Springer Publishing.

Partusch, M. (2007). Assessment and evaluation strategies. In B. A. Moyer & R. A. Wittmann-Price (Eds.), *Nursing education: Foundations of practice excellence* (pp. 213–227). Philadelphia, PA: F. A. Davis.

Paul, R., & Elder, L. (2007). Critical thinking: The nature of critical and creative thought. *Journal of Developmental Education, 32*(2) 34–35.

Pearson, A., Wiechula, R., Court, A., & Lockwood, C. (2007). A reconsideration of what constitutes "evidence" in the healthcare professions. *Nursing Science Quarterly, 20,* 85–88.

Philipin, S. M. (1999). The impact of project 2000 educational reforms on the occupational socialization of nurses: An exploratory study. *Journal of Advanced Nursing, 29*(6), 1326–1331.

Philpott, J., & Batty, H. (2009). Learning best together: Social constructivism and global partnerships in medical education. *Medical Education, 43*(9), 923–924.

Piaget, J. (1972). *The psychology of the child.* New York, NY: Basic Books.

Popil, I. (2011). Promotion of critical thinking by using case studies as teaching method. *Nurse Education Today, 31*(2), 204–207. doi:10.1016/j.nedt.2010.06.002

Ramsden, P., & Entwistle, N. J. (1981). Effects of academic departments on students' approaches to studying. *British Journal of Educational Psychology, 51,* 368–383.

Romeo, E. M. (2010). Quantitative research on critical thinking and predicting nursing students' NCLEX-RN, performance. *Journal of Nursing Education, 49*(7), doi:10.3928/01484834-20100331-05

Rose, S. (2011). Academic success of nursing students: Does motivation matter? *Teaching and Learning in Nursing, 6*(4), 181–184. DOI: 10.1016/j.teln.2011.05.004

Russell, S. S. (2006). An overview of adult learning. *Urologic Nursing, 26*(5), 349–370.

Schaefer, J. J., Vanderbilt, A. A., Cason, C. L., Bauman, E. B., Glavin, R. J. Lee, F. W., & Navedo, D. D. (2011). Literature review: Instructional design and pedagogy science in healthcare simulation. *Simulation in Healthcare, 6*, S30–S41.

Scheffer, B. K., & Rubenfield, M. G. (2000). A consensus statement on critical thinking in nursing. *Journal of Nursing Education, 39*(8), 352–359.

Squire, K. (2006). From content to context: Videogames as designed experience. *Educational Researcher, 35*(8), 19–29.

Society for Simulation in Healthcare (SSH). (2014). *Certified healthcare simulation educator handbook.* Retrieved from http://ssih.org/certification/handbook

Stillman, P. L., Ruggill, J. S., Rutala, P. J., & Sabers, D. L. (1980). Patient instructors as teachers and evaluators. *Journal of Medical Education, 55*, 186–193.

Swanson, D. B., & Stillman, P. L. (1990). Use of standardized (simulated) patients for teaching and assessing clinical skills. *Evaluation & the Health Professions, 13*(1), 79–103.

Tyler, R. W. (1949). *Basic principles of curriculum and instruction.* Chicago, IL: University of Chicago Press.

Vaihinger, H. (1927). *The philosophy of the as-if system of the theoretical, pragmatic, and religious fictions of mankind based on an idealistic positivism.* Aalen, Germany: Scientia.

Van Heukelom, J. N., Begaz, T., & Treat, R. (2010). Comparison of postsimulation debriefing versus in-simulation debriefing in medical simulation. *Simulation in Healthcare, 5*, 91–97.

Vroom, V. (1964). *Work and motivation.* New York, NY: Wiley.

Vygotsky, L. S. (1978). *Mind in society: The development of higher mental processes.* Belmont, CA: Wadsworth.

Walker, S. (2003). Active learning strategies to promote critical thinking. *Journal of Athletic Training, 38*(3), 263–267.

Walton, J., Chute, E., & Ball, L. (2011). Professional nurse: The pedagogy of simulation: A grounded study. *Journal of Professional Nursing, 27*, 299–310.

Wang, E. E. (2011). Simulation and adult learning. *Disease-a-Month, 57*, 664–678. doi:10.1016/j.disamonth.2011.08.017

Watson, G., & Glaser, E. M. (1964). *Critical thinking appraisal.* Orlando, FL: Harcourt, Brace & Jovanovich.

Wittmann-Price, R. A., & Fasolka, B. (2010). Objectives and outcomes: The fundamental difference. *Nursing Education Perspective, 31*(4), 233–236. doi: 0.1043/1536-5026- 31.4.233

Wittmann-Price, R. A., & Godshall, M. (2009). Strategies to promote deep learning in clinical nursing courses. *Nurse Educator, 34*(5), 214–216.

Wong, C. K., & Driscoll, M. (2008), A modified jigsaw method: An active learning strategy to develop the cognitive and affective domains through curricular review. *Journal of Physical Therapy Education, 21*(3), 15–23.

Wortham, S. (2011). What does philosophy have to offer education, and who should be offering it? *Educational Theory, 61*(60), 727–741.

Implementing Simulation in the Curriculum

NINA MULTAK

Education is simply the soul of a society as it passes from
one generation to another.
—G. K. Chesterton

> This chapter addresses Content Area 2: Demonstrate Knowledge
> of Simulation Principles, Practice, and Methodology (Society for
> Simulation in Healthcare [SSH], 2014).

LEARNING OUTCOMES

- Discuss the principles of integrating simulation into a curriculum
- Describe the variety of content areas to which simulation can be applied
- Discuss the need to use resources effectively and efficiently

Issenberg, McGaghie, Petrusa, Gordon, and Scalese (2005) describe the best practices of simulation in their critical review of simulation-based healthcare education. Curricular integration rated highly among the dozen best practices noted as being essential for the effective use of simulation. It is widely accepted that simulation-based learning is most effective when integrated with other learning events and focused on specific learning outcomes. Additionally, simulation-based healthcare education is identified as being complementary to clinical education.

Healthcare educators should understand the principles of integrating simulation into a curriculum and identify the curricular areas in which simulation can be effectively implemented. Resources should be used effectively and efficiently. Simulation-based healthcare education and evaluation need to be planned, scheduled, and carried out with consideration given to the entire curriculum (Scalese & Issenberg, 2008). Simulation should involve all educational stakeholders and garner the necessary administrative support, including funding and materials (Issenberg et al., 2005).

DEVELOPMENT OF A CURRICULUM

When developing a health education curriculum, the final step of the process of educational curricula development is the actual implementation of the project (Kern, Thomas, & Hughes, 2009). The steps of curriculum development according to Kern and colleagues are as follows.

- The first step in the model of Kern and colleagues identifies problem development with a subsequent needs assessment. This should include an evaluation of the problem, identifying both the current educational approach and the ideal educational approach.
- The next step includes a focused assessment of the learners and the most ideal learning environment. For simulation-based healthcare education, the educator should decide in which of the following environments the information would best be learned: a simulation lab, a classroom, or in situ.

The Certified Healthcare Simulation Educator™ (CHSE™) should analyze the current educational approach along with practitioners and the healthcare educational system to address the current educational needs. The difference between the ideal approach and current approach represents a gap and is identified by the general needs assessment. A targeted needs assessment should include an assessment of

- The needs of one's specific learner group
- The healthcare institution and specific learning environment, which may differ from the needs of the specific student population (Kern et al., 2009)

Setting goals and objectives serves as a basis for assessment, and specific measureable learning objectives should be considered. This includes

- Cognitive (knowledge)
- Affective (attitudinal)
- Psychomotor (skill and behavioral; Kern et al., 2009)

Educational strategies considered should be specific to learners and content of the curriculum.

Implementation of simulation in a curriculum requires consideration of many specific issues. Considerations for implementation include

- Obtaining political support
- Identifying and procuring resources
- Identifying and addressing barriers to implementation

- Introducing the curriculum (piloting or phasing-in)
- Administering the curriculum and refining the curriculum over successive cycles

The final step in the model of Kern and colleagues includes evaluation and feedback. This can be used to drive ongoing support, justify additional resources, and answer research questions about the effectiveness of specific curriculum elements. Table 7.1 outlines the model's steps and acknowledges the actual work needed to complete the steps.

TABLE 7.1
Steps to Curriculum Development According to the Model of Kern and Colleagues

STEPS	WORK NEEDED TO COMPLETE THE STEPS
Step 1: Problem identification and general needs Assessment - Identify the problem or educational gap - Identify the current approach (who is doing what, when, how; resource limitations) - Identify the ideal approach - Ideal − current approach = general assessment	Work for Steps 1 and 2 - Systematic review of literature - Needs assessment report - Assessment tool
Step 2: Needs analysis of targeted learners - Identify the learners, level of training, previous experience, current performance, learning styles and preferences - Identify barriers or enabling factors - Identify the available resources for this group (simulation, faculty, clinical experiences) - Identify multiple ways to obtain information/needs assessment (Kern et al., 2009)	
Step 3: Goals and objectives - Review types and levels of objectives - Learning domains: cognitive, psychomotor, affective - Review Bloom's taxonomy of educational objectives - Write specific, measurable, achievable, relevant, timely objectives	Work for Steps 3 and 4 - Identification of a new educational tool or method - Development of simulation scenarios - Research on the merits of educational processes or tools

(continued)

TABLE 7.1
Steps to Curriculum Development According to the Model of Kern and Colleagues
(*continued*)

STEPS	WORK NEEDED TO COMPLETE THE STEPS

Step 4: Educational strategies
 	
• Use multiple educational methods and match methods to objectives
• Review/discuss pros and cons of different methods
• Choose methods that are feasible in terms of resources
• Consider different simulation options:
  • Computer-based virtual patients
  • Role-playing
  • Standardized (simulated) patients
  • Task trainers or models
  • Virtual reality simulators
  • Mannequin simulators
  • Hybrid simulation
  • Group-learning projects
  • Supplemental interactive activities	

Step 5: Implementation • Consider resources: personnel, time, facilities, funding/costs • Administration and operations • Piloting, phasing-in, full implementation	Work for Steps 5 and 6 • Descriptive study of curriculum implementation • Cost-effective analysis report • Assessment tool
Step 6: Evaluation and feedback • Identify users and use (formative, summative), resources for evaluation, questions to ask, evaluation design • Select measurement method • Assess ethical issues • Data collection and analysis • Identification of results	

Adapted from Kern et al. (2009).

A needs assessment for a curriculum can be accomplished by many methods, including

- Informal discussions
- Questionnaires
- Surveys
- Interviews

- Focus groups
- Observations
- Tests
- Literature review
- Available published documents

DELIBERATE PRACTICE

Simulation-based learning can be applied to many areas in a healthcare curriculum. Research on expert performance has transformed the way healthcare educators approach how clinicians acquire clinical competence and how expertise is defined (Ericsson, 2004, 2008). The concept of deliberate practice, where education is focused on improving particular tasks, has been essential to the development of the simulation-based experiential learning paradigm and has been implemented by healthcare educators across many disciplines (Ericsson, 2008).

LEARNING DOMAINS

Simulation can measure outcomes in the cognitive, affective, and psychomotor domains (Kardong-Edgren, Adamson, & Fitzgerald, 2010). Cognitive domain learning may include the acquisition and recall of facts and figures, concepts, and principles. Cognitive learning outcomes have been identified as a basic strategy for the assessment of student learning. A traditional lecture followed by a multiple-choice or short-answer exam is an example of cognitive evaluation. Healthcare simulation offers an opportunity for teaching and evaluation of higher level cognitive functions, such as the application, synthesis, and evaluation of healthcare knowledge (Kardong-Edgren et al., 2010).

Learning in the affective domain includes the values, attitudes, and beliefs that are essential for a healthcare provider. Assessment of the affective domain requires educators to identify and verify that healthcare learners have absorbed the values, attitudes, and beliefs essential for a healthcare provider and that these are reflected in their professional practice. Mannequin simulation allows opportunities for learners to reveal their competency in the affective domain through participation in simulation scenarios.

Technical skill performance is an example of the assessment of psychomotor learning. Using task trainers, virtual reality simulators, and mannequin simulators, the CHSE can assess the acquisition of technical skills (Jeffries & Norton, 2005). Using a case scenario to evaluate technical skills allows CHSEs to teach and evaluate psychomotor skills in a setting that is more realistic than a traditional skills station (such as suturing on a task trainer or starting an intravenous [IV] line using a simulated IV arm) and much safer than an actual patient care setting, such as a live patient in an emergency department. Evaluation instruments that measure pre-established outcomes may be used for a comprehensive evaluation of learning (Kardong-Edgren et al., 2010).

INTEGRATING SIMULATION

Simulation training can be implemented in various components of a curriculum.

- Basic science courses can effectively use simulation modalities. Pharmacologic effects can be simulated on a mannequin for usual dosage ingestion or overdose. Medication effects can also be taught in code or advanced cardiac life support scenarios.
- Simulators can be used to teach vitals sign assessment as well as evaluation of cardiac and pulmonary conditions to healthcare learners.
- Crisis management training can be implemented with consideration of complex details of realistic case scenarios.

Effectively directing simulation resources can result in an educator's ability to implement simulation successfully in the educational curriculum. These resources are shown in Figure 7.1.

FIGURE 7.1 Resources needed to include simulation in a curriculum.

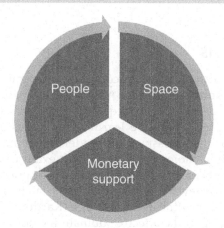

Organizational barriers can hinder the implementation of simulation-based education in the curriculum (McGaghie, Issenberg, Petrusa, & Scalese, 2010). Scheduling trainees to attend simulation activities can be a challenge. It is suggested that leaders in the institution support simulation programming by encouraging faculty to become involved and avoid learner scheduling and space issues. Faculty and financial resources can also be supported by administrative personnel (McGaghie et al., 2010).

EVIDENCE-BASED SIMULATION PRACTICE (EBSP) 7.1

Research suggests that the pressure of clinical responsibilities, clinical workload, and the perception that direct clinical experience is always more valuable than simulation-based education can adversely affect scheduled training sessions. These misperceptions can also affect student practice time, which may result in outcomes that are less effective than anticipated or that are delayed (McGaghie et al., 2010).

SIMULATION CONCEPTS

Establishing the best approach to integrating simulation in a curriculum can be determined by the institution as well as by the discipline and can address the potential effect of combining simulation-based healthcare education with other educational strategies (McGaghie et al., 2010).

Simulation-based education considerations prior to curricular implementation are

- **Realism:** Educational goals should match simulation type. Task trainers should be used for procedural skills, whereas complex events should involve a high-fidelity mannequin simulator (McGaghie et al., 2010).

- **Reliability (e.g., assessment tools, implementation process):** The development of effective evaluation tools should follow an organized process with a clearly defined endpoint (Kardong-Edgren et al., 2010).

- **Validity (e.g., content, construct):** Ideally, simulation evaluation instruments validly measure each of the three domains of student performance: cognitive, psychomotor, and affective. Several types of validity need to be considered when using tools for evaluation, including

  - Content validity—refers to the appropriateness of each item and comprehensiveness of the measurement.

  - Construct validity—refers to the process of establishing that an action accurately represents the concept being evaluated (Kardong-Edgren et al., 2010).

  - Face validity—does the evaluation tool appear to be measuring the concept it is supposed to measure?

  - Predictive ability—is there a correlation between the responses and an expectation? (Zheng & Agresti, 2000)

- **Feasibility (e.g., efficient, effective, achievable):** There should be possibilities for replication of some or nearly all of the essential aspects of a clinical situation so that the situation can be readily understood and managed when it occurs in actual clinical practice (Cant & Cooper, 2010).

- **Learner-centered education:** Students can use deliberate practice in a focused manner to master skills at their own pace (Ericsson, 2004).

- **Interprofessional education:** Interprofessional education (IPE) has been recognized by various international professional societies (e.g., World Health Organization, Institute of Medicine) and accreditation organizations as foundational to achieving safe, high-quality, accessible, patient-centered care.

- **Teamwork:** Critical teamwork competencies should be identified and used as a focus for training content; teamwork to be designed to improve team processes (Salas, Diaz-Granados, Weaver, & King, 2008).

> **Simulation Teaching Tip 7.1**
> Simulation program development should occur in conjunction with other curriculum programming. Simulation can be used for both formative and summative assessments and therefore is most valuable when integrated throughout the training curriculum. Involving faculty in the development of assessment tools enables more faculty involvement in simulation programming.

- **Human factors:** Engaging learners in repetitive practice is suggested as a primary factor in studies showing skill transference to real patients. With increased simulator availability, learning curves are shortened, which leads to faster skill automaticity. Simulators must be made available at a convenient location that accommodates learners' schedules (Issenberg et al., 2005).

- **Patient safety:** Simulation is an important educational technique for improving clinical training and patient safety (Wang, 2011).

SUMMARY

Simulation-based educators should highlight evidence-based information, which supports the best practices of simulation (McGaghie et al., 2010). Implementing simulation in the curriculum is among the top in the best practice list according to research. Other best practices noted in this research include feedback, deliberate practice, outcome measurement, appropriate fidelity, attention to skill acquisition and maintenance, mastery in learning, transference to practice, team training, high-stakes training, instructor training, and appropriate educational and professional context.

CASE STUDY 7.1

Faculty colleagues suggest that simulation programming is time-consuming and uses many resources. They suggest that implementation of simulation in the curriculum is not necessary because the current method of education, which has been in place for many years, produces learners who pass their certification exams. The faculty members also suggest that simulation would require additional faculty support and they do not wish to volunteer for additional educational projects.

In order to convince colleagues that simulation would be an effective educational modality, the faculty member interested in implementing simulation in the curriculum should highlight to the colleagues that simulation can be used for both formative and summative components of healthcare education training. With recent advances in the development of simulator technologies, assessment opportunities in healthcare professions education have expanded significantly. Although more traditional forms of assessment, such as multiple-choice questions, continue to be used, simulation-based assessments have gradually become common in the evaluation process, both formatively, as part of training and educational activities (Katz, Peifer, & Armstrong, 2010; Rudolph, Simon, Raemer, & Eppich, 2008; Steadman et al., 2006), and in a summative situation, such as a component of the certification and licensure process (Berkenstadt, Ziv, Gafni, & Sidi, 2006; Boulet, Smee, Dillon, & Gimpel, 2009; Dillon, Boulet, Hawkins, & Swanson, 2004; Hatala, Kassen, Nishikawa, Cole, & Issenberg, 2005).

Additionally, simulation-based learning includes the acquisition of technical skills, and it may also incorporate cognitive and affective learning (Jeffries & Norton, 2005). Through the incorporation of simulation into a healthcare education curriculum, CHSEs can readily teach and evaluate psychomotor skills in a setting that is more realistic than a traditional skills station, yet safer than live patient care where a patient may be acutely ill.

PRACTICE QUESTIONS

1. Which of the following is well established regarding integrating simulation into the curriculum?

   A. Integrate with other learning events
   B. Simulation can be substituted with lectures
   C. Clinical experience can substitute for immersive simulation
   D. Educational objectives are not required for case scenarios

2. Which of the following best describes a complete needs assessment?

   A. Identify the problem or educational gap
   B. Identify the current approach (who is doing what, when, how, resource limitations)
   C. Identify the ideal approach
   D. Ideal – current approach = general assessment

3. Which of the following learning domains is not evaluated through simulation?

   A. Affective
   B. Constructive
   C. Psychomotor
   D. Cognitive

4. Realism for technical skill assessment would be best assessed by which of the following?

   A. Full-body mannequin
   B. Standardized patient
   C. Task trainer
   D. Computer-based interactive activity

5. Which of the following organizational barriers can prevent simulation implementation in the curriculum?

   A. Lack of administrative support
   B. No dedicated space for simulation
   C. No time in the curriculum
   D. All of the above

6. In which step of the educational model of Kern and colleagues (2009) should the faculty member "identify the learners, level of training, previous experience, current performance, learning styles and preferences"?

   A. Step 1
   B. Step 2
   C. Step 3
   D. Step 4

7. "Deliberate practice" as discussed by Ericsson is best described as which of the following in simulation?

   A. Practice once per week with an instructor
   B. Practice in class only
   C. Practice until competency is achieved
   D. Practice scheduled for student

8. Which type of validity best describes the process of establishing that an action accurately represents the concept being evaluated in simulation?

   A. Construct validity
   B. Content validity
   C. Objective validity
   D. Implementation validity

9. Which of the following is a primary benefit of assessing technical skills using simulation modalities?

   A. Shorter time
   B. Patient safety
   C. Cost efficient
   D. Faculty training time

10. Simulation can be effectively integrated into the curriculum in which of the following areas?

    A. Basic sciences
    B. Basic clinical assessment
    C. Crisis management training
    D. All of the above

REFERENCES

Berkenstadt, H., Ziv, A., Gafni, N., & Sidi, A. (2006). The validation process of incorporating simulation-based accreditation into the anesthesiology Israeli national board exams. *Israel Medical Association Journal, 8*, 728–733.

Boulet, J. R., Smee, S. M., Dillon, G. F., & Gimpel, J. R. (2009). The use of standardized patient assessments for certification and licensure decisions. *Simulation Health, 4*, 35–42.

Cant, R., & Cooper, S. (2010). Simulation-based learning in nurse education: Systematic review. *Journal of Advanced Nursing, 66*(1), 3–15.

Dillon, G. F., Boulet, J. R., Hawkins, R. E., & Swanson, D. B. (2004). Simulations in the United States Medical Licensing Examination (USMLE). *Quality Safe Health Care, 13*, i41–i45.

Ericsson, K. A. (2004). Deliberate practice and the acquisition and maintenance of expert performance in medicine and related domains. *Academic Medicine, 79*(10), S70–S81

Ericsson, K. A. (2008). Deliberate practice and acquisition of expert performance: A general overview. *Academic Emergency Medicine, 15*(11), 988–994.

Hatala, R., Kassen, B. O., Nishikawa, J., Cole, G., & Issenberg, S. B. (2005). Incorporating simulation technology in a Canadian internal medicine specialty examination: A descriptive report. *Academic Medicine, 80*, 554–556.

Issenberg, S. B., McGaghie, W. C., Petrusa, E. R., Gordon, D. L., & Scalese, R. J. (2005). Features and uses of high-fidelity medical simulations that lead to effective learning: A BEME systematic review. *Medical Teacher, 27*, 10–28.

Jeffries, P. R., & Norton, B. (2005). Selecting learning experiences to achieve curriculum outcomes. In D. M. Billings & J. A. Halstead (Eds.), *Teaching in nursing: A guide for faculty* (2nd ed., pp. 187–212). St. Louis, MO: Elsevier.

Kardong-Edgren, S., Adamson, K. A., & Fitzgerald, C. (2010). A review of currently published evaluation instruments for human patient simulation. *Clinical Simulation in Nursing, 6*, e25–e35.

Katz, G. B., Peifer, K. L., & Armstrong, G. (2010). Assessment of patient simulation use in selected baccalaureate nursing programs in the United States. *Simulation in Healthcare, 5*, 46–51.

Kern, D. E., Thomas, P. A., & Hughes, M. T. (2009). *Curriculum development for medical education: A six step approach* (2nd ed.). Baltimore, MD: Johns Hopkins University Press.

McGaghie, W., Issenberg, S. B., Petrusa, E. R., & Scalese, R. J. (2010). A critical review of simulation-based medical education research: 2003–2009. *Medical Education, 44*, 50–63

Rudolph, J. W., Simon, R., Raemer, D. B., & Eppich, W. J. (2008). Debriefing as formative assessment: Closing performance gaps in medical education. *Academic Emergency Medicine, 15*, 1010–1016.

Salas, E., Diaz-Granados, D., Weaver, S. J., & King, H. (2008). Does team training work? Principles for health care. *Academic Emergency Medicine, 11*, 1002–1009.

Scalese, R. J., & Issenberg, S. B. (2008). Simulation-based assessment. In E. S. Holmboe & R. E. Hawkins (Eds.), *Practical guide to the evaluation of clinical competence* (pp. 179–200). Philadelphia, PA: Mosby Elsevier.

Society for Simulation in Healthcare (SSH). (2014). *Certified healthcare simulation educator handbook.* Retrieved from http://ssih.org/certification/handbook

Steadman, R. H., Coates, W. C., Huang, Y. M., Matevosian, R., Larmon, B. R., McCullough, L., & Ariel, D. (2006) Simulation-based training is superior to problem-based learning for the acquisition of critical assessment and management skills. *Critical Care Medicine, 34*, 151–157.

Wang, E. (2011). Simulation and adult learning. *Disease of the Month, 57*, 664–678.

Zheng, B., & Agresti, A. (2000). Summarizing the predictive power of a generalized linear model. *Statistics in Medicine, 19*, 1771–1781.

Ethical, Legal, and Regulatory Implications

in Healthcare Simulation

BONNIE A. HAUPT AND COLLEEN H. MEAKIM

*Excellence calls for character . . . integrity . . . fairness . . .
honesty . . . a determination to do what's right.
High ethical standards, across the board.*
—Price Pritchett

This chapter addresses Content Area 2: Demonstrate Knowledge
of Simulation Principles, Practice, and Methodology (Society for
Simulation in Healthcare [SSH], 2014).

LEARNING OUTCOMES

- Discuss the regulatory requirements and issues that affect simulation practice
- Discuss the ethical and legal implications associated with healthcare simulation
- Discuss the case studies and practice questions as they relate to legal, ethical, and regulatory issues that may arise during simulation scenarios

Simulation use in healthcare education was developed to improve patient safety, enhance professional performance, reduce errors, and improve overall patient outcomes. Calhoun, Boone, Miller, and Pian-Smith (2013) believe that simulation permits consequences of errors from real-life events to be studied and recreated without causing patient harm. Simulation education must not only focus on creating a safe learning environment to protect patients from harm but it should also protect learners. Establishing trust in the learner–educator relationship is crucial to implementing successful simulation experiences. This chapter explores the importance of ethical, legal, and regulatory implications in healthcare simulation education, including the role of simulation in the development of the learner's personal professional integrity.

HISTORY

What thoughts come to mind when you hear the word "Tuskegee"? Do you think of the famous Tuskegee airmen, the African Americans who were trained to maintain and fly combat planes (Tuskegee Airmen, 2013)? Or do you think of the 1932–1972 United States Public Health Service Syphilis Study at Tuskegee (Centers for Disease Control, 2012)? The researchers involved in the study caused distress and pain for African Americans and their families by withholding treatment of those who had the disease. Are you familiar with the name Henrietta Lacks? In 1951, Ms. Lacks's cells were used without her permission or knowledge. The cells were used by the scientific community to develop cloning, gene mapping, and other historical research (Skloot, 2010). Ethical dilemmas created in the scientific community have led to changes in research involving human subjects to prevent ethical and moral harm. A code of ethics was developed by the American Educational Research Association (AERA) in 2011. This code governs the ethical standards and principles for researchers working in education (AERA, 2013). Hundreds of books and articles have been published to guide educators in educational ethics.

EVIDENCE-BASED SIMULATION PRACTICE (EBSP) 8.1

In order to develop a safe learning environment and protect the Certified Healthcare Simulation Educator™ (CHSE™), Auburn University in Auburn, Alabama, developed evidence-based job descriptions for simulation learning coordinators (SLCs) by using information from the International Nursing Association for Clinical Simulation and Learning (INACSL). Having an SLC assists faculty with appropriate, state-of-the-art simulation and debriefing teaching methods (Gore & Schuessler, 2013).

CREATING A SAFE ENVIRONMENT

In 2011, the Agency for Healthcare Research and Quality (AHRQ) recognized simulation as an educational tool to enhance skills and allow healthcare providers to test new clinical procedures in a safe learning environment. According to Truog and Meyer in 2013, for simulation to be credible, it must be developed on a strong foundation of safety and trust. Globally, simulation centers are developing standards and guidelines to create a safe environment focusing on creating protection of learners' ethical, legal, and regulatory rights. A review of simulation centers within universities and healthcare institutions found specific guidelines, including

• Codes of conduct and confidentiality guidelines
• Learner evaluation processes
• Recording and photo use consent forms in release contracts

Codes of Conduct and Confidential Guidelines

Codes of conduct and confidential guidelines developed by simulation centers stress the importance of abiding by the Health Insurance Portability and Accountability Act of 1996 (HIPAA) regulations during simulation scenarios. Simulation experiences are to be considered as real-life events. Learners are expected

- To act in a professional manner
- Be prepared to participate
- Not discuss the information outside of the simulation center

Sharing of information could impede the confidentiality of participants or affect other participants' learning opportunities.

> **Simulation Teaching Tip 8.1**
> Many simulation centers ask learners to sign a contract letter prior to courses, agreeing to the confidentiality of the simulation experience, thereby creating an ethical environment for all learners.

Learner Evaluations

How learners are evaluated has received a great deal of interest from simulation educations and learners alike. Elfrink, Nininger, Rohig, and Lee (2009) define formative evaluation as evaluations that occur during the learning activity or program with a goal to reach objectives focusing on the current course and occur no later than midcourse. The purpose of formative evaluations is to promote self-assessment through providing learners with feedback (Jeffries & McNelis, 2010). Summative evaluations are those that take place at the end of a grading period, course, or for a competency-related situation (Elfrink, Nininger, Rohig, & Lee, 2009). Jeffries and McNelis (2010) noted that summative evaluations are used to award a grade, or degree, or certify competency, using a standardized criteria. When evaluating learners, they must be informed as to whether they are participating in a formative or summative simulation experience. When developing scenarios, CHSEs should take into consideration

- The goals of the simulation
- The use of the appropriate evaluations for the content

Recording and Photo Use

Wang (2011) believes learners can be guided by CHSEs during debriefing in reviewing learner objectives and performances. Recording of simulation experiences for debriefing purposes is widely used in healthcare simulation education. Cantrell (2008) highlights that video recording use during scenarios captures learner performance, which can be viewed with learners after the experience. Video recording may provide a moment of clarity for the learner during a debriefing session. Recording can recall precise interactions during the simulation to focus on what went well and what needs improvement, to allow for critical reflection. Recording consents and releases should emphasize

- How long the material(s) will be stored
- Purposes of the recording
- That participants have no compensation rights

Simulation centers are also challenged with issues regarding religious objections to being recorded, and, in some instances, standardized (simulated) patients (SPs) who are members of the Screen Actors Guild who decline recording and photographs.

> **Simulation Teaching Tip 8.2:**
> Having a policy "up front" about expectations regarding video recording and picture taking will allow learners, SPs, and CHSEs to decide whether they can meet the learning outcomes or expectations of the experience if recorded debriefing is not done.

PROFESSIONAL DEVELOPMENT THROUGH SIMULATION

Part of the simulation process includes the development of the individual learner's understanding of the chosen profession's value system. Therefore, initially learners and CHSEs must come to a common understanding of what the group's professional value system entails. In the broadest sense, professionalism includes requirements for practitioners to be honest and responsible, which ultimately can lead to a sense of professional integrity (Weisman, Haynes, & Solicitor, 2013).

However, both learners and educators share responsibility for the learning activities associated with simulation. Both must participate in preparation for simulation, as well as identifying knowledge gaps and strategizing to address these gaps. If these activities are integrated throughout the curriculum and constructed based on the profession's code of conduct, this process can lead to an enhanced moral reasoning process (Gillespie, 2005; Wiseman, Haynes, & Solicitor, 2013). If learners can develop their own personal and social responsibility within the simulated clinical environment, they should be more able to reflect and analyze situations to assist in clinical decision making (Wiseman, Haynes, & Solicitor, 2013).

Educators have a key role in the process of developing learners' moral and ethical reasoning processes. There are varieties of ways that moral and ethical situations can be woven into simulation activities, including simulations with overriding issues that have these components embedded in them. Scenarios focusing on specifically complex healthcare issues can include

- Informed consent
- Patient confidentiality
- End-of-life care
- Care of vulnerable populations
- Genetic and reproductive issues
- "Do not resuscitate" orders

Such simulations can generate critical thinking, enhance communication, and allow for consideration of complex ethical issues from various participants. Participation in a mock ethics committee, in which learners assume various roles as committee or family members, is another example of an activity that can teach participants about communication-related issues for both medical personnel and families (Gisondi, Smith-Coggins, Harter, Soltysik, & Yarnold, 2004; Gropelli, 2010; Rostain & Parrott, 1986).

SUMMARY

Simulation experiences were created to improve patient safety, enhance professional performance, reduce errors, and improve overall patient outcomes. However, it is extremely important to remember that protection of human rights applies to the learners as well. When developing simulation experiences, not only should there be an emphasis on objectives, methods, and outcomes, but CHSEs must also consider the importance of ethical, legal, and regulatory concerns when developing these experiences.

CASE STUDY 8.1

Review the following case study and answer questions 1 and 2.

The healthcare simulation team is excited to have received funding and equipment to develop a simulation training center. The group has worked tirelessly on developing and coordinating the first simulation scenario that will be piloted this fall with undergraduate learners. The scenario objectives, methods, and outcomes focusing on a failure-to-rescue case will be presented. The simulation environment consists of high-fidelity mannequins, in which learners will be recorded during each session. The team has decided not to inform learners of the recording or that the findings of the scenario will be shared with administrators and could potentially cause learners to be removed from the program.

1. Reflect on what major ethical, legal, and regulatory implications the simulation training center team has overlooked in their planning phases for the simulation experience.
2. The simulation team wants to try a new product during a simulation scenario. Would the team need to obtain learner consent to participate?

PRACTICE QUESTIONS

1. A learner is of a religious belief that does not allow video recording, and all other learners have agreed to recording for debriefing purposes. The simulation educator should

   A. Explain to the learner that it will be destroyed after debriefing
   B. Make an exception and not video record the learner, but ask the learner to write a summary reflection
   C. Explain to the learner that the learner cannot meet course objectives and will not pass the scenario
   D. Explain to the learner it is for educational purposes only

2. The simulation educator overhears learners talking outside the simulation room about the scenario, using information specific to the diagnosis, treatment, and outcomes. The first action the simulation educator should take is

A. Arrange a meeting with the participants in a private place and discuss the situation
B. Inform the participants they have failed the scenario due to unprofessional behavior
C. Give the participants a written warning for unprofessional behavior
D. Ask the participants to immediately stop the conversation and address the unprofessionalism

3. Following a formative simulation session, the team identifies a mechanical issue that did not allow the session to be video recorded. The simulation educator planned to use the video recording as part of the debriefing. What action should the simulation educator take now?

A. Cancel the debriefing because there is no recording
B. Conduct the debriefing without the video
C. Present the key points of the simulation to the participants
D. Reschedule the session when the mechanical issue has been fixed

4. A participant arrives to the simulation lab late after the session has begun without having completed the preclass assignment. The simulation lab policy states that all readings must be completed before class. The best action for the simulation educator is to

A. Allow the learner to participate and require the learner to complete an additional simulation assignment
B. Allow the learner to participate and extend the session to make up the time
C. Not allow the learner to participate and agree to discuss alternatives after the session
D. Not allow the learner to participate until the preclass assignment is completed

5. A journalist requests to observe, record, and interview participants in the simulation lab. Your institution does not have a policy regarding outside observers. The best response by the simulation educator to this request is

A. "No, but I will be willing to give you a tour and answer any questions."
B. "Yes, this is a summative evaluation, and I will need to get permission from the participants to be recorded."
C. "Yes, but you will need to come back next week after our policy is finalized."
D. "Yes, absolutely; here is a list of simulations that would be best for your report."

6. The simulation lab's policy states that videos will be destroyed after 5 days unless necessary for a research project approved by the institutional review board (IRB). To protect the learners, videos are stored on a secure password-protected server. A faculty member contacts the simulation team and asks to save a class simulation video for a future class scheduled in 14 days. The faculty member has spoken with all of the participants and has received verbal consent to use the video. Which of the following is the best response to the request?

    A. Because the video was an excellent example to use in the classroom, an exception to the policy will be made.

    B. The participants have all given verbal consent; therefore, the video will be saved for the faculty member.

    C. The video can only be used for the next 10 days, and then it will be deleted.

    D. The video was created to use in the classroom only, and it will be deleted per policy.

7. A simulation evaluation that is used to assess learners' competency for a degree, award, or against a criteria is called

    A. Formative evaluation

    B. Cumulative evaluation

    C. Peer evaluation

    D. Summative evaluation

8. A simulation evaluation that is used to promote self-assessment, guide learners, clarify misconception, and provide feedback is called

    A. Formative evaluation

    B. Cumulative evaluation

    C. Peer evaluation

    D. Summative evaluation

9. A benefit for healthcare simulation educators when using formative evaluation in simulation-based learning (SBL) is to

    A. Improve the learner's performance

    B. Determine whether the competency was achieved

    C. Assign a final grade

    D. Require the learner to figure out the scenario independently

10. While conducting team simulation activities, communication, collaboration, and trust of the teams may be enhanced during the session when

    A. The same team leader is used every time

    B. Learners are criticized for their mistakes

    C. A safe learning environment is created

    D. Learners are encouraged to practice in silos

REFERENCES

Agency for Healthcare Research and Quality (AHRQ). (2011). *Improving patient safety through simulation research.* Retrieved from http://www.ahrq.gov/research/findings/factsheets/errors-safety/simulproj11/index.html

American Educational Research Association (AERA). (2013). Retrieved from http://www.aera.net

Calhoun, A. W., Boone, M. C., Miller, K. H., & Pian-Smith, M. C. (2013). Using simulation to address hierarchy issues during medical crises. *Simulation in Healthcare, 8*(1), 13–19.

Cantrell, M. A. (2008). The importance of debriefing in clinical simulations. *Clinical Simulation in Nursing, 4*(2), e19–e23. doi:10.1016/j.ecns.2008.06.006

Centers for Disease Control and Prevention. (2012). *U.S. public health service syphilis study at Tuskegee.* Retrieved from http://www.cdc.gov/tuskegee

Elfrink, V. L., Nininger, J., Rohig, L., & Lee, J. (2009). Case for group planning in human patient simulation. *Nursing Education Perspectives, 30*(2), 83–86.

Gillespie, M. (2005). Student–teacher connection: A place of possibility. *Journal of Advanced Nursing, 52*(2), 211–219.

Gisondi, M., Smith-Coggins, R., Harter, P. M., Soltysik, R. C., & Yarnold, P. R. (2004). Assessment of resident professionalism using high-fidelity simulation of ethical dilemmas. *Academic Emergency Medicine, 11*(9), 931–937.

Gore, T., & Schuessler, J. B. (2013). Simulation policy development: Lessons learned. *Clinical Simulation in Nursing, 9*(8), e319–e322.

Gropelli, T. M. (2010). Using active simulation to enhance learning of nursing ethics. *Journal of Continuing Education in Nursing, 41*(3), 104–105.

Jeffries, J. R., & McNelis, A. M. (2010). Evaluation. In W. M. Nehring & F. R. Lashley (Eds.), *High-fidelity patient simulation in nursing education* (pp. 405–424). Sudbury, MA: Jones and Barlett.

Pritchett, P. (2013). *Finest quotes. Ethics quotes.* Retrieved from http://www.finestquotes .com/select_quote-category-Ethics-page-0.htm

Rostain, A. L., & Parrott, M. C. (1986). Ethics committee simulations for teaching medical ethics. *Journal of Medical Education, 61*(3), 178–181.

Skloot, R. (2010). *The immortal life of Henrietta Lacks.* New York, NY: Broadway Paperbacks, Random House.

Society for Simulation in Healthcare (SSH). (2014). *Certified healthcare simulation educator handbook.* Retrieved from http://ssih.org/certification/handbook

Truog, R. D., & Meyer, E. C. (2013). Deception and death in medical simulation. *Simulation in Healthcare, 8*(1), 1–3.

Tuskegee Airmen Inc. (2013). *A brief history.* Retrieved from http://tuskegeeairmen.org /explore-tai/a-brief-history/

Wang, E. E. (2011). Simulation and adult learning. *Disease a Month, 57*(11), 664–678. doi: 10.1016/j.disamonth.2011.08.017

Wiseman, A., Haynes, C., & Solicitor, S. H. (2013). Implementing professional integrity and simulation-based learning in health and social care: An ethical and legal maze or a professional requirement for high-quality simulated practice learning? *Clinical Simulation in Nursing, 9*(10), e437–e443. Retrieved from http://dx.doi.org/10.1016/j .ecns.2012.12.004

Human Patient Simulator Simulation

CAROL OKUPNIAK

Simulation is fiction—your decisions are real.
—John Cornele

This chapter addresses Content Area 2: Demonstrate Knowledge of Simulation Principles, Practice, and Methodology (Society for Simulation in Healthcare [SSH], 2014).

LEARNING OUTCOMES

- Discuss the principles of human simulator simulation learning in healthcare education
- Describe the variety of methodologies for the use of human simulator simulation
- Describe the principles of interprofessional team work

When considering the incorporation of human simulator simulations for the education of healthcare professionals, it is important to understand the principles, practice, and methodologies necessary for a successful simulation experience. Included in this understanding is knowledge of the relationship between the learner and the environment and how healthcare decisions will be assessed and evaluated. When using human simulators as an educational tool, the designer of the simulation scenario incorporates learning methodologies into the process of planning, implementation, and evaluation of the learning that takes place with human simulator simulation experiences. Among the outcomes measured during simulation scenarios are participation, attitude, knowledge, and skills (Issenberg, McGaghie, Petrusa, Gordon, & Scalese, 2005).

SIMULATION PRINCIPLES

Simulation-Based Learning

Simulation-based learning (SBL) is a process that occurs in a safe and carefully controlled setting that enhances skill acquisition and training using a simulated environment as the platform for learning (Lateef, 2010). Many healthcare institutions and academic settings are using SBL to educate and evaluate healthcare professionals and those in educational programs to become future healthcare professionals. Simulation is a technique that replicates real-life experiences with scenarios that immerse the learner in an environment that attempts to closely duplicate the clinical environment (Lateef, 2010). In addition to task and technical skills, SBL can also be used to identify problem-solving and decision-making skills. Team education, communication, and interpersonal skills are evaluated during SBL. To use simulation effectively, sound teaching–learning principles are needed. Without sound principles and planning, adverse consequences can easily occur during a simulation experience. For example, Lateef (2010) has identified common problems detected during simulation scenarios involving teams.

- Group does not understand that each team member has a unique role, especially in interdisciplinary teams
- Lack of clear role definition resulting in role confusion
- No plan in place to use when mistakes or errors occur
- No method to measure individual or team performance

The success of using simulator scenarios to educate healthcare professionals should be measured in relationship to the improvement in clinical competence and the potential or actual impact on patient safety and outcomes.

Deliberate Practice

Using human simulator experiences gives the learner an opportunity to practice and acquire clinical skills without practicing on live human patients (McGaghie, Issenberg, Petrusa, & Scalese, 2010). A core principle of human simulator education is the concept of *deliberate practice*. Deliberate practice is defined as a learner's endeavor to practice for the purpose of improving a task or skill beyond the current level of proficiency (Clapper & Kardong-Edgren, 2012). Using the concept of deliberate practice, simulation can improve the effectiveness of the learning experience. An integral component of deliberate practice is *critical reflection*. A learner must recognize a deficit in knowledge in an effort to seek learning opportunities to narrow this gap in knowledge. With the assistance of a Certified Healthcare Simulation Educator™ (CHSE™), the learner becomes actively engaged in practicing and improving a task, skill, or decision-making process. When a learner engages in deliberate practice, feedback from the CHSE is necessary to communicate improvement and identify areas that continue to need refinement (Ericsson, 2008).

Team Training

Many events in a healthcare environment require a cohesive team to accomplish their tasks (Andreatta, Bullough, & Marzano, 2010). Like a real clinical environment, human simulator scenarios most often include a small group of participants rather than just an individual learner. Knowing how to incorporate principles

EVIDENCE-BASED SIMULATION PRACTICE (EBSP) 9.1

Sawatsky, Mikhael, Punatar, Nassar, and Argwal (2013) used deliberate practice with first-year residents to study its effectiveness in teaching handoff communication. The study focused on the accuracy of information being provided in handoffs, the time it took the resident to give a handoff, and the residents' comfort and perceived efficiency in giving handoffs. Practices improved significantly with deliberate practice. This study indicated a change in skill and knowledge (6.31 to 7.64, $p < .001$).

of team education and crisis resource management (CRM) into a scenario involving more than one learner will build this competency. The first step in team education in simulation is to articulate the specific competencies targeted toward acquiring team-building skills (Salas, Rosen, & King, 2009). Once these competencies are recognized, a level of measurement can be calculated to guide the debriefing process.

Simulation Teaching Tip 9.1
If at all possible, when assigning learners to teams, make every team diverse. Diversity in race, gender, as well as role should be considered for every interprofessional team in order to teach cultural awareness and sensitivity as well as group collaboration.

Whether a team of learners from the same discipline or an interprofessional group, the principles of team training can be applied to human simulator education. A framework for building teams was developed by the Agency for Healthcare Research and Quality (AHRQ) called Team Strategies and Tools to Enhance Performance and Patient Safety or TeamSTEPPS® (AHRQ, 2013). This process of team training is designed for healthcare professionals to improve patient safety and achieve better patient outcomes. Simulation aids the acquisition of team skills by allowing the learner to practice in a simulated, safe environment. Using TeamSTEPPS in simulation is one way to aid in the design, measurement of objectives, and evaluation of team training (Table 9.1).

Within TeamSTEPPS training is a principle known as CUS, which stands for

- "I am **C**oncerned!
- I am **U**ncomfortable!
- This is a **S**afety issue!" (AHRQ, 2013).

The purpose of CUS is to empower individuals to speak up if they are concerned about an actual or potential breach in safety. Included in the CUS course of action is a two-challenge rule (AHRQ, 2013). Under this rule, if individuals feel that their concern has not been recognized, they should

- Verbalize this concern at least twice. If, after the second exchange, the team member concludes that the response is not acceptable, the team member is expected to take a different, more assertive course.
- This alternate course may include following the chain of command to insure a safe environment.

TABLE 9.1
Components of Team Training in Human Simulator Simulations

Leadership	Delegation of tasks to other team members, planning, organizing, and motivating other team members
Peer observation	A shared understanding of group dynamics and team roles; ability to recognize errors and openly communicate ideas and suggestions for correction
Flexibility	Ability to adapt or change as the scenario unfolds or the group dynamics change
Group membership	Recognition that the work of the team is paramount and individual goals are secondary
Balance	The workload of all team members should be balanced and match the knowledge and skills of each individual
Trust	An atmosphere of mutual trust should exist in which individuals are able to share knowledge and speak about errors in judgment and action and accept constructive feedback
Communication	All members of the team are able to openly communicate, confirm that their message was heard and understood, and clarify if necessary

The use of the CUS rule can be employed during a simulation scenario and measured as part of the evaluation criteria.

Crisis Resource Management

Another method of assessing teams is through a process of CRM. When CRM began in the aviation industry, it was originally titled "crew resource management." CRM has been incorporated throughout healthcare education (Cheng, Donoghue, Giffoyle, & Eppich, 2012). A team is identified as two or more individuals with specific roles and tasks who make decisions by interacting and coordinating with one another (Baker, Gustafson, & Beaubien, 2010). The key principles of CRM are

- Having a clear leader and well-defined roles
- Knowing your environment and resources
- Having a plan and sharing and adapting the plan as needed
- Requesting help early
- Distributing the work and supporting all members of the team
- Prioritizing and delegating tasks to others (Joshi, 2013)

Using the principles of CRM within a simulation scenario will help the team perform in a co-ordinated and efficient manner in the care of the simulated patient.

Closed-Loop Communication

When communicating to members of the team during simulator simulations, it is imperative that each individual's message is heard and understood. *Closed-loop* communication is a method of communication in which there is a sender and receiver of a specific message. The receiver of the message confirms the message that was communicated by the sender, thereby ensuring that the message was received and understood (Hunt, Shilkofski, Stavroudis, & Nelson, 2007).

EXHIBIT 9.1

Closed-Loop Communication

- A sender delivers a message to a receiver.
- The receiver of the message acknowledges that the message was received and ascribes meaning to the message.
- The sender communicates with the receiver to ensure that the expected meaning was conferred through the message.
- If the sender does not feel that the message was interpreted as intended, the conversation continues until the loop is closed.

SBAR Communication

The acronym SBAR stands for situation, background, assessment, and recommendation. SBAR communication is an organized, structured method of two-way communication in a healthcare setting. The person conferring the information provides

- S = A short, but relevant summary of the current situation
- B = The background of the patient relevant to the information exchange
- A = Important assessment findings
- R = A recommendation for action on the part of the receiver of the information

In many simulator simulations, it is expected that the participants communicate with each other, other disciplines, and those outside of the simulated environment using SBAR communication.

SIMULATION METHODOLOGY

Experiential Learning

A methodology is the theoretical analysis of the body of methods and principles associated with a body of knowledge. Kolb's model of experiential learning is often applied to simulation learning (Kolb & Fry, 1975). Kolb's model places the learner into one of four learning styles. These styles are converger, diverger, assimilator, and accommodator (D'Amore, James, & Mitchell, 2012).

- Convergers are best at problem solving and making decisions.
- Divergers are more creative and are able to form new ideas.
- Assimilators apply inductive reasoning to a situation.
- Accommodators are those who are actively engaged and are able to adapt quickly when the situation changes.

Each of these learning styles can be an asset during a simulation scenario (D'Amore, James, & Mitchell, 2012).

Because the learners are living the experience during simulation, they have the ability for increased engagement. Due to the reality of the setting, the learner is more engaged and interacts more fully in the activity. The goal of experiential learning is to gain new knowledge and understanding of key concepts or principles. During experiential learning, learners are asked to perform within a defined role in an activity that has context and meaning for the learners.

Adult Learning

Simulation is a technique that uses a guided experience to replicate the real world in a manner that is thoroughly interactive (Gaba, 2004). Within the simulated environment, the adult learner practices using the concepts of andragogy or the teaching of adults. The work of Malcolm Knowles (1950) centers on the topic of andragogy. Adult learners are self-directed and independent and consider that they are responsible for their own learning (Wang, 2011). Adult learners also have experience and previously learned knowledge that can be used as a resource for future learning (Zigmont, Kappus, & Sudikoff, 2011). Ensuring a proper environment for learning is another principle of adult learning. This is also the basis of using simulation to educate healthcare professionals.

Because simulation allows adults to practice skills and behaviors in a team environment, it has the ability to motivate adults to learn (Zigmont, Kappus, & Sudikoff, 2011). Adult learners expect confidentiality of their performance after a simulation is concluded. This is especially challenging when both the simulation and the debriefing are group experiences. The simulation educator, while providing a safe, rich learning environment, must maintain respect and support for the adult learner during simulation and maintain confidentiality of all involved. In addition, the participants of the simulation must also respect the need to maintain confidentiality of the actions during the simulation scenario and debriefing to protect the privacy of all participants.

There are additional concepts related to adult learners not originally considered by Knowles (1950). Not all adults learn in the same way. Learning is situation specific, and there are many factors that affect the adult learner. One important factor of adult learning is how a person's culture affects learning (Clapper, 2010). It is also assumed that adults experience information overload and are not capable of additional learning. It has been found that adults who perceive themselves as overloaded will continue to learn if they consider the activity an important and meaningful part of their development (Clapper, 2010). The challenge for educators using simulation is to convey the importance and value of the experience for the adult learner.

Situational Awareness

Situational awareness is a method of continuous assessment of the environment. A construct of situational awareness in team activities is to inform all members about the individual's perception of the situation and environment so that everyone has the same understanding (Hunt, Shilkofski, Stavroudis, & Nelson, 2007). This shared cognizance helps each team member see the larger picture during a simulation scenario rather than concentrating only on an individual task. When situational awareness is employed during a scenario, all team members are kept informed and updated on the plan of care and all new developments in patient status.

Perfect Practice

A novel approach to simulation learning is a methodology termed *perfect practice* or *do overs*. This process allows the learner to complete a human simulator simulation, discover new knowledge from the debriefing session, and return to the simulated environment to repeat the same simulation with the new insight gained from the debriefing. Ishoy, Epps, and Packard (2010) found increased learner satisfaction and improved self-confidence when learners are permitted to repeat the simulation and are given the opportunity to provide feedback on their repeat performance.

HIGH-FIDELITY SIMULATION

The concept of simulation is not new in medical education. However, the use of high-fidelity simulators used in healthcare provider education has been a relatively new phenomenon. *Fidelity* is the measure to which the simulator or the simulation match the real environment the scenario is attempting to simulate (Maran & Glavin, 2003). Due to significant advancements in simulator technology, it is now possible to create a simulated environment using many high-fidelity strategies to construct a setting very close to the real world. Today's high-fidelity mannequins are capable of a multitude of physiologic functions. In addition to mannequin fidelity, there is also physical, functional, psychological, and task fidelity that adds to the realism for the learner. The higher the fidelity of the simulation, the more human and physical recourses and time are needed when preparing and executing the simulator scenario (Alinier, 2011).

Current high-fidelity mannequins are available in models representing different stages of the life span from fetal and neonatal through adult. High-fidelity mannequins can be used for specific tasks, such as central line placement, or whole-body mannequins can be used to respond with complex, multisystem, physiologic adaptation to the learner's actions or inactions. Advancement in the science of designing high-fidelity human simulators continues as technology improves. What is available today may seem primitive in only a few years as improvements in computerization, robotics, and materials science improve our ability to create a more realistic human simulator.

Functional Fidelity

Functional fidelity is the degree of accuracy in the operation of the simulated system. When operating a computerized, high-fidelity mannequin, the physiologic manifestations should be as close as possible to how a real person would respond. Responses to medication administration, oxygen delivery, and other treatments should be manifested in the mannequin as in a real human. An important consideration is the training of the simulator operator. Adequate training is imperative to be able to present a mannequin with high functional fidelity to the learner.

Task Fidelity

Task fidelity is the measure of how authentic the simulated task is to the real task. It is important to match the task to the knowledge of the learner. During simulation, learners should not be expected to perform a task for which they have not been educated or that is outside of their scope of practice. Using complex simulators to educate a novice in basic skills is not necessary and may not be appropriate (Maran & Glavin, 2003). When using a simulator to learn a skill, the task fidelity should be very close to what the learner will experience within a real setting to avoid transferring negative motor skills and to promote transferring positive motor skills (Maran & Glavin, 2003).

Physical Fidelity

Physical fidelity refers to the environment where the simulation takes place. This includes the visual, auditory, kinesthetic or tactile, and spatial surroundings. When able, the setting should resemble the real clinical structures as closely as possible. Equipment and furnishings within the setting should be fully functioning. Attention to detail is an important part of physical fidelity. Some simulation centers take every aspect of the physical environment into consideration when preparing for a simulation scenario. Changing the room temperature, changing time on the clocks, and adding authentic odors are some examples of increasing the physical fidelity of a simulation scenario.

Psychological Fidelity

Psychological fidelity is the degree to which the learner perceives the scenario as real. This aspect of simulation fidelity is not always easy to secure. Simulations ask the learner to forget temporarily that the scenario is not real and engage in the activity, believing in its authenticity. It can take great effort to plan the physical, functional, and task fidelity, but it is up to the learner to consider the psychological fidelity of the scenario.

> **CASE STUDY 9.1**
>
> John is the CHSE and he is running an interprofessional high-fidelity simulation experience that involves learners of medicine, nursing, respiratory therapy, and unlicensed assistive personnel (UAP). The scenario involves a patient with sepsis whose respiratory and circulatory status is declining to the point of circulatory collapse, and a "code" is initiated. During the code, the medical learner shouts orders to the other members and the nursing learners who are having difficulty finding the equipment in the "code cart" where it should be. The respiratory therapist is asking for guidance as to what he should be doing for the team effort. The UAP is recording the times of events. If you were the CHSE, how would you handle this situation? What aspects of team collaboration need to be emphasized? How would you prepare the next interprofessional team for the simulation experience?

PRACTICE QUESTIONS

1. Which of the following best describes SBAR communication?

   A. A concise method of documenting the current status of a patient's condition
   B. A communication technique that evokes the two-challenge rule when one party is in disagreement with the intended action
   C. A dialogue between physicians and nurses
   D. A brief two-way exchange of information that includes a recommendation for action

2. When a learner puts a tourniquet on a simulator and the simulated blood vessel becomes engorged with fluid, what type of fidelity is this associated with?

   A. Functional fidelity
   B. Task fidelity
   C. Physical fidelity
   D. Psychological fidelity

3. A technique that replicates real-life experiences with scenarios that immerse the learner in an environment that attempts to closely duplicate the clinical environment best describes

   A. SBL
   B. Perfect practice
   C. Deliberate practice
   D. Adult learning theory

4. Simulation principles include principles of adult learning theory proposed by Malcolm Knowles (1950), also known as

   A. Pedagogy
   B. Deliberate practice
   C. Andragogy
   D. Team training

5. During a simulation scenario a learner informs the group that she is applying a nonrebreather oxygen mask to the patient at 10 L/minute and reports that the pulse oximetry improved from 92% to 96%. This is an example of

   A. Perfect practice
   B. Closed-loop communication
   C. Adult learning theory
   D. Situational awareness

6. When a member of the healthcare team communicates information to another team member and is unsatisfied with the response, the next step is to

   A. Document the incident in the medical record
   B. Invoke the two-challenge rule
   C. Follow the chain of command
   D. Complete the action on his own

7. Having a high-fidelity mannequin make vomiting sounds during a simulator simulation is an example of what kind of fidelity?

   A. Physical fidelity
   B. Functional fidelity
   C. Task fidelity
   D. Psychological fidelity

8. Simulation learners are using deliberate practice on a task training to learn intubation, and one learner keeps repeating the same mistakes. The appropriate instructions to the learner by the simulation educator would be

   A. "Keep trying to do the skill until you are successful."
   B. "Review the physiology of the trachea before you try again."
   C. "What part of the procedure do you find is difficult for you and why?"
   D. "Please stop, and you should watch your colleagues before trying again."

9. An adult learner in a simulation experience is most apt to

   A. Understand the pathophysiology behind a skill.
   B. Demonstrate exact skill execution.
   C. Be hesitant to perform a skill.
   D. Understand the need for being successful at a skill.

10. During a team simulation exercise, one learner provides another healthcare learner with information about the patient. The other learner does not acknowledge the information. The first learner tells the team member who is role-playing the nursing supervisor that critical information is missing. The learner playing the nursing supervisor should

    A. Reprimand the learner who did not acknowledge the information.
    B. Repeat the information to all the learners.
    C. Stop the scenario and restart with clearer ground rules.
    D. Tell the learner to repeat the information a second time.

REFERENCES

Agency for Healthcare Research and Quality (AHRQ). (2013). *TeamSTEPPS®: National implementation*. Retrieved from http://teamstepps.ahrq.gov/about-2cl_3.htm

Alinier, G. (2011). Developing high-fidelity health care simulation scenarios: A guide for educators and professionals. *Simulation Gaming, 42*(9), 9–26. doi:10.1177/1046878109355683

Andreatta, P. B., Bullough, A. S., & Marzano, D. (2010). Simulation and team training. *Clinical Obstetrics and Gynecology, 53*(3), 532–544. doi:10.1097/GRF.0b13e3181ec1a48

Baker, D. P., Gustafson, S., & Beaubien, J. M. (2010). *Medical teamwork and patient safety: The evidence-based relation*. Rockville, MD: Agency for Healthcare Research and Quality (AHRQ). Retrieved from www.ahrq.gov/research/findings/final-reports/medteam/references.html

Cheng, A., Donoghue, A., Giffoyle, E., & Eppich, W. (2012). Simulation-based crisis resource management training for pediatric critical care medicine: A review for instructors. *Pediatric Critical Care Medicine, 13*(2), 197–204.

Clapper, T. C. (2010). Beyond Knowles: What those conducting simulation need to know about adult learning theory. *Clinical Simulation in Nursing, 6*(1), e7–e14. doi:10.1016/j.ecns.2009.07.003

Clapper, T. C., & Kardong-Edgren, S. (2012). Using deliberate practice and simulation to improve nursing skills. *Clinical Simulation in Nursing, 8*(3), e109–e113. doi:10.1016/j.ecns.2010.12.001

D'Amore, A., James, S., & Mitchell, E. K. L. (2012). Learning styles of first-year undergraduate nursing and midwifery students: A cross-sectional survey utilizing the Kolb learning style inventory. *Nurse Education Today, 32*(5), 506–515. doi:10.1016/j.nedt2011.08.001

Ericsson, K. A. (2008). Deliberate practice and acquisition of expert performance: A general overview. *Society for Academic Emergency Medicine, 15*(11), 988–994. doi:10.11/j.1553-2712.2008.00227.x

Gaba, D. M. (2004). The future vision of simulation in health care. *Quality and Safety in Health Care, 13*, i2–i10. doi:10.1136/qshc.2004.009878

Hunt, E. A., Shilkofski, N. A., Stavroudis, T. A., & Nelson, K. L. (2007). Simulation: Translation to improved team performance. *Anesthesiology Clinics, 25*, 301–319. doi:10.1016/j.anclin.2007.03.004

Ishoy, B., Epps, C. D., & Packard, A. (2010). "Do-overs" and double debriefing: A pilot study evaluating a different design for student simulation experiences. *Clinical Simulation in Nursing, 6*(3), e117. doi:10.1016/j.ecns.2010.03.041

Issenberg, S. B., McGaghie, W. C., Petrusa, E. R., Gordon, D. L., & Scalese, R. J. (2005). Features and uses of high-fidelity medical simulations that lead to effective learning: A BEME systematic review. *Medical Teacher, 27*(1), 10–28. doi:10.1080/01421590500046.924

Joshi, N. (2013). Crisis resource management. *Academic life in emergency medicine*. Retrieved from http://academiclifeinem.com/crisis-resource-management

Knowles, M. S. (1950). *Informal adult education: A guide for administrators, leaders, and teachers*. New York, NY: Association Press.

Kolb, D. A., & Fry, R. (1975). Toward an applied theory of experiential learning. In C. Cooper (Ed.), *Theories of group process*. London, UK: John Wiley.

Lateef, F. (2010). Simulation-based learning: Just like the real thing. *Journal of Emergencies, Trauma, and Shock, 3*(4), 348–352. doi:10.4103/0974-2700.70743

Maran, N. J., & Glavin, R. J. (2003). Low- to high-fidelity simulation—A continuum of medical education? *Medical Education, 37*, 22–28. doi:10.1046/j.1365-2923.37.s1.9.x

McGaghie, W. C., Issenberg, S. B., Petrusa, E. R., & Scalese, R. J. (2010). A critical review of simulation-based medical education research: 2003–2009. *Medical Education, 44*, 50–63. doi:10.1111/j.1365-2923.2009.03547.x

Salas, E., Rosen, M. A., & King, H. B. (2009). Integrating teamwork into the "DNA" of graduate medical education: Principles for simulation-based training. *Journal of Graduate Medical Education, 1*(2), 243–244. doi:10.4300/JGME-D-09-00074.1

Sawatsky, A. P., Mikhael, J. R., Punatar, A. D., Nassar, A. A., & Argwal, N. (2013). The effects of deliberate practice and feedback to teach standardized handoff communication on the knowledge, attitudes, and practices of first-year residents. *Teaching and Learning in Medicine, 25*(4), 279–284.

Society for Simulation in Healthcare (SSH). (2014). *Certified healthcare simulation educator handbook.* Retrieved from http://ssih.org/certification/handbook

Wang, E. E. (2011). Simulation and adult learning. *Disease a Month, 57*(11), 664–678. doi: 10.1016/j.disamonth.2011.08.017

Zigmont, J. J., Kappus, L. J., & Sudikoff, S. N. (2011). Theoretical foundations of learning through simulation. *Seminars in Perinatology, 35,* 47–51. doi:10.1053/j.semperi.2011 .01.002

Moulage in Simulation

JOHN T. CORNELE

I hear and I forget. I see and I remember. I do and I understand.
—Confucius

This chapter addresses Content Area 2: Demonstrate Knowledge of Simulation Principles, Practice, and Methodology (Society for Simulation in Healthcare [SSH], 2014).

LEARNING OUTCOMES

- Discuss the value of realism and the use of moulage in simulation
- Describe the established methods of creating simulated injuries and medical conditions
- Discuss the sources of moulage materials and possibilities of adding moulage to simulation sessions

Moulage is a French term that means casting or molding; today, it is the art of applying mock injuries for the purpose of training healthcare personnel. The formal practice dates back to the 18th century, when wax figures and castings of body parts were used for this purpose. The concept of using models in education can also be seen in early Greek culture. Thus, the use of simulated injuries and illnesses or moulage to educate healthcare practitioners is not new, but its utilization in modern education is expanding.

This chapter provides an overview of moulage and its use in casualty and illness simulation. The chapter discusses makeup as well as an indication of the educational basis for its choice as a tool for use in simulation. Several broad areas are addressed, covering ideas involving the use of moulage in specific situations, with human patient simulators (HPS) or mannequins and with standardized patients (SPs), setting the stage by adding props and standardized participants (confederates), and some of the specific techniques as well as the process of cleanup. The more advanced concept of making your own moulage supplies and materials are also addressed. The chapter outline includes

- Educational basis for moulage
- Basic moulage supplies
- Actors and makeup—moulage for SPs
- Mannequins and makeup—moulage for HPS
- Special effects basics—creating props and setting the stage
- Striking the set—cleanup and resetting

The use of moulage in a simulation scenario is limited only by the scenario developer's imagination and expertise. Care must be taken, however, to keep this imagination from running wild as excessive or inappropriate moulage or makeup can detract from the simulation or provide incorrect cues to the learners.

EDUCATIONAL BASIS FOR THE USE OF MOULAGE IN SIMULATION

Although there is a paucity of actual research on the use of moulage and makeup in educational simulation, anecdotal reports are plentiful. It seems logical that when speaking of simulation as an experiential learning tool, anything that enhances the reality of the learning environment is supportive to the learner's experience. Moulage, then, is one more tool that the educator can use to enhance the reality of the learning environment (Figure 10.1).

Caution should be exercised though, as improperly done moulage can detract from the experience. The choice to use or not use moulage should be driven by the objectives of the simulation and not solely by the expertise of the moulage artist. Makeup and props used for their own sake or to surprise or deliberately confuse or trick the learner will not support the learning outcomes and may send the learners down a false path by providing incorrect cues or information. This is not to say that moulage cannot be used as a distractor to add a higher level of difficulty to a scenario, but just that caution should be used. In fact, the use of varying complexities of moulage can quite nicely adjust the presentation to create several different versions of the same scenario, altering the amount and consistency of wound drainage, for example, leading the learners in one case to deal with an uncomplicated postoperative wound

> **Simulation Teaching Tip 10.1**
> In a study of critical care simulations for undergraduate nursing learners, Mould, White, and Gallagher (2011) were able to show that high-fidelity simulations increased both the confidence and competency of the learners. Although Mould et al. does not specifically mention moulage or makeup, the concept of increased realism is explored and found to be beneficial.

> **Simulation Teaching Tip 10.2**
> A word of caution: This is quite a captivating component of simulation and the more that you find yourself involved with moulage, the more tricks you will collect and the larger your makeup kit will grow until you find yourself pushing it around on a cart.

FIGURE 10.1 The Drexel University simulation lab.

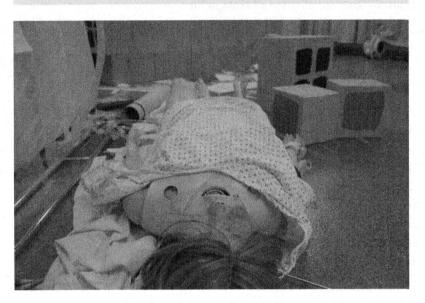

and in another with a grossly infected one. One must remember to match the need and type of moulage with the learning outcomes for the scenario.

BASIC MOULAGE SUPPLIES

Assembly of a good basic moulage kit does not have to be time-consuming or expensive. It is best to start small and keep the kit consistent with the state of one's moulage skills. In the beginning, you may only be focusing on one or two items or appliances, such as

- A few application sponges
- A color wheel of makeup
- Some glycerin and water
- A premolded commercial wound

Simulation Teaching Tip 10.3
An easy recipe for sweat or diaphoresis is to mix approximately one-third glycerin and two-thirds water by volume in a bottle with a spray attachment. This allows easy application on either SP actors or mannequins. The more glycerin used, the more the solution will bead on the skin. Some experimentation may be needed to get a mixture that works just the way that you want it to. As a caution, the glycerin does tend to build up and get gooey and sticky if not cleaned thoroughly at the end of the day. Soap and water are usually all that is necessary for cleanup. As always, care should be taken around the eyes when working with actors.

In the beginning, some sweat, vomit, bleeding, and a wound or two may be all you need.

Table 10.1 contains a short list of some equipment you might start with.

TABLE 10.1
Suggested Basic Supplies for a Moulage Kit

SUPPLIES	POSSIBLE SOURCES
Makeup (a bruise wheel and burn wheel) Sponges (application) Sponges (stipple) Cotton-tipped applicators (lots) Makeup brushes (inexpensive to start) Liquid latex Spirit gum Cold cream Glycerin Petroleum jelly Tongue depressors (lots) Stage blood, both thick and thin Cleanup products Baby wipes Tissues	Halloween stores, theatrical supply stores, online ordering, makeup counters, drug stores, etc.

As experience increases, the materials used to create injuries and illnesses become more varied. Advanced materials may include

- Liquid latex
- Silicone
- Gelefects and molding wax

PREPARING SUBSTANCES

When trying a new product, be sure to review its properties and characteristics before using it in an actual simulation. Working with a platinum silicone rubber compound is quite different when compared with a liquid latex preparation with regard to setting time and compatibility with plastics. Whatever you choose to work with, time should be set aside well in advance of the event to allow for familiarization with the product and the techniques needed to produce a realistic result. Substances that need time to dry or set may change your preparation timeline; moulage of the mannequins may need to be started hours or even days ahead of the simulation event. If using actors, in addition to the need for more time for application, new materials require a reassessment of sensitivities and allergies. The time to find out that the blood doesn't "run" correctly or that the pus is the wrong color or that the adhesive you chose makes the actor itch and break out in a rash is not when students are in the scenario. Gauging the effect of moulage in a scenario is part of the testing process that should be done with any new or revised scenario.

MOULAGE FOR SPs

Using moulage with an SP can produce a greatly enhanced learning experience for the learner. The combination of the natural conversational interaction with a person as a patient coupled with properly applied makeup or an appliance can produce a very realistic environment. As Garg (2009) noted in a study of second-year medical students, simulation education improved the learner's ability to correctly recognize skin lesions as well retain the clinical skill longer. The quality of the makeup used can have an impact on this process; the better the makeup or appliance (prosthetic), generally, the better the result.

> **Simulation Teaching Tip 10.4**
> As you are learning moulage techniques, remember to take pictures of your work. This will show you your progression and hopefully your improvement.
> At times, a static picture and quiet reflection by the moulage artist can reveal inconsistencies in technique as well as outright errors. In addition, this process will build a portfolio of your work as well as provide a reminder of past solutions to moulage challenges.

MAKEUP

Although it is generally true that makeup used in simulations does not need to be expensive, a modest increase in investment can have a positive impact. A higher quality of theatrical-grade makeup from manufacturers, such as Ben Nye or Mehron to name but two, will produce more consistent results and be easier to work with. Frequently, companies such as these will package makeup in wheels or stacks that have colors grouped for specific purposes; bruise or burn wheels, for example. This makes the challenge of choosing the correct colors for the desired illness or injury easier. Makeup that is designed and tested to be used on people also can have a lower risk of allergic or sensitivity reactions. Quite a few of the commercial products are manufactured with this in mind, but it is always prudent to check using small amounts and allowing time for any reaction. Good-quality makeup can also be obtained from the obvious sources of makeup counters and drugstores; however, at times, the color selection for illness and injury can be a bit sparse. Although there are many good-quality sources of makeup available, determining what works best requires trial and error, and in the end, choices are frequently made by personal preference. The application of moulage on a live person will produce more satisfactory results mostly due to the fact that makeup blends better on the skin of the actor, and this process allows for more natural coloration and appearance. Materials that are designed for use on the skin work best in that environment. SPs are favorable to work with for several reasons.

- Generally it is easier to produce more realistic results
- Makeup blends more easily and consistently
- Most human-approved adhesives work better
- SPs can be taught to care for or refresh the makeup, shortening the reset time between encounters
- They can assist with cleanup and removal of appliances

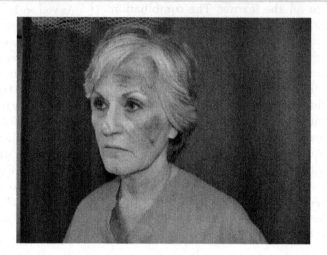

FIGURE 10.2 The application of moulage to a live person will produce more satisfactory results. The makeup blends better on the skin of the actor, allowing for more natural coloration and appearance.

Some drawbacks to working with live actors are that

- They move (sometimes a lot)
- They have to go to the restroom (sometimes a lot)
- They may have allergies
- They are sometimes fussy
- It is sometimes difficult to get them to sit still for hours

It can be frustrating for the moulage artist if after an hour of constructing a realistic wound, the patient returns from the restroom and states that the wound "just fell off." Patience is one other key ingredient that should be stocked in any makeup case (see Figure 10.2).

MANNEQUINS AND MAKEUP: MOULAGE FOR HPS

Applying moulage to mannequins can be quite a challenge and produce widely varied results especially when one compares the results achieved with live actors. The variation of the types of plastics that are found in the construction of most mannequins makes it difficult to have a standard approach to the application of makeup or appliances. Some of the issues encountered when working with mannequins and makeup are

- Blending of the makeup is more difficult and the results look less realistic at times.
- Some types of makeup can stain easily; this calls for all newly used makeup to be tested on a sample mannequin part or hidden area in advance. Generally, the softer and more porous the plastic, the greater the chance that staining may occur.

FIGURE 10.3 The Drexel University simulation lab.

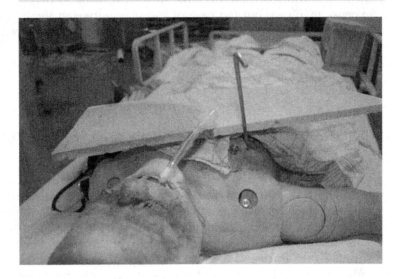

- When attaching appliances, some may not fit well unless specifically made for use with the mannequin in question.

A concern that many people have when using makeup on mannequins is the fear that it will stain or permanently mark the mannequin. Although this is a valid concern, much of the higher quality makeup is useable with mannequins. Of course, the mannequin's manufacturer recommendations should be followed to take the most care. Cautious testing in an area that won't be seen if there is staining can produce favorable results and show which makeup can best be used (Figure 10.3). Testing on the reverse of the mannequin's chest skin or behind a removable leg pad or skin and then cleaning the area not only lets you know how the makeup behaves on the plastic, but also what is the best product to use for cleanup.

Another problem is the compatibility of the plastics with both the makeup that you are using as well as with the different types of plastics and adhesives that are used together. Care must be taken when combining plastics of different types as some will inhibit the curing of some adhesives, leaving the appliance sliding off the mannequin. In addition, not all adhesives are created equal and do not stick to all plastics. One solution is to use a sheet of plastic material as a base, especially if it has some adhesive properties; a clear occlusive dressing comes to mind. At times, the challenge is finding an adhesive that has good sticking ability to keep wound appliances in place, but not so good that it forms a permanent bond or else you may end up with an unintentionally dedicated trauma mannequin.

> **Simulation Teaching Tip 10.5**
> Recycling of old mannequin arms, legs, and so on, can produce parts with wounds that can be swapped out after the session.

Some mannequin manufacturers will produce wound sets that will fit onto their mannequins. These may not look as realistic as they should, and there is expense involved, but the ease of use may outweigh the investment. The realism can be enhanced with some makeup and a drizzle of blood. And if the part is repeatedly used in the same type of scenario, minimal staining may not be an issue. As with all moulage, some experimentation is needed to be sure what you implement is what you intended.

SPECIAL EFFECTS BASICS: CREATING PROPS AND SETTING THE STAGE

Many items needed for a simulation may be created as well as purchased. One is only limited by resources and imagination. Sometimes simply changing the mannequin's clothes, moving it from a bed to a stretcher, and adding a code cart will add the impression that care is being delivered in an emergency department. In the movie industry, this is called *setting the stage* or dressing the set. This should not be a daunting task or involve a great expense. Most often, the supplies that you need you can find in your environment or around you with only a bit of looking. A good source of wardrobe items for your mannequins may be only as far away as the local thrift store or an e-mail to your faculty and staff requesting old cast-off clothing. Perhaps a short trip to a local beauty supply store or wig shop for some new hair will really change the character of the patient: add a pair of glasses, a sweater, and a purse; and Mrs. Jones begins to emerge.

Empty cardboard boxes painted gray and black can make passable cinder blocks that can be used for the wall that will fall on the SP at the end of the disaster providing yet one more victim; the best part is that they fold flat for storage, ready for use in future scenarios. Foam blocks painted gray will work as well but are more challenging to store. Making props and scene decorations can be fun and creative. Using props to add realism to the scenario makes it a much richer experience for the learners. All components should support the story and be logical additions that reinforce the reality for the learners. Props, however, should not get in the way or cause distractions, causing the learners to commit errors due to the incorrect representation of the scene. Therefore, it would seem that we need to construct completely realistic environments that use only real equipment and materials. That is not necessarily true; a fabricated prop can be valuable and inexpensive as long as it gives the proper and correct clue to the learner in the simulation. A cardboard box with the image of the front panel of a fetal monitor and actual monitoring strips pulled from the opening can assist the suspension of disbelief and provide information that the learner needs to navigate through the scenario. With props, as with moulage, if the learner spends more time trying to guess what he or she is looking at than getting useful information to use in the scenario, you have missed the mark.

> **Simulation Teaching Tip 10.6**
> When designing the scenario, the character of the room should not be forgotten; it is as important to moulage the room as it is to moulage the patient.

FIGURE 10.4 Striking the set; cleanup and resetting.

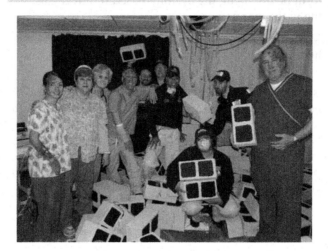

STRIKING THE SET: CLEANUP AND RESETTING

The session isn't over until the cleanup is done, and this can be one of the more challenging aspects of using moulage. It is wise to check materials used in moulage beforehand for ease of cleanup (Figure 10.4). Essentially, *striking the set* is a theater term that means to put the performance space back to the condition in which you found it. This means not only cleaning the mannequin and the simulation space, but also putting all the appliances and props away. If a logical and protective system is designed to store these materials when not in use, it will extend the useful life of the items. For example, the useable life of silicone- or latex-molded wounds can be extended if they are cleaned properly, removing excess adhesive and makeup, and stored in an air-tight container with a light dusting of talcum powder. Proper care of moulage supplies will ensure they will be available for many more uses. Props and wardrobes of both the mannequin and the SP should be stored in a way that will make them easily accessible for the next session. One method is to create a scenario container to house all the essentials for that scenario; this will help to keep all materials in one place, and if the storage container is portable, it may be taken to the location of the mannequin or actor during setup.

Cleaning materials needed for after the sessions are not much different than those needed for daily cleanup in the simulation laboratory. Sponges and non-bleach-containing wipes are staples. Attention should be paid to items that can be used on humans, gentle cleansing wipes and makeup remover, cold cream, and the like. Mannequins may need some additional help, adhesive removers and alcohol, for instance. Some common needs for cleanup are as follows.

- **Baby wipes:** These are particularly helpful when working with actors and for keeping your hands clean during the makeup process.

- **Alcohol:** Any strength is good, but if you are working with liquid silicone compounds, you will need at least 90% as it does a better job of cleaning up the unreacted material.

- **Adhesive removers:** When using adhesive removers, start with the mildest form before using the acetone-based removers, as these may remove the coloring in the mannequin.

- **Makeup remover or cold cream:** This does work best on SP actors, and they can help with the cleanup. Some products can be used on mannequins as well.

It is important to follow the mannequin manufacturer's guidelines on products used for cleanup. And it is always a good practice to test all cleaning materials on a small nonobvious area of the mannequin before large-scale use. Sometimes it is a good idea to put a barrier material on the mannequin to make cleanup of makeup easier. Plastic wraps or adhesive clear dressings work well. Some experimentation may be needed to see what method fits your expertise and budget.

SUMMARY

Moulage is a great art to add to simulation and encourage realism. Moulage is an art that calls for creativity and practice, and developing authenticity. Moulage can be applied to both the human simulation instrument and the environment to better assist healthcare learners to understand patient care.

CASE STUDY 10.1

You are setting up a trauma scene for interprofessional healthcare providers. You need to transform a large room into a car accident scene in which four teenagers are involved. One is thrown from the car and has a compound femur fracture. The driver has a head injury. The third has an abdominal wound, and the fourth has a lacerated arm. What materials would you use to set the stage? How would you develop the wounds to produce realism? Where would you place the victims in the environment?

PRACTICE QUESTIONS

1. A new simulation coordinator has recently read an article on the use of moulage in simulation and intends to incorporate it into upcoming scenario events. The coordinator realizes that the most important consideration to implementing moulage as a methodology is

   A. The additional expense and justification that must now be incorporated into the cost of the simulation
   B. Breaking the news to the SPs that they will now be wearing makeup and responsible for cleanup
   C. Performing an inventory of the types of mannequins to ensure compatibility of moulage and plastics
   D. Adjusting the timing of the simulation sessions to include the preparation time needed for moulage

2. The best makeup to use on a mannequin is

   A. A product that has a low concentration of parabens as a base
   B. A product that has been tested on a hidden area of mannequin skin
   C. A product that mixes well with an even base of petroleum jelly
   D. A product that uses a small amount of red dye number 4

3. A simulation educator and moulage proponent is hired and states that at her previous place of employment they sculpted and molded their own wounds. You know that the current staff does not have the skillset to accomplish this, the department does not have the materials on hand, and acquiring them will incur an additional expense; therefore, your best answer is

   A. We can review the possibility after considering the costs of materials and training.
   B. Our budget and current staffing doesn't allow for onsite manufacturing or construction.
   C. It is a questionable prospect because we do not have sculptors on staff.
   D. The store-bought wounds and sticky notes work just fine.

4. A faculty member has just returned from a moulage conference and is very excited about a new recipe that she has learned for creating pus and infection. She wants to add an infected wound to an upcoming end-of-life simulation to see how the students will react. She feels that it will have a big impact, especially if she can add the right odors. The best response to her would be

   A. That is a great idea, but only if it is very realistic and we add treatment materials.
   B. The suggested moulage does not support nor is it indicated by the objectives of the case.
   C. Putting makeup on actors carries too much risk of allergic reaction and staining.
   D. It is not a good idea as it will add expense to the scenario and cause excessive cleanup.

5. A simulation educator who has been in his role for several years indicates that he does not have a good understanding of the educational theories supporting the use of moulage in simulation with the following comment

   A. "Simulation is a fabrication and not real; so the environment is not important as long as the students are successful."
   B. "The students do not know the difference; regardless of how the simulation is laid out, we just need to keep the process moving."
   C. "Adding a realistic vague distracting wound to the simulation keeps the students on their toes."
   D. "As simulation is a representation of a realistic event, the more realistic the simulation, the more impact there is on the learning process."

6. A novice simulation educator needs more mentoring when she tells you

   A. "Simulation is just as effective without using moulage."
   B. "Moulage adds to the learners' perception of the situation."
   C. "Moulage is part of simulation preparation."
   D. "SPs are effective with moulage."

7. It is important to have an SP understand the importance of protecting the moulage that was done on him because

A. It is costly.
B. It is a work of art that should not be destroyed.
C. Many students can learn from one moulaged SP.
D. It is time-consuming.

8. When unsure of the type of material a high-fidelity mannequin is made of, which needs to be made up for a scenario, the best method is to

A. Apply the makeup lightly.
B. Test a small section.
C. Use a plastic cover.
D. Provide pictures of a person around the mannequin.

9. A simulation educator requests a budget to buy moulage supplies, but only half of the finances are received. The best action would be to

A. Try again in the following year's budget to secure the money.
B. Use no moulage.
C. Buy supplies and wait for reimbursement.
D. Use inexpensive makeup for the fiscal year.

10. Understanding moulage is important, and applying appropriate moulage to the simulation scenario should be guided by

A. The equipment being used
B. The financial status of the laboratory
C. The learning objectives
D. The artist's capability

REFERENCES

Garg, R. (2009). Modeling and simulation of two-phase flows. *Graduate theses and dissertations.* Paper 10657. Retrieved from http://lib.dr.iastate.edu/etd/10657

Mould, J., White, H., & Gallagher, R. (2011). Evaluation of a critical care simulation series for undergraduate nursing students. *Contemporary Nurse: A Journal for the Australian Nursing Profession, 38*(1/2), 180–190.

Society for Simulation in Healthcare (SSH). (2014). *Certified healthcare simulation educator handbook.* Retrieved from http://ssih.org/certification/handbook

Simulation Principles, Practice, and Methodologies for Standardized Patient Simulation

LINDA WILSON AND SAMUEL W. PRICE

A mind is a simulation that simulates itself.
—Erol Ozan

This chapter addresses Content Area 2: Demonstrate Knowledge of Simulation Principles, Practice, and Methodology (Society for Simulation in Healthcare [SSH], 2014).

LEARNING OUTCOMES

- Discuss the history of standardized patient (SP) simulation
- Describe the process for SP simulation case development, implementation, and evaluation

SPs were introduced into medicinal training in a limited fashion in the 1960s, but it took almost 30 years for the concept to enter the fields of nursing education and research (Barrows, 1993; Bolstad, Xu, Shen, Covelli, & Torpey, 2012). Initial objections toward using SPs included the high cost of implementation (hiring and training SPs, videotaping experiences), the so-called "Hollywood"-ization of the hard sciences, and a skepticism that an actor, not a trained healthcare professional, could correctly help assess a learner's skills (Bolstad, Xu, Shen, Covelli, & Torpey, 2012; Wallace, 1997). Yet, SPs are not necessarily all trained actors and have been found to have lower levels of unreliability and bias than nursing instructor observation or preceptor input (Bolstad, Xu, Shen, Covelli, & Torpey, 2012). Overcoming this original skepticism and proving their usefulness, reliability, and consistency in a healthcare education setting, SP experiences have greatly increased in popularity, and for good reason, because they offer a safe environment for learners.

The realism of the SP encounter relies on effective case writing by the Certified Healthcare Simulation Educator™ (CHSE™) and precise training by either the CHSE or the specific SP trainer. The training is based around measurable learning outcomes, but not every single question or reaction that the SP might encounter during a day of work can be preemptively trained for, but an SP can be given guidelines, direction, and may even use his or her own personal background in some situations. A well-trained SP will react naturally, determined by the role he or she is playing that day. It is also important that the CHSE keeps the personality, attributes, and capabilities of the SP in mind when writing the scenario. It would not make much sense to write the case with a gender-specific problem if the available SPs are not all the same gender.

Flexibility is another benefit of working with SPs. During an SP experience, students practice communication, history-taking, and physical examination skills (Rutherford-Hemming & Jennrich, 2013). Different cases may emphasize certain illness manifestations, complications, or ethical challenges. The SP can even be instructed to emphasize his or her "attitudes toward the medical profession" (Wallace, 2007). This attitude could range from a healthy skepticism to mild verbal aggression to contempt. The SP can be trained to propose a number of challenging situations that the student might face with a real patient, and the entire class can undergo the same experience because of the consistency and standardization provided by the SP.

SP CASE DEVELOPMENT

The SP case development begins with the identification of the simulation objectives or educational goals and setting for the simulation scenario (Olive, Elnicki, & Kelly, 1997). It is very important to be clear on the setting of the scenario to help the students understand their role and what is expected of them during the simulation scenario. In an SP simulation scenario, the SP can have the role of a symptomatic patient, a nonsymptomatic patient, a psychiatric patient, an emotionally hysterical patient, a severely depressed patient, or any type of patient you need; the sky is the limit because of the SP being a real person—anything is possible (Wilson & Rockstraw, 2012; Gorter et al., 2000). A well-written simulation scenario includes clear objectives; training materials, including a detailed script; and clear descriptions of medical details that are appropriately described for the SP's use, along with enough background to describe the complexity of the patient (Wallace, 2007).

TIMING OF THE SIMULATION SCENARIO

When planning the simulation scenario, you must consider the timing of the scenario. This is important for planning and scheduling the participant for the experience. The entire simulation encounter includes the following: (a) total time the student has to work with the patient; (b) time for the patient to complete the student observation checklist; (c) time for the patient to provide feedback to the student; (d) time after the encounter if you want the participant to do documentation, or a survey or a posttest; and (e) time for the SP to prepare for the next student. Many SP simulation scenarios do not include anything after the encounter. So, for example, if you are planning for the student to be with the patient for a maximum of 15 minutes, and you are going to allow 5 minutes for the SP to complete the checklist, 7 minutes for the feedback session, and 3 minutes for the patient to prepare for the next student—each total encounter will take 30 minutes.

Example 1:   Time with patient = 15 minutes
Checklist time = 5 minutes
Feedback time = 7 minutes
Turnaround time = 3 minutes
Total encounter time = 30 minutes

Example 2:   Time with patient = 30 minutes
Checklist time = 10 minutes
Feedback time = 15 minutes
Turnaround time = 5 minutes
Total encounter time = 60 minutes

This will assist you with planning the scheduling of the simulation experience, also taking into consideration the number of simulation rooms you have available and the number of students who have to complete the simulation experience.

IDENTIFY THE SETTING

The setting is a very important part of scenario planning. Where is your scenario taking place? Is it taking place in a physician's office, in an emergency department, in a medical surgical unit, in a critical care unit, in the community, in a patient's home, or in a clinic? Ideally, the simulation room should depict this environment or if that is not possible, a sign should be clearly posted to remind the student of the environment where the scenario is taking place.

SP ROLE

The role of the SP must be clearly identified. The SP can portray a patient, a family member, a student, or any other role imagined.

SP POSITION AND ATTIRE

As part of the scenario development, you must also identify the position of the patient when the student enters the room and the attire the patient should be wearing.
Position examples

- Sitting in the chair
- Sitting on the exam table
- Walking back and forth in room
- Pacing anxiously in room

Attire examples

- Wearing a patient gown, with underwear on
- Wearing a patient gown, no underwear
- Wearing regular clothes
- Wearing a gown, with pants on

EVIDENCE-BASED SIMULATION PRACTICE (EBSP) 11.1

Hawk, Kaeser, and Beavers (2013) used SPs to increase confidence in chiropractic learners when they had to confront patients about smoking cessation. Using SPs to demonstrate the interaction needed to put the five "A's" of smoking cessation (ask, advise, assess, assist, arrange) in place, 81% of learners ($N = 68$) said it increased their confidence, and 77% said they would now be comfortable using it in future practice.

STUDENT ROLE

The role of the student participant should also be very clear. Is the student working in a new graduate nurse role, a physician role, a physician assistant role, or an advanced practice nurse role? The students should be reminded of their roles in the simulation instructions and door sign so that they function within their scope of practice.

IDENTIFY THE FOCUS AND OBJECTIVES

The SP simulation scenario has to have a clear focus and objectives. Is the scenario going to be based on a specific medical diagnosis (asthma, congestive heart failure, shortness of breath, abdominal pain), a mental illness (psychosis, hearing voices), psychosocial challenges (depression, anxiety), ethical situations (do not resuscitate [DNR], organ donation, assisted suicide), or another scenario? This selection will be the basis for writing your case. It is important to include clear information about the selected condition/situation in the case for the education of the SPs.

Next, what are the objectives or educational goals for the student completing this scenario? For example, if you are working with undergraduate nursing students, objectives could include

1. Obtaining a complete history from the patient
2. Completing a focused physical exam based on the patient diagnosis
3. Providing patient education based on educational needs identified during the time with the patient

Another example, if you are working with medical students or advance practice nurses, objectives could include

1. Obtaining a complete history from the patient
2. Completing a focused physical exam based on the patient diagnosis
3. Identifying patient diagnosis
4. Ordering diagnostic tests as appropriate
5. Providing patient with appropriate information and plan of care

The objectives are also linked to the specific course or educational program of the student. It is important that the student be aware of the required objectives or educational goals for the simulation experience.

SP QUESTIONS AND ANSWERS

The SP case should also include any questions the student may ask during the scenario and the response the patient is supposed to provide to the student. Any questions specific to the diagnosis or condition of the patient will need a specific answer, such as symptoms and medications, for example. For other questions that do not have a direct impact on the direction of the scenario, you may have the patients use their own information and not require a specific answer. Depending on the complexity of the case, one must be realistic as to how many specific lines or questions the SP can memorize and portray.

DOOR SIGN

The door sign is the sign that will be posted outside the simulation room to provide information to the student (see Exhibit 11.1). The door sign should include

- Information about the scenario
- What you expect the student to do in the scenario
- How much time the student has to complete the scenario

EXHIBIT 11.1

Door Sign Examples

DOOR SIGN EXAMPLE 1

Mr./Mrs. Pat Foles came to the emergency room with complaints of increased thirst, increased urination, and hunger and is now admitted to the medical–surgical unit. You have 40 minutes to complete a history, focused physical exam, and appropriate patient teaching.

DOOR SIGN EXAMPLE 2

Mr./Mrs. Fran Victorino has been in the hospital for the past week and was diagnosed as having HIV. The patient is preparing to be discharged from the hospital. You are to give the patient discharge instructions, including the important steps to prevent transmission of HIV to others, such as measures for safe sex, and so on. The discharge instructions have already been prepared for you by the doctor and are provided in the patient chart. You have 15 minutes to complete this encounter.

STUDENT CHECKLIST

The student checklist is a detailed checklist of what you expect the student to do during the scenario. In most institutions, this checklist is completed by the SP immediately after the completion of the scenario and before the patient provides feedback to the student. Depending on how you decide to design your checklist, you can choose to separate the checklist items by categories, such as communication, physical exam, patient teaching, diagnostic tests, or other categories. If a checklist item is subjective, it can be helpful to put a descriptor to provide information on how to evaluate that checklist item. For example, in Table 11.1 you will see a checklist item "good eye contact," and the descriptor explains that if the students have good eye contact at least half of the time, they will get credit for that checklist item. It is also important to remember—the longer the checklist, the longer time you have to allow for the SP to complete the checklist.

> **Simulation Teaching Tip 11.1**
> If there is a checklist item that has more than one part—where a student could possibly do one part correctly and one part incorrectly, such as listening to the lungs—it is helpful to separate that into two separate checklist items as you will see in the example checklist in the following text.

TABLE 11.1 Example Checklist Items	
COMMUNICATION	**PHYSICAL EXAM**
Introduces self (name and title)	Washed hands before examination
Checked patient's ID band	Explained to me what she or he was doing with each step of exam
Good eye contact (50% or greater of the time)	Helped to position me
Speaks clearly in terms the patient can understand	Was professional in manner
Active listener	Maintained modesty during exam
Asked patient's age or date of birth	Checked blood pressure in both arms
Asked about patient's marital status	Blood pressure sitting or lying down
Asked about patient's work history	Blood pressure standing
Askedabout previous hospitalizations	Counted my pulse
Asked about allergies	Counted my respiratory rate
Asked about past medical history	Listened to my heart in at least four places on skin
Asked about current medications	Listened to my lungs in at least four places (two pairs) anterior and posterior on skin
Asked about a history of chest pain	
Asked about a history of palpitations	
Asked about smoking history	
Asked about alcohol history	
Asked about diet	
Asked about exercise	
Asked about stresses in life	
Created an atmosphere that put the patient at ease	

STUDENT EVALUATION CRITERIA AND PASSING SCORE

There are many ways to evaluate the student checklist items. Some of the common evaluation methods include

- Done/Not Done/NA
- Done/Not done/Done but not correctly
- Likert scale rating

Your simulation program may select one way to evaluate all of your simulation experiences or they may be different based on a specific program or course.

If the simulation is a "high-stakes testing" simulation in which the student has to achieve a specific score to pass, you must also pick a passing score. Many programs will pick the score for a grade of "C" at their school. Or the specific score might be mandated by your licensing agency.

Another aspect to consider is the value of each checklist item. Is each checklist item of equal value, or are some checklist items worth more points than others? You can also identify specific patient safety checklist items that are critical—if the student misses that checklist item, he or she automatically fails the experience— such as checking the patient's identity or ID band.

Exhibit 11.2 demonstrates two SP simulation cases, including the student checklist. The first case is an ethical dilemma case and the second case is a hypertension case.

EXHIBIT 11.2

SP Simulation Cases and Student Checklists

Case 1
Case—DNR (Do Not Resuscitate) Ethical Dilemma—Mini Case—Passing Score 76%

Length of time for the encounter: 15 minutes
Checklist time: 5 minutes
Feedback time: 7 minutes
Turnaround time: 3 minutes

NAME: Fran Victorino

SETTING: Inpatient room

SCENARIO: Your mother, Isabelle Victorino, is 86 years old, has metastatic liver cancer, and was found on the floor at home unconscious.

DOOR SIGN: The person in the room is the daughter/son of your patient. This family member is very upset by the information received from the other nurse, who told them their family member is a DNR. The family member wants to speak with you since you are the current nurse for the patient. Your assignment is to talk with this family member. You have 15 minutes for the encounter.

OPENING LINE: "I'm so glad you're here. I need to talk to you about my mother. What does "DNR" mean? The other nurse just told me my mom has been made DNR. Exactly what does that mean?"

You have been out of town and your sister, who lives with your mother, called you this morning and told you your mother had to be taken to the hospital. You are now at the hospital in the intensive care unit's waiting room after seeing your mother. You just found out from the other nurse that your mother has a DNR

(continued)

EXHIBIT 11.2 (continued)

order, which was given by your sister. You do not understand what DNR means and want "everything done" for your mother. You are a little bit anxious, a little upset, and are pacing a bit in the room. When the nurse arrives, you ask the nurse, "What does 'DNR' mean anyway?" "Who made my mother a DNR?" You add, "My mother, if she could speak for herself, would want everything done...she wants to live!"

TRAINING QUESTIONS:

What do you think "DNR" means? It means you don't do anything. Right?

Do you understand what it means to resuscitate someone in your mother's advanced age and deteriorated condition? Not really.

Do you understand what is involved in the resuscitation? No.

Have you ever discussed this topic (DNR) with your mother? No, but I am sure she would want to live. I'm sure she would want everything done.

Do you know whether or not your mother has a living will? I'm not sure.

Do you understand what a "living will" is? No.

Do you have power of attorney over your mother's medical conditions? No, my sister does.

Have you spoken to your sister? No.

Do you think it would be wise to talk to your sister? Yes, perhaps I need to.

Would you like to speak to your mother's physician? Yes.

Would you like us to arrange a family meeting? Yes.

Would you like to speak to a hospital counselor or a clergy member? Yes, could I see a clergy member?

Challenge: "Are you sure this DNR is for my mom? I can't imagine my sister would do something like that."

Student Checklist (Done/Not Done/NA)

Did the student establish eye contact?

Did the student establish a rapport?

Did the student allow you to speak without interruption?

Did the student tell you about the DNR in a sensitive, informative way?

Did the student try to find out what you know and your perceptions, e.g., what do you think DNR is?

Did the student acknowledge your emotion?

Was the student professional in manner?

Was the student supportive?

Was the student an attentive listener?

Did the student exhibit comforting body language?

Did the student use silence appropriately?

Did the student determine what your support systems are?

EXHIBIT 11.2 (*continued*)

Did the student explain what DNR means?

Did the student verify the DNR order in the chart?

Did the student explain to you how a DNR order is obtained?

Did the student suggest speaking to your sister or suggest a family meeting?

Did the student offer to call the primary doctor to discuss the situation?

Did the student offer to call someone for you for support?

SP will also provide feedback

Case 2
Case Hypertension—Passing Score 76%

Length of time for the encounter: 40 minutes

Checklist time: 7 minutes

Feedback time: 10 minutes

Turnaround time: 3 minutes

NAME: Fran Jackson

SETTING: Medical–Surgical Unit (inpatient hospital room)

SCENARIO: The patient has a 2-day complaint of severe headache. On arrival to the emergency room, the patient was diagnosed with severe hypertension. The patient's initial blood pressure in the emergency department was 200/120. BACK-GROUND: The patient had been to the emergency department about 6 months ago with a similar complaint and was diagnosed with hypertension at that time. The patient was given a prescription for a hypertension medication, Lopressor. The patient was taking the medication as prescribed until he/she went to a health fair at the church about 1 week ago. The blood pressure at the health fair was "normal." Since the blood pressure was normal and the patient was feeling great, the patient decided to just stop taking the medication. Plus the medication was very expensive and the patient can certainly use that money for something else. The patient started getting a severe headache about 2 days ago and thought he/she should get checked at the emergency department (ED). Patient is pleasant and talkative.

DOOR SIGN: Mr./Mrs. Fran Jackson was admitted to the medical surgical unit from the ED day. The patient has a 2-day complaint of severe headache. On arrival at the emergency room, the patient was diagnosed with severe hypertension. Do a complete history, focused physical exam, and appropriate patient teaching. You have 40 minutes for the encounter.

OPENING LINE:
This is a(n) (use your own age) patient who has been admitted to the medical–surgical unit (an inpatient room) from the ED.

(continued)

EXHIBIT 11.2 (*continued*)

CHALLENGE QUESTIONS:

The blood pressure medicine that the doctor had me on . . . can you tell me how that medication works?
The medication acts on certain receptors in the body and decreases blood pressure and heart rate.

Why was my blood pressure normal at the health fair?
The medication was working or was in you system so that made your blood pressure within normal range when you went to the health fair.

TRAINING QUESTIONS:

What is your date of birth? Use your own

Are you married? Use yourself

Occupation? Worked in a factory (or store or office, etc.), left on disability due to back injury. Currently under a lot of stress because having a difficult time making "ends meet" on the income you are receiving.

When did the severe headache start? Two days ago.

Does anything make it worse? No. I don't think so.

Does anything make it better? No. I tried the usual over-the-counter medication that I take for headache but it did not help at all.

Have you had any fever or chills? No, not that I know of, but I haven't taken my temperature.

Have you ever had anything similar in the past? Yes, I came to the emergency department about
6 months ago with a similar headache. At that time, they said I had high blood pressure. They gave me a prescription for a blood pressure medication called Lopressor.

Have you ever used any recreational drugs? No.

Have you ever been hospitalized? No (or use your own if necessary but nothing related to current complaint).

Have you ever had surgery? Use yourself.

Have you ever been pregnant? Use yourself.

Do you have any chronic illnesses? Yes, I guess the high blood pressure could be considered a chronic illness, but I did not think I had it anymore.

Are you taking any medications? Yes, I was taking a medication after my last visit to the emergency department. It was a medication for my high blood pressure. I stopped taking the medication after I had my blood pressure checked at the health fair at church. My pressure was normal when they took it there; so I knew I did not need the medication any longer. I also felt great! Plus that medication was very expensive!

How is your father? Died from a stroke a few years ago. Father also had hypertension.

How is your mother? Alive if appropriate, or deceased.

How is/are your sibling(s)? Healthy.

Past health history (none or your own)

Neurological (none)

Cardiovascular (high blood pressure)

EXHIBIT 11.2 (*continued*)

Respiratory (none)

Gastrointestinal (none)

Genitourinary (none)

Gynecological (none)

Obstetrical (use yourself)

Diet (I eat anything I want. I love potato chips, dill pickles, I love anything that tastes salty)

Medications

Prescription medications (I was taking Lopressor once a day when I had the high blood pressure, but prior to coming to the ER today, I was not taking any medications)

Over-the-counter medications (none or your own)

Medication Allergies (none)

Seasonal allergies (use your own)

Psychosocial history

Smoking history (yes, smoked one pack a day for as long as I can remember)

Alcohol history (like to have a few beers with my friends on the weekend)

Recreational drug history (none)

Sexual history (use your own)

Stressors—(stressed about finances—difficulty making ends meet on disability salary)

You should be in a hospital gown, bra and underwear okay, sitting on the edge of the table.

STUDENT CHECKLIST (Done/Not Done/NA)

COMMUNICATION

Introduces self (name and title)

Checks patient's ID band

Good eye contact (50% or greater of the time)

Speaks clearly in terms the patient can understand (three-strikes rule)

Active listener

Asked patient's age or date of birth

Asked about patient's marital status

Asked about patient's work history

Asked about previous hospitalizations

Asked about allergies

Asked about your past medical history

Asked about your family's past medical history

Asked about current medications

Asked about a history of chest pain

Asked about a history of palpitations

(continued)

EXHIBIT 11.2 (continued)

Asked about smoking history

Asked about alcohol history

Asked about my diet

Asked about exercise

Asked about stresses in life

Created an atmosphere that put the patient at ease

Answered patient's question about blood pressure medication: Lopressor

Answered patient's question about why BP was normal at the health fair

PHYSICAL EXAM

Washed hands before examination

Explained to me what she/he was doing with each step of exam

Helped to position me

Was professional in manner

Maintained modesty during exam

Checked blood pressure in both arms

Blood pressure sitting or lying down

Blood pressure standing

Counted my pulse

Counted my respiratory rate

Took my temperature

Listened to my heart in at least four places anterior on skin

Listened to my lungs in at least four places (two pairs) bilateral anterior on skin

Listened to my lungs in at least four places (two pairs) bilateral posterior on skin

PATIENT TEACHING

Discussed the importance of taking meds as prescribed

Discussed the importance of a low-salt diet

Discussed the importance of exercise

Offered information or suggested some options for stress management

Offered information or suggested some options for smoking cessation

SP will also provide feedback

SP FEEDBACK

Another important aspect of the case development is planning for the SP feedback at the end of the simulation experience. A common type of feedback is for the patient to provide interpersonal feedback on how the student made him or her feel as a patient. The feedback can be either very specific or general (see Chapter 16 for extensive information on SP feedback).

Examples of an SP case template and a blank SP case template are provided in Exhibit 11.3.

EXHIBIT 11.3

Standardized Patient Case Template

Communication

1. Introduces self with name and title
2. Checks patient ID band
3. Good eye contact (at least 50% of the time)
4. Was professional in manner
5. Speaks clearly in terms the patient can understand (three-strikes rule)
6. Active listener
7. Asked about
8. Asked about
9.
10.

Physical Exam

1. Washes hands before the exam
2. Explained to me what he/she was doing with each step of the exam
3.
4.
5.
6.
7.
8.
9.
10.

Patient Education
1. Discussed the importance of
2. Discussed the danger signs of
3. Offered information or suggested some options for
4.
5.
6.
7.
8.
9.
10.

SP will also provide feedback

STANDARDIZED PATIENT CASE BLANK TEMPLATE

Title of case:

Patient name:

Length of time for the encounter (max time student can be in the room is 15 min/30 min/45 min):

Checklist time:

Feedback time:

(continued)

EXHIBIT 11.3 (continued)

Turnaround time:

Setting:

Overview of scenario/scenario background for patient:

Instructions/door sign (Information for student to see prior to experience that includes what is to be done during the experience and ends with how many minutes the student has to complete the experience.):

Mr./Mrs. . . . . . . came to the . . . . . . for . . . . . .
You have . . . . . . minutes to . . . . .

Opening line (what you want the patient to say at the beginning of the experience):

Patient position at start of scenario (sitting on table/sitting in chair):

Patient dress at start of scenario (regular clothes/patient gown):

Challenge question (question patient is to ask the student during the experience plus the answer to the question):

Questions during the experience (training questions) (Identify questions the student may ask during the experience that *require a specific answer*. List the question below and the answer to the question. For all other questions, the patient can "use his or her" information):

Please delete/change/add to the list below

What is your age?
Are you married?
Occupation?

EXHIBIT 11.3 (continued)

Have you ever had anything similar in the past?
Have you ever used any recreational drugs?
Have you ever been hospitalized?
Have you ever had surgery?
Have you ever been pregnant?
Do you have any chronic illnesses?
Are you taking any medications?
How is your father?
How is your mother?
How is/are your sibling(s)?
Past health history:
Immunizations up to date?
Diet/activity/exercise:
Medications
Prescription medications:
Over-the-counter medications:
Medication allergies:
Seasonal allergies:
Psychosocial history:

Checklist items (items used to evaluate the student during the experience—each of these items will be marked with one of the following: Done/Not done/ NA):
Passing score:

Communication
1.
2.
3.
4.
5.
6.
7.
8.
9.
10.

Physical Exam
1.
2.
3.
4.
5.
6.
7.
8.
9.
10.

(continued)

EXHIBIT 11.3 *(continued)*

Patient Education
1.
2.
3.
4.
5.
6.
7.
8.
9.
10.

SP will also provide feedback

ORIENTATION, EDUCATION, AND TRAINING OF SPs

The SP case scenario written by the CHSE is explained to the SPs during the SP training session before the simulation experience begins, and ideally in advance of the day of the simulation experience. If the training is taking place on the day of the simulation experience, it is important that the students do not interact with the SPs before the experience to keep the level of realism as high as possible.

Depending on the SP experience the instructor has crafted, "Training for a standardized patient involves, for example, learning what history questions to listen for or how the physical examination should be done" (Errichetti, Gimpel, & Boulet, 2002, p. 627). Along with describing the direction that the case is supposed to take, the CHSE will also explain the objectives of the scenario.

The training of the SP begins with the specifics of the simulation case, including

- Name of the patient
- Role of the patient (patient, family member, etc.)
- Setting of the scenario (e.g., medical–surgical unit, emergency department, etc.)
- Background of the scenario (i.e., why the patient came in)
- The information the learner will know before beginning the scenario (such as the door sign)
- An opening line or lines to begin the scenario (if included in the scenario)
- Challenge questions (i.e., a specific question about the condition or chief complaint about the SP's condition if included in the scenario)

> **Simulation Teaching Tip 11.2**
> If you are new to writing SP case scenarios, when you have finished your first case, and start your next case, just do a "save as" and start with your original case as a baseline.

- Training questions (what questions the students might ask and what answer is required)
- Checklist items
- Feedback

Along with the education about the case itself, the SP must also be clear on the student checklist and how it should be completed. After the scenario, the SP will complete the student checklist prior to the feedback session. Through observation, the SP completion of the checklist contributes to the student evaluation, which is formally done by the CHSE.

After reviewing the case and the checklist, the SPs can ask questions, discuss strategies, or practice through role-playing. The goal of the SP's training and education on the case is that the SP enters the role "so carefully coached . . . that the simulation cannot be detected by a skilled clinician" (Barrows, 1993, p. 444).

> **Simulation Teaching Tip 11.3**
> When using SPs for simulation learning experiences, it is best to use a consistent set of actors who work routinely at your institution because they become part of the "culture of learning" at your educational organization.

SP's ROLE IN LEARNER EVALUATION AND FEEDBACK

For an SP scenario, the SP can be clearly instructed on how to complete the student checklist. The SP's training is directly related to the accuracy of the SP's completion of the checklist (Wallace, 2007). In addition, for the results of the checklists to be valid, how the checklist is created is crucial to the validity and reliability of the checklist (Gorter et al., 2000). As mentioned previously, the SP's completion of the checklist contributes to the student evaluation, which is formally done by the CHSE.

SPs have a unique role in postscenario feedback. The feedback time can be a heightened time of awareness for the student, and information provided to the student at that time can make a lasting impression. Many students, after completing the SP simulation experience, state "I will never forget what that patient told me!" or "The SP feedback was the best part of the experience." The role of SPs in healthcare simulation education is depicted in Figure 11.1.

FIGURE 11.1 SP's role in healthcare simulation education.

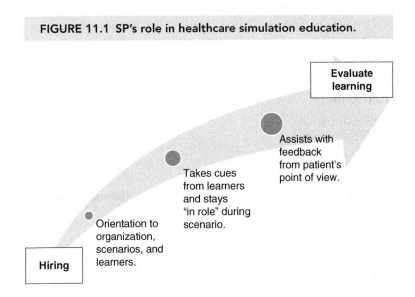

HYBRID SIMULATION USING SPs AS CONFEDERATES

Many simulation scenarios find it optimal to combine both the human-patient simulator (HPS) and SPs in a simulation scenario. When SPs are used in this fashion, it is referred to as "hybrid simulation" or the SP can be referred to as a "confederate" in the simulation scenario (see Chapter 12 for extensive information on hybrid simulation).

SUMMARY

SPs are a very important aspect of healthcare simulation education! To have a successful SP simulation experience, the case development must be accurate and comprehensive. In addition to the carefully developed case scenario, SP training is equally important. The SP completion of the checklist must be accurate and consistent. The SP feedback has to be carefully structured because it can have a lasting impression on the student. SP simulation provides the opportunity for the most realistic simulations in a safe environment. In the future, SP simulation will be an expected standard in every simulation program.

CASE STUDY 11.1

A medical learner during an SP simulation scenario leaves the examination room without fully interviewing the SP. The learner comes out and tells the CHSE that this is difficult for her because the SP "looks exactly like" her mother who died less than a month ago. The SP also leaves the examination room and comes out to the desk to discuss the situation with the CHSE. How would the CHSE best handle this specific situation?

PRACTICE QUESTIONS

1. A simulation educator is planning to start using SP simulation in the simulation lab. Where should the educator look to find SPs?

   A. Advertise for SPs through the school website
   B. Contact another simulation center in the area for advice
   C. Check with the drama department at the university
   D. All of the above

2. When an SP is used with an HPS scenario, this type of simulation is often referred to as

   A. SP simulation
   B. HPS simulation
   C. Hybrid simulation
   D. Double simulation

3. When developing an SP simulation scenario, the maximum time limit for the length of the scenario is

   A. Fifteen minutes
   B. Thirty minutes
   C. Forty-five minutes
   D. There is no maximum time limit

4. What is the best method for SP training?

   A. Review of the case scenario
   B. Demonstrate the assessment techniques
   C. Role-playing
   D. All of the above

5. During a simulation scenario, the student, completing the assessment, proceeds to examine the patient's eye with the otoscope. The patient should

   A. Not do anything.
   B. Tell the student the wrong scope is being used.
   C. Scream
   D. State, "I do not want you to examine my eyes."

6. During an SP scenario, the SP notices the student looking at a piece of paper in her pocket. After the session is over, the SP should

   A. Do nothing.
   B. Make a note on the student checklist.
   C. Ask the student about the note.
   D. Notify the simulation educator.

7. After an SP simulation experience, a student comes out of the room crying. The simulation educator should

   A. Do nothing.
   B. Wait until after the feedback session and approach the student.
   C. Take the student aside and speak to the individual in a private area.
   D. Ask the student to leave the simulation lab.

8. The SP role in the evaluation of students is

   A. To grade the student
   B. To complete the checklist to document what the student did and did not do
   C. The SP has no involvement in student evaluation
   D. To compare the student performances against each other

9. The acronym SP stands for standardized patient. What other word is sometimes substituted for the word "standardized"?

   A. Super
   B. Stupendous
   C. Simulated
   D. Steadfast

10. The simulation educator wants the SP to have a blood pressure of 190/100 for the scenario. How can the educator make this happen?

    A. Have the SP drink a lot of caffeine before the scenario.
    B. It is not possible.
    C. Have the SP hand a Post-it note with the words "BP 190/100" to the student after the student takes the blood pressure.
    D. Have the SPs do a strenuous exercise class prior to the scenario.

REFERENCES

Barrows, H. S. (1993). An overview of the uses of standardized patients for teaching and evaluating clinical skills. *Academic Medicine, 68*(6), 443–451.

Bolstad, A. L., Xu, Y., Shen, J. J., Covelli, M., & Torpey, M. (2012). Reliability of standardized patients used in a communication study on international nurses in the United States of America. *Nursing & Health Sciences, 14*(1), 67–73.

Errichetti, A., Gimpel, J., & Boulet, J. (2002). State of the art in standardized patient programs: A survey of osteopathic medical schools. *Medical Education, 102*(11), 627–631.

Gorter, S., Rethans, J. J., Scherpbier, A., van der Heijde, D., Houben, H., van der Vleuten, C., & van der Linden, S. (2000). Developing case-specific checklists for standardized-patient-based assessments in internal medicine: A review of the literature. *Academic Medicine, 75*(11), 1130–1137.

Hawk, C., Kaeser, M. A., & Beavers, D. V. (2013). Feasibility of using a standardized patient encounter for training chiropractic students in tobacco cessation counseling. *Journal of Chiropractic Education, 27*(2), 135–140. doi:http://dx.doi.org/10.7899/JCE-13-2

Olive, K. E., Elnicki, D. M., & Kelley, M. J. (1997). A practical approach to developing cases for standardized patients. *Advances in Health Sciences Education, 2*(1), 49–60.

Rutherford-Hemming, T., & Jennrich, J. A. (2013). Using standardized patients to strengthen nurse practitioner competency in the clinical setting. *Nursing Education Perspectives, 34*(2), 118–121.

Wallace, P. (1997). Following the threads of an innovation: The history of standardized patients in medical education. *Caduceus, 13*(2), 5–26.

Wallace, P. (2007). *Coaching standardized patients.* New York, NY: Springer Publishing Company.

Wilson, L., & Rockstraw, L. (2012). *Human simulation for nursing and health professions.* New York, NY: Springer Publishing Company.

· · · 12 · · ·

Hybrid Simulation

ANTHONY ERRICHETTI

The whole is greater than the sum of its parts.
—Aristotle

This chapter addresses Content Area 3: Educate and Assess
Learners Using Simulation (Society for Simulation in Healthcare
[SSH], 2014).

LEARNING OUTCOMES

- Discuss an overview of patient simulation modalities
- Compare hybrid patient simulations—varieties and possibilities
- Describe how to develop mannequin-based and human hybrid simulations
- Describe documents to create mannequin-standardized participant scenarios
- Discuss preparing the standardized participant for hybrid simulations
- Discuss issues of simulation fidelity

Artistotle's maxim about how complexity is created from simplicity holds true for hybrid patient simulations, the use of two or more patient simulation modalities simultaneously or sequentially. For example, when mannequin simulators are combined with standardized patients (SPs), there is an advantage gained that neither of the two could offer alone. Hybrid patient simulations combine a mixture of simulation modalities, learning strategies, and professionals into a powerful platform for teaching and assessing clinical competencies. However, the complexity of combining multiple simulation modalities—from the artificial to the human—requires planning and cooperation.

Simulation is an aid to the imagination for both the educator and learner. "It allows us to create, populate and activate possible futures, and explore ramifications of these developed scenarios" (Vincenzi, Wise, Moulana, & Hanock, 2009, p. ix). The "willful suspension of disbelief," a concept described by the poet Samuel Taylor Coleridge (1817), is directly applicable to simulation learning.

If writers could combine "human interest with a semblance of truth" (Coleridge), then readers could overlook a story's implausibility (Barth, 2001). Indeed the first task for simulation educators is to get learners to "buy into" a scenario that all know is a construction, a representation of reality. Hybrid patient simulation is an approach that combines various elements of "constructed reality"—live, computerized, and mechanical—used in an environment that looks and sounds real. Live participants can be incorporated into a scenario and be given distinct roles to create that "semblance of truth" (Coleridge) that makes learning compelling.

FOUNDATIONS OF PATIENT SIMULATIONS

The use of simulation to teach essential skills is widespread and deeply embedded into human culture. We seem to be "hardwired" to substitute the authentic with constructed reality. From infancy, we practice sucking and rooting reflexes through a pacifier, essentially a part-task trainer that simulates a mother's nipple (Moroney & Lilienthal, 2009).

The military has used war simulation for millennia. The ancient Hindu game *Chaturanga* and the Chinese *Go* were used to practice strategic thinking, and large-scale "war games" replicated battlefield conditions (Allen, 1987). The Roman Jewish historian Flavius Josephus (1981) notes that the Roman general Tiberius conducted war games that were "bloodless battles" to prepare for actual battles that were "bloody drills" (Josephus, 1981).

Aviation has long been at the forefront of using simulation to teach core competencies in our era, and its use has been a model for healthcare simulation (Friedrich, 2002; Gaba & DeAnda, 1988). The Wright Brothers used a "kiwi bird" simulator in 1910 to teach flight control using a defunct Wright Type B Flyer (Bernstein, 2000). The Antoinette Trainer (circa 1910; Figure 12.1) was a barrel split in half with short wings, allowing students to practice banking and turning while an instructor, pushing or pulling on the wings, simulated turbulence. Such simulators

Figure 12.1 Antoinette Trainer.

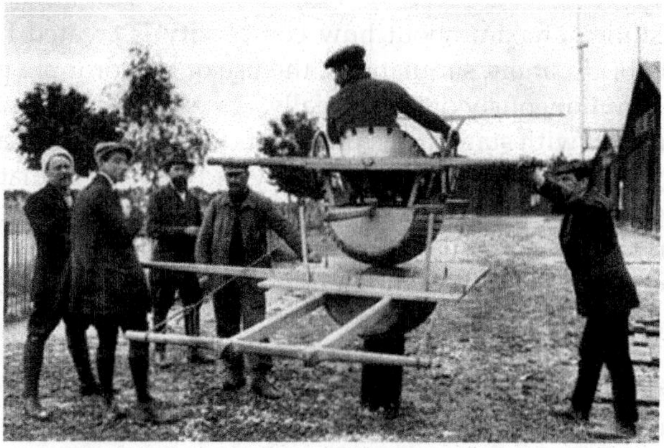

Used with permission from flightsimulationmuseum.org.

were hybrids combining task trainers with an instructor acting as a "standardized participant," that is, an individual who plays a role in a simulation to add realism and to move critical action forward.

Human-patient simulation today has two roots, computerized mannequins and SPs. SimOne, the first computer-controlled mechanical patient simulator was developed at the University of Southern California in 1967 by a team led by Stephen Abrahamson and Judson Denson (Abrahamson, 1997). In the late 1960s, the Harvey simulator, a hybrid between a cardiac task trainer and computer-enhanced mannequin simulator, integrated the bedside findings and realistically reproduced both common and rare cardiac diseases (Gordon, 1974).

SPs, introduced by Howard Barrows in 1963 at the University of Southern California, have long been used to teach clinical skills and are the foundation for performance-based assessment (Harden & Gleeson, 1979).

EVIDENCE-BASED SIMULATION PRACTICE (EBSP) 12.1

SPs—highly trained professionals—are now used in high-stakes licensure examinations (Dillon, Boulet, Hawkins, & Swanson, 2004). Used in formative assessment exercises, most commonly in one-on-one encounters, SPs portray patients, document and assess skills, and provide feedback to learners.

TYPOLOGY AND MODES OF SIMULATION

Simulations can be divided into four types (Andrews, Brown, Byrnes, Change, & Hartman, 1998).

1. *Live*—learners interacting with real systems or people, for example, evaluating patients as SPs or customer exercises in which actors, playing patients, assess reception office staff

2. *Virtual*—learners interacting with simulated systems, for example, training on a computer-based virtual reality (VR) surgical simulation (Gallagher et al., 2005)

3. *Constructive*—learners interacting with simulated systems and simulated people, for example, operating room team training using VR in which simulated participants substitute for actual participants (Baydogan, Belfore, Scerbo, & Mazumbar, 2009)

4. *Hybrid*—combining live, virtual, and constructive modes of simulation in different combinations

There are four kinds of simulated patients used by healthcare educators for teaching and skills evaluation

1. Part-task trainers
2. Humans (SPs and standardized participants)

3. Computerized mannequins

4. Virtual (computer-based) patients

The following summarizes their utilization and features, with examples of combining the modes into hybrid simulations.

Part-Task Trainers

Resusci Anne, a plastic mannequin, was introduced in 1960 to teach cardiopulmonary resuscitation (Grenvik & Schaefer, 2004), and thus began the advent of commercially available part-task trainers. Today, a wide variety of trainers is available to practice airway management, vascular access, echocardiography, cardiovascular assessment, and many others tasks.

> **Simulation Teaching Tip 12.1**
> Part-task procedures can also be practiced using common objects, for example, using an orange to practice injection or using a pig's foot to practice suturing.

Part-task trainers replicate the anatomy, for example, the skin, head, upper and lower extremities, esophagus, and thorax; and in some cases, the physiology of a part of the human body. This allows learners and professionals to practice specific tasks or technical procedures (Aggarwal, Moorthy, & Darzi, 2004) without harming or hurting an actual patient. Parts of the whole task are used to prepare the learner for the whole task (Sinz, 2004). Part-task procedures can improve learning efficiency because a specific skill can be practiced multiple times until mastered. They can also reduce training costs because the learner would not participate in a full simulation exercise until a particular skill is mastered. Examples of part-task trainers, which are hybrids, are

- Starting an intravenous (IV) line on an arm attached to an SP
- Suturing a leg wound attached to an SP
- Using a pelvic trainer with an SP
- Performing a urinary catheterization on a part-task trainer with an SP
- Doing a rectal exam on a part-task trainer with an SP

Human-Patient Simulations

Although SPs are used mostly to teach and assess individual clinician competencies, they can be combined with standardized participants, sometimes referred to as confederates, who portray nonpatient roles. Also, standardized participants are increasingly incorporated into mannequin-based hybrid scenarios. They are scripted into a simulation to add realism and provide additional challenges and information to learners. They can portray, for example, a patient's (mannequin) family member, a healthcare team member, or any other role required by the scenario. They can be "programmed" to portray distinct personality "types" and emotionally complex and nuanced roles that correspond to the learning objectives of a learning module. Standardized participants can also be used to assess skills (e.g., to determine whether procedures are used in a correct and timely manner, assess team communication, etc.) and provide feedback during the postencounter debriefing. Standardized participants, like SPs, require training for whatever roles they take on. Examples of how to use SPs or standardized participants with hybrid simulation are

- Learner interacts with an SP, and a standardized participant is a healthcare team member
- Learner must provide "bad news" to a distraught family member after examining an SP who portrays an end-of-life patient

Mannequin-Based Simulations

Mannequin-based simulations are used primarily for training and assessing healthcare teams. Depending on the model, these computerized, mechanical high-fidelity mannequins represent patients at various developmental stages (infant, child, adult) and are used for different purposes (e.g., anesthesia training, birthing simulations, and with programmable cardiovascular, respiratory, and neurological responses to clinical interventions). Depending on the model, the ingenuity of the simulation technician, and the condition of the patient, all mannequins can have a "voice." Talking through a microphone and listening though headphones, the patient's voice is usually that of a standardized participant placed away, for example, behind a one-way mirror and whose role is to answer questions as a patient would. Examples of SPs or standardized participants with hybrid mannequins are

- Learners interact with both the SP and the mannequin because they are portraying the same patient
- Standardized participants are used as
  - Mannequin's voice
  - A family member
  - A healthcare team member

VR and Computer-Based Simulations

Computer-based simulations using videos, drawings, and animation used to represent the patient have shown promise in developing clinical reasoning skills (Cook & Triola, 2009). Learners interact with the patient by asking questions (typing or speaking); by viewing data from monitors, labs, or x-rays; and by performing diagnostic or therapeutic actions (typically by making choices with the mouse).

At a much higher technology level, VR systems allow learners to become immersed in a computer-generated environment with individuals or groups of individuals (Schmorrow et al., 2009). One purpose of VR is to immerse the user in a computer-generated environment (Pimentel & Teixeria, 1992). The cost of VR systems, however, is high, making their use impractical at this time for most users. Below are examples of hybrid VR, and Chapter 17 provides in-depth information on VR.

- A computer program simulates a living condition of a patient before the learner interacts with the SP or mannequin in the simulation laboratory
- Use of real-time VR with a group of learners and multiple SPs

THE ROLE OF THE SIMULATION EDUCATOR IN HYBRID SIMULATION

Arguably, the most common hybrid simulation involves mannequins and standardized participants. Such hybrids involve four simulation education roles. However, the practicality of the simulation lab functioning is that there is a great deal of overlap in the following functions that may be performed by one or more people with multiple responsibilities.

1. **Mannequin-patient simulation specialist:** Preferably an individual with a clinical background, for example, physician, nurse, or paramedic. This individual designs healthcare team educational and assessment programs, constructs mannequin patient scenarios, and participates in debriefing and feedback.

2. **Mannequin-patient technician:** An individual with both mechanical and computer skills is desirable. The technician works with the specialist to prepare the mannequin for the encounter, troubleshoots mannequin technical/mechanical problems, keeps the mannequins in good repair, and occasionally functions as the mannequin voice or standardized participant. Often, the specialist doubles as the technician.

3. **SP educator:** Working with the simulation specialist, the SP educator advises how to use people effectively in a scenario, writes standardized participant training notes, and trains them for the scenario.

4. **Psychometrician:** Designs assessment rubrics, and collects, analyzes, and reports performance data.

Simulation educators have a number of functions in this resource-intensive process, which are outlined here.

Stakeholder Education

One of the most important roles is to educate stakeholders (e.g., learners and clinical faculty) about how patient simulations are used as an educational strategy. Learning topics include

- Simulation as an educational strategy
- Adult learning principles
- Simulator applications
- Logistics
- Developing scenarios
- Assessing performance
- Debriefing and feedback

Faculty development can take many forms, for example, seminars, webinars, and discussion of articles. One of the most powerful ways to educate faculty about how simulation works is to take them through actual encounters, experiencing the simulation, assessment, and debriefing process as the learner would. This step helps faculty understand the needs of learners and the strengths and limitations of simulation learning. Faculty need to understand the curricular, technical, and logistical issues involved in developing simulations to facilitate effective educational programs. These issues become more complicated when developing hybrid scenarios.

Curriculum Development

Development of the educational curriculum with its various goals, objectives, methods, and intended outcomes is the first step in developing a program. Done in conjunction with clinical faculty, educators determine what skills are best taught and practiced through simulations and at the appropriate learner level. They have to decide what simulation modalities are best suited to the educational plan and be creative when the desired modality is not available, lacks fidelity, or is in short supply.

Scenario Development

Simulation scenarios are vehicles for assessing skills. All simulations are an opportunity to provide learners a formative or summative assessment and help faculty self-assess the quality of their clinical education. The patient simulation scenario is a plan indicating how a program will unfold, how the mannequin will be programmed or operated remotely, and how standardized participants will be part of the scenario. An example of information supplied to a standardized participant to prepare for role portrayal is shown in Table 12.1.

Standardized Participant Training

Standardized participants can have a number of functions that require preparation, training, and rehearsal. Scenario notes that guide role portrayal, like SP cases, must be written down and modified as needed. Training "on the fly" should be avoided, especially when assessing and comparing the performance of groups. All simulation scenarios have the ability to be "standardized" (as in standardized test) if the conditions of testing are standardized.

- Training objectives
- Setting, scenario (the vehicle for assessing skills)
- Types of simulators used
- Timing
- Equipment
- Performance assessment and debriefing/feedback

The following list is an outline of required training for standardized participants depending on how extensive their role will be in the simulation.

TABLE 12.1
Hybrid Mannequin With Standardized Participant

Scenario Summary

1. Scenario name
2. Patient's name, age, gender (mannequin)
3. Scenario setting
4. Condition of the patient at scenario start
5. Educational plan

- Learner level
- Program goals
- Program learning objectives
- Methods—e.g., types of simulators used
- Intended outcomes
- Challenges to the learner

Standardized Participant Information

1. Standardized participant's name(s) and relationship to the patient.
2. Narrative—Describe the scenario, what the standardized participant will know about the patient's condition at the start of the scenario, how the SP will interact with the health team, and how the SP will act.

Patient Information (Mannequin)

List information the family member(s) will be able to give team members if requested.
NOTE: Write the answers to the following information as the family member would give it. Avoid jargon.

- Patient's overall health:
- Past medical history:
- Patient's medications and why taken:
- Past surgical history:
- Health risk behaviors
  - Exercise:
  - Diet:
  - Tobacco use:
  - Alcohol use:
  - Substance use:
- Other pertinent information:

- *Portraying a nonclinical role*: Standardized participants can be trained for a number of roles, such as patient (as part of a two-part sequential simulation [e.g., a live patient who "becomes" a mannequin patient]) a family member, or other auxiliary role required of the scenario (e.g., a bystander in a simulation taking place in the field).

- *Portraying a clinical role*: A clinician can enter a simulation as a standardized participant playing a clinical role he or she can perform with credibility. This adds verisimilitude to the simulation because the clinician can realistically participate and further the action from the inside out. Standardized participants can also "fill in" as simulated team members or clinicians, but their participation will be limited to whatever part they can play realistically.

- *Skills assessment*: Standardized participants, both clinical and nonclinical, can be trained to document when procedures are done in a timely and correct manner (e.g., correctly intubating a mannequin patient or part-task trainer). It is recommended that all charged with this task practice the skill being assessed until mastered, and practice observing, assessing the skill, and remembering it for later documentation during practice encounters. Clinical experience and performance assessment experience are two separate skill domains.

- *Assessing team communication skills*: Standardized participants are arguably in the best position to assess team communication because they are participating from within. Their roles may also require them to challenge learners, for example, to be a demanding family member or an incompetent team member. Such challenges are dictated by the training objectives. They are therefore part of their training notes, and they can then judge how well the learners respond to their challenges. Team communication is best assessed through the use of an assessment rubric.

- *Debriefing and feedback*: Standardized participants, who are clinicians, as well as simulation specialists/facilitators, are in the best position to explore clinical decision-making issues and identify "performance gaps" during debriefing (Rudolph, Simon, Rivard, Dufresne, & Raemer, 2007). Their clinical knowledge and understanding of the teaching objectives can create a climate of trust and learner engagement. Both clinical and nonclinician standardized participants who have been charged with assessing communication have a role in debriefing communication. Their role may be to challenge learners to maintain both interpersonal and team communication throughout the encounter.

Issues of Hybrid Simulation and Patient Fidelity

Simulation "fidelity" refers to the extent to which a simulation or device replicates the environment or a patient's physiological condition (Alessi, 1988). All simulation modalities have "fidelity issues," that is, they are more or less realistic, possessing a "degree of similarity" to actual patients (Hays & Singer, 1989). In general, the more "standardized" or replicable the simulation is, the less realistic it may seem because of the need to standardize testing conditions for all. One advantage of hybrid simulations is that higher fidelity simulators (e.g., high-end mannequins and SPs) can balance out the less realistic, low-fidelity simulators. But the so-called "high-fidelity" mannequin simulators only come alive when used with human simulations, for example, by adding a human voice or using standardized participants.

Applying the general simulation fidelity classifications of Yaeger, and colleagues (2004), hybrid simulation can be labeled in the following manner.

- *Low-fidelity* simulations using part-task trainers that focus on single skills and permit learners to practice in isolation

- *Medium-fidelity* simulations that employ "full-body" mannequins, hybrid simulations, or SPs, but in a setting that lacks sufficient cues for the learner to be fully immersed in the situation

- *High-fidelity* simulations that allow for full immersion in settings that could potentially be used for actual patient examination or treatment

> **Simulation Teaching Tip 12.2**
> Combining simulators and manipulating the environment, when done well, has the potential to add realism to a scenario and deflect artificiality.

The preceding items focus on mechanical or "physical fidelity," that is, how closely a simulator resembles the thing being simulated physically and kinesthetically (Salas, Bowers, & Rhodenizer, 1998). By this definition, SPs have the highest fidelity. But from a training perspective, the issue is more complex. A training system is a series of episodes or experiences that systematically build key skills from basic to more complex adaptive skills (Kozlowski, 1998). Low-fidelity simulation, therefore, can be a building block toward higher level functioning that can be practiced and assessed through higher fidelity hybrid simulations.

One goal of simulation training, regardless of the simulators used, is to achieve "psychological fidelity," that is, a situation in which the risks and rewards of learner participation correspond in a convincing way to real-world risks and rewards (Ranney, 2011). Indeed, patient simulations reach their full potential as teaching and assessment opportunities when learners suspend disbelief, immerse themselves in the scenario, and perform as they would in a real-world situation. This can only be achieved with the expertise of the simulation educator who has the ability to construct a realistic work setting from simulation devices, humans, hybrids, environmental cues, and the judicious use of imagination.

SUMMARY

Hybrid simulation is limited only by the imagination. Combining the best methods of simulation to achieve the learning outcomes is the goal of simulation educators. Hybrid simulation methods provide flexibility and realism to help learners achieve their learning outcomes.

CASE STUDY 12.1

As an experienced simulation educator, you would like to teach fourth-year healthcare students the following learning objectives.

- Discuss methods of attaining sobriety with the patient and family
- Recognize the symptoms of alcohol withdrawal
- Implement treatment measures to minimize the effect of alcohol withdrawal
- Communicate the prognosis of esophageal cancer that has metastasized to other organs

Choose two different hybrid methods that could be used to accomplish these learning outcomes and explain how to do it.

PRACTICE QUESTIONS

1. The goal of using hybrid simulation is to
   A. Assess student learning
   B. Develop different modalities of teaching
   C. Construct reality for practice
   D. Assist in programmed evaluation

2. A discipline that used simulation effectively and was a forerunner of healthcare simulation efforts included

   A. Medicine
   B. Architecture
   C. Automobile companies
   D. Aviation

3. An appropriate role for a standardized participant would be

   A. A prisoner who is brought to the emergency room with appendicitis
   B. A mother who is in labor
   C. A child having an asthma attack
   D. A sitter watching a patient with Alzheimer's

4. A simulator that represents part of the human anatomy would best fit the description of

   A. Virtual
   B. Simulator
   C. Human
   D. Task trainer

5. Students are being taught to deal effectively with end-of-life issues in an intensive care unit (ICU). In order to best facilitate their learning, the simulation educator must develop

   A. Constructed reality
   B. Physical fidelity
   C. Environmental fidelity
   D. Psychological fidelity

6. The highest fidelity constructed is portrayed in which of the following situations by using

   A. A part-task trainer to learn Foley catheter insertion in a simulated hospital room
   B. VR to perform a delicate laparoscopic procedure
   C. SP to portray a patient in drug withdrawal in a simulated clinical examination room
   D. An obstetrical emergency with a mannequin in an actual labor suite in a hospital

7. The first consideration to incorporating simulation into a curriculum is

   A. Developing the teaching strategies
   B. Deciding on the simulation equipment
   C. Developing the learning outcomes
   D. Financing the simulation laboratory

8. Research is being conducted using two groups; one group of learners is using a mannequin with an SP to learn suturing, and the other group is using a part-task trainer. The person entering the data into the spreadsheet should be a(n)

   A. Mannequin-patient simulation specialist
   B. Mannequin-patient technician
   C. SP educator
   D. Psychometrician

9. Healthcare team training is best accomplished by using

A. VR
B. Mannequins
C. Part-task trainers
D. Role-play

10. During a scenario, the mannequin malfunctions. The best person to address the technical problems would be a(n)

A. Mannequin-patient simulation specialist
B. Mannequin-patient technician
C. SP educator
D. Psychometrician

REFERENCES

Abrahamson, S. (1997). Sim one: A patient simulator ahead of its time. *Caduceus, 13*(2), 29–41.

Aggarwal, R., Moorthy, K., & Darzi, A. (2004). Laparoscopic skills training and assessment. *British Journal of Surgery, 91,* 1549–1580.

Alessi, S. M. (1988). Fidelity in the design of instructional simulations. *Journal of Computer-Based Instruction, 15*(2), 40–47.

Allen, T. B. (1987). *War games.* New York, NY: McGraw Hill.

Andrews, D. H., Brown, J., Byrnes, J., Chang, J., & Hartman, R. (1998). *Enabling technology: Analysis of categories with potential to support the use of modeling and simulation in the United States air force.* Air Force Research Lab, Mesa, AZ. Human Effectiveness Directorate.

Barth, J. (2001). *The symbolic imagination.* New York, NY: Fordham.

Baydogan, E., Belfore, L. E., Scerbo, M., & Mazumdar, S. (2009). Virtual operating room team training via computer-based agents. *International Journal of Intelligent Control and Systems, 14,*(1), 115–122.

Bernstein, M. (2000). *Grand eccentrics: Turning the century: Dayton and the inventing of America.* Wilmington, OH: Orange Frazer Press.

Coleridge, S. T. (1817). *Biographia literaria.* Princeton, NJ: Princeton University Press.

Cook, D. A., & Triola, M. M. (2009). Virtual patients: A critical literature review and proposed next steps. *Medical Education, 43*(4), 303–311.

Dillon, G. F., Boulet, J. R., Hawkins, R. E., & Swanson, D. B. (2004). Simulations in the United States Medical Licensing Examination (USMLE). *Quality & Safe Health Care, 13*(Suppl. 1), i41–i45.

Friedrich, M. J. (2002). Practice makes perfect: Risk-free medical training with patient simulators. *Journal of the American Medical Association, 288*(22), 2808, 2811–2812.

Gaba, D., & DeAnda, A. (1988). A comprehensive anesthesia simulation environment: Re-creating the operating room for research and training. *Anesthesiology, 69*(3), 387–394.

Gallagher, A. G., Ritte, E. M., Champion, H., Higgins, G., Fried, M. P., Moses G, Smith, C. D., & Satava, R. M. (2005). Virtual reality simulation for the operating room: Proficiency-based training as a paradigm shift in surgical skills training. *Annals of Surgery, 241*(2), 364–372.

Gordon, M. S. (1974). Cardiology patient simulator. Development of an animated manikin to teach cardiovascular disease. *American Journal of Cardiology, 34,* 350–355.

Grenvik, A., & Schaefer, J. J. (2004). From Resusci-Anne to Sim Man: The evolution of simulators in medicine. *Critical Care Medicine, 32,* S56–S57.

Harden, R. M., & Gleeson, F. A. (1979). Assessment of clinical competence using an objective structured clinical examination (OSCE). *Medical Education, 13,* 41–54.

Hays, R., & Singer, M. (1989). *Simulation fidelity in training system design: Bridging the gap between reality and training.* New York, NY: Springer-Verlag.

Josephus, F. (1981). *The Jewish war* (G. A. Williamson, Trans). New York: NY: Penguin.

Kozlowski, S. W. J. (1998). Training and developing adaptive teams: Theory, principles, and research. In J. A. Cannon-Bowers & E. Salas (Eds.), *Decision making under stress: Implications for training and simulation* (pp. 115–153). Washington, DC: APA Books.

Moroney, W. F., & Lilienthal, M. G. (2009). Human factors in simulation and training: An overview. In D. Vincenzi, J. Wise, M. Mouloua, & P. A. Hancock (Eds.), *Human factors in simulation and training*. Boca Raton, FL: Taylor and Francis CRC Press.

Pimentel, K., & Teixeria, K. (1992). *Virtual reality: Through the new looking glass*. New York, NY: McGraw-Hill.

Ranney, T. A. (2011). Psychological fidelity: Perception of risk. In D. L. Fisher, M. Rizzo, J. Caird, & J. D. Lee (Eds.), *Handbook of driving simulation for engineering, medicine and psychology*. Boca Raton, FL: Taylor and Francis CRC Press.

Rudolph, J. W., Simon, R., Rivard, P., Dufresne, R. L., & Raemer, D. B. (2007). Debriefing with good judgment. *Anesthesiology Clinics, 15,* 361–376.

Salas, E., Bowers, C. A., & Rhodenizer, L. (1998). It's not what you have but how you use it: Toward a rationale use of simulation to support aviation training. *International Journal of Aviation Psychology, 8*(3), 197–208.

Schmorrow, D., Nicholson, D., Stephanie, J., Lackey, S. J., Allen, R. C., Norman, K., . . . Peter, A. (2009). Virtual reality in the training environment. In D. Vincenzi, J. Wise, M. Mouloua, & P. A. Hancock (Eds.), *Human factors in simulation and training*. Boca Raton, FL: Taylor and Francis CRC Press.

Sinz, E. (2004). Partial-task-trainers and simulation in critical care medicine. In W. F. Dunn (Ed.), *Simulators in critical care and beyond* (pp. 33–41). Des Plaines, IL: Society of Critical Care Medicine.

Society for Simulation in Healthcare (SSH). (2014). *Certified healthcare simulation educator handbook*. Retrieved from http://ssih.org/certification/handbook

Vincenzi, D. A., Wise, J. A., Moulana, M., & Hanock, P. A. (2009). In *Human factors in simulation and training*. Boca Raton, FL: Taylor and Francis CRC Press.

Yaeger, K. A., Halamek, L. P., Coyle, M., Murphy, A., Anderson, J., Boyle, K., . . . Smith, M. D. (2004). High-fidelity simulation based training in neonatal nursing. *Advances in Neonatal Care, 4*(6), 326–331.

Part-Task Trainers

DEBORAH S. ARNOLD AND RUTH A. WITTMANN-PRICE

Practice does not make perfect.
Only perfect practice makes perfect.
—Vince Lombardi

This chapter addresses Content Area 3: Educate and Assess
Learners Using Simulation (Society for Simulation in Healthcare
[SSH], 2014).

LEARNING OUTCOMES

- Identify the principles behind choosing an appropriate task trainer
- Compare different types of task trainers
- Review practice questions as they relate to task trainers

Part-task trainers (PTTs) are probably among the oldest types of healthcare simulations known to professions besides practicing skills on one another. PTTs have been used successfully for years to teach "healthcare skills" and are still a valuable part of the simulation education services.

Simulation education using task trainers allows learners to obtain and/or enhance clinical skills and processes in a safe learning environment. Task trainers can be incorporated into all levels of education from novice to expert. The ability to practice high-risk, low-volume skills can enhance the confidence of individuals and teams and assist them to think critically and respond appropriately individually as well as within a team. Practicing skills deliberately helps learners know how to respond when a complex emergency occurs (Issenberg et al., 1999). The comprehensive use and worth of task trainers cannot be understated. Spooner, Hurst, and Khadra (2012) state, "Task trainers are fundamental in the teaching of anatomic landmarks and in enabling learners to acquire, develop, and maintain the necessary motor skills required to perform specific tasks" (p. 59).

Their vital impact on quality patient care and safety is likely to become more prominent as learners are able to demonstrate enhanced psychomotor and cognitive thinking skills. Choosing to use a PTT allows the faculty to validate a skill prior to performing a skill on a real patient. Task trainers are affordable, easy to move, skill specific, and allow for standardization of a process.

SIMULATORS, FIDELITY, PTTs, AND COMPLEX TASK TRAINERS

Simulator refers to a physical object or a representation of the full or part task to be replicated. It is used by some specifically to refer to technologies that recreate the full environment in which one or more targeted tasks are carried out. This can also be called fully immersive simulation (Cooper & Taqueti, 2008).

Fidelity is the principle that a simulator is able to realistically imitate true physiological realism. *Fidelity* can be defined as the degree to which the appearance and capabilities of the simulator resemble the appearance and function of the simulated system (Maran & Glavin, 2003). Low fidelity is the farthest from realism, showing no physiological change, movement, animation, or progression. High fidelity is the closest to realism, showing physiological change, movement, animation, and progression.

PTTs are devices that replicate limited aspects of a task, but do not present an integrated experience (Gaba, 2004). Examples of PTTs are provided in Exhibit 13.1.

EXHIBIT 13.1
Examples of Part-Task Trainers
Intubation mannequins Intravenous (IV) arms Female pelvises (Galloway, 2009)

They are used in healthcare education and include the anatomical segment relevant to a particular procedural skill. Cost, size, and risk of simulation equipment is considered when selecting resources. They are used to teach novices the basics of psychomotor skills and allow for maintenance and fine-tuning of expert skills. PTTs can be used in situ in a real clinical environment or set up in a simulated learning environment. The benefit of portability adds value to just-in-time education, education that takes place in relation to a decrease in census and downtime. PTTs minimize wear and tear of high-fidelity mannequins and are more cost-effective when used for acquisition of skills.

PTTs range in complexity from using a piece of fruit to teach injections to a torso to teach central line placement and care. They typically do not include patient feedback. An important trend is the combination of PTTs with either standardized patients (live actors) or full-mannequin simulators to allow for task completion in a more fully immersive environment (Kyle & Murray, 2008).

It is often difficult to suspend disbelief with PTTs, but they are often used in hybrid formats to increase realism if that is essential to the learning outcomes (Beaubien & Baker, 2004). An example is placing a task trainer arm for an intravenous (IV) line in the shirt sleeve of a standardized patient while the actual arm is concealed under a hospital gown. This can prevent pain while the learner is practicing an IV procedure on the task trainer. Chapter 12 explains the hybrid concept more completely.

Complex PTTs increase the fidelity in the learning experience by allowing the learner to use a PTT along with a computer-simulated environment (Galloway, 2009). Examples are provided in Exhibit 13.2.

EXHIBIT 13.2

Examples of Complex Part-Task Trainers

- Surgical skills
- Central line catheterization
- Scopes, such as bronchoscopes (Galloway, 2009)
- Chest tube insertion
- Ultrasound techniques (Spooner, Hurst, & Khadra, 2012)

Complex task trainers represent both virtual reality and haptic technology in healthcare education using computer-based technology. This equipment tends to be more expensive. Complex task trainers work better in a simulated learning environment related to portability. "Haptic" refers to the sense of touch and the meaning of touch (Orledge, Phillips, Murray, & Lerant, 2012). This type of trainer allows the faculty to clearly see where the learner is applying touch and the amount of pressure applied as well to as assess whether a thorough exam has been done (Durham & Alden, 2008). Complex task trainers are used in combination with PTTs so that physical interaction can occur within the virtual reality environment. This may be referred to as box-type simulation trainers. They can be used for surgical techniques, such as laparoscopic surgery.

An example used in our lab is an IV task trainer that is attached to a computer program. The learner must demonstrate knowledge of the correct procedure on the computer for the PTT to respond to the tourniquet and the arm vein to protrude to accommodate an IV insertion. Often complex PTTs provide the learner with the texture of the simulated anatomical body part (Spooner, Hurst, & Khadra, 2012).

Simulation Teaching Tip 13.1
Learners can often practice on part- and complex task trainers independently if the protocol for the procedure has been taught and is written out. This assists learners in providing self-directed deliberate practice and in being accountable for the learning before it is time for evaluation of knowledge.

Simulation Teaching Tip 13.2
There is increasing research using PTTs to promote better patient outcomes. Posner and Hamstra (2013) studied groups of medical students ($N = 145$) using a PTT (female pelvis) with and without a hybrid component (standardized patient). The study observed communication skills in randomized groups of students. The results showed no significant difference in communication skills, but technical skill was increased in the group that performed on the PTT without the standardized patient. This study indicates that PTTs are effective for skill practice.

CURRICULUM DEVELOPMENT USING PTTs

Educational goals and simulation tools go hand in hand when thinking about the type of simulator equipment to use. The educator needs to have the end in mind. What will the learner achieve at the end of this learning encounter? Whether there is financial value in using a high-fidelity mannequin for the placement of an IV line or practice of chest tube insertion when the consumable costs are much higher with higher fidelity simulation equipment should be identified. Faculty should weigh the benefits of using a PTT for individual educational encounters against the benefits of using a high-fidelity simulator to place a second line during a critical event in immersive team simulation education training. Using technology to provide hands-on experience guided by proven educational principles, we can provide the very best evidence-based learning environment for our future caregivers (Kyle & Murray, 2008).

PTTs are an invaluable asset when setting up a simulation experience for a group of learners. PTTs can be used as an "unmanned station" for learners to practice as long as they are properly prepared. Chapter 18 discusses setting up stations for learner practice in depth.

Additional studies are needed that focus on the evaluation of a learned skill on a PTT and the performance of that skill in actual practice (Boulet, Jeffries, Hatala, Korndorffer, Feinstein, & Roche, 2011).

EVIDENCE-BASED SIMULATION PRACTICE (EBSP) 13.1

Nitsche, McWeeney, Schwendemann, Rose, Davies, Watson, and Brost (2009) successfully developed their own low-cost task trainers to teach in utero, urinary tract, stenting procedures. They used gravid pig uteruses and changed the amount of fluid and substances to teach the procedure.

ADVANTAGES OF PTTs

Of all the simulation methods, PTTs are probably the least expensive. Once the equipment is bought, it can usually be used over and over with very little maintenance.

Table 13.1 provides examples of PTTs developed as cost-effective teaching tools to assist healthcare learners reach their learning goals.

Simulation Teaching Tip 13.3
Care of PTTs is important. Follow the manufacturer's instructions on cleaning and storing to increase the usability and shelf life of PTTs.

SUMMARY

PTTs are among the first-used simulation modalities and are still very effective for student learners when used alone and in a hybrid format. PTTs are cost-effective and can be used by learners independently as well as with the guidance of a simulation educator. Everyone working in the field of simulation should become broadly familiar with the technologies, pedagogies, and research methods in each domain to better inform strategies and tactics for application and diffusion of simulation in healthcare education, training, and research (Cooper & Taqueti, 2008).

TABLE 13.1
Examples of Part-Task Trainers Use

AUTHOR	USE OF PTTs
Steehler et al. (2012, 2013)	Developed task trainers to teach endoscopic sinus surgery skills; the PTTs were validated and inexpensive
Zerth, Harwood, Tommaso, and Girzadas (2012)	Developed a cost-effective PTT to teach pericardiocentesis, a procedure done using ultrasound guidance
Sprick, Owen, Hein, and Brown (2011)	Used a PTT to teach endotracheal intubation
Owen, Follows, Reynolds, Burgess, and Plummer (2002)	Used a PTT to teach the proper application of cricoid pressure needed for patient procedures
Hein and Owen (2006)	Used a PTT for learning to intubate

CASE STUDY 13.1

A learner is using an IV task trainer that is hybrid and uses a computer to run through the procedure.

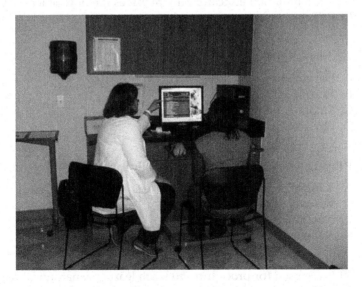

The learner does well on the IV insertion on the PTT, but states, "I know this is not how it is really going to be with patients." As the simulation educator, how would you respond?

PRACTICE QUESTIONS

1. The novice simulation educator needs more mentoring when he states

   A. "The students learn better when they use the mannequin."
   B. "The learning outcomes should guide the equipment we use."
   C. "Keeping the part-task training in a climate-controlled room is important,"
   D. "Being available at all times to assist and watch students using the part-task trainer (PTT) is important."

2. PTTs can be used in a hybrid format with other modalities. To teach communication skills, the best method would be to use a PTT with

   A. Virtual reality
   B. A standardized patient
   C. A mannequin
   D. Another PTT

3. PTTs can be all of the following except

   A. Manufacturer made
   B. Developed by the simulation educator
   C. Made from household items
   D. Part of a high-fidelity mannequin

4. When using learning stations in the simulation laboratory

   A. PTTs should not be used.
   B. Stations should each have a debriefing.
   C. The simulation educator only oversees the flow of learners.
   D. PTTs can be peer supervised.

5. Adding texture to the PTT adds

   A. Developmental fidelity
   B. Psychological fidelity
   C. Emotional fidelity
   D. Physical fidelity

6. PTTs that are called "complex" usually include a PTT coupled with

   A. A high-fidelity mannequin
   B. Virtual reality
   C. A standardized participant
   D. A standardized patient

7. PTTs are used for procedures to teach learners anatomical placements and

   A. Landmarks
   B. Neurological responses
   C. Correct pressure to apply
   D. Patient sensitivity

8. When using PTTs that depict severe traumatic wounds or burns, it would be important to

    A. Allow the students to orient to the PTT.
    B. Make sure the student treats the PTT as if real.
    C. Make sure the students do not act surprised when they view the PTT.
    D. Cover the PTT until it is time to use it.

9. Having students practice a procedure over and over on a PTT is subscribing to the concept of

    A. Behaviorism
    B. Surface learning
    C. Multitasking
    D. Deliberate practice

10. Using the lowest fidelity equipment to facilitate learning outcomes effectively can be viewed as

    A. Lack of equipment
    B. Cost-effective learning
    C. Scaffolding
    D. Leveled learning

REFERENCES

Beaubien, J., & Baker, D. (2004). The use of simulation for training teamwork skills in health care. *How low can you go? Quality and Safety in Health Care, 13*(Suppl. 1), 51–56.

Boulet, J. R., Jeffries, P. R., Hatala, R. A., Korndorffer, J. R., Feinstein, D. M., & Roche, J. P. (2011). Research regarding method of assessing learning outcomes. *Simulation in Healthcare, 6,* S48–S51.

Cooper, J. B., & Taqueti, V. R. (2008). A brief history of the development of mannequin simulators for clinical education and training. *Postgraduate Medical Journal, 84*(997), 563–570.

Durham, C., & Alden, K. (2008). Enhancing patient safety in nursing education through patient simulation. In R. G. Hughes (Ed.), *Patient safety and quality: An evidence-based handbook for nurses* (pp. 1–40). Retrieved from http://www.http/ahrq.gov

Gaba, D. M. (2004). The future vision of simulation in health care. *Quality and Safety in Health Care, 13*(Suppl. 1), i2–i110.

Galloway, S. J. (2009). Simulation techniques to bridge the gap between novice and competent healthcare professionals. *The Online Journal of Issues in Nursing, 14*(2). Retrieved from http://www.nursingworld.org/MainMenuCategories/ANAMarketplace/ANA Periodicals/OJIN/TableofContents/Vol142009/No2May09/Simulation-Techniques .aspx

Hein, C., & Owen, H. (2006). Learning endotracheal intubation: Failings of current part-task trainers proceedings title. *Journal of Emergency Primary Health Care, 4*(3), 9–10.

Issenberg, S. B., McGaghie, W. C., Hart, I. R., Mayer, J. W., Felner, J. M., Petrusa, E. R., . . . Ewy, G. A. (1999). Simulation technology for healthcare professional skills training and assessment. *Journal of the American Medical Association, 282,* 861–866.

Kyle, R. R., & Murray, W. B. (2008). *Clinical operations, engineering and management.* London, UK: Elsevier/Academic Press.

Maran, N. F., & Glavin, R. F. (2003). Low to high fidelity simulation a continuum of medical education. *Medical Education, 37*(Suppl. 1), 22–28.

Nitsche, J. F., McWeeney, D. T., Schwendemann, W. D., Rose, C. H., Davies, N. P., Watson, W., & Brost, B. C. (2009). In-utero stenting: Development of a low-cost high-fidelity task trainer. *Ultrasound in Obstetrics & Gynecology, 34*(6), 720–723.

Orledge, J., Phillips, W. J., Murray, W. B., & Lerant, A. (2012). The use of simulation in health-care: From systems issues, to team building, to task training, to education and high stakes examinations. *Current Opinion in Critical Care, 18*(4), 326–332.

Owen, H., Follows, V., Reynolds, K. J., Burgess, G., & Plummer, J. (2002). Learning to apply effective cricoids pressure using a part task trainer. *Anaesthesia, 57*(11), 1098–1101.

Posner, G. D., & Hamstra, S. J. (2013). Too much small talk? Medical students' pelvic examination skills falter with pleasant patients. *Medical Education, 47*(12), 1209–1214.

Spooner, N., Hurst, S., & Khadra, M. (2012). Medical simulation technology: Educational overview, industry leaders, and what's missing. *Hospital Topics, 90*(3), 57–64. doi: 10.1080/00185868.2012.714685

Sprick, C., Owen, H., Hein, C., & Brown, B. (2011). A new part task trainer for teaching and learning confirmation of endotracheal intubation. *Studies in Health Technology & Informatics, 163*, 611–615.

Society for Simulation in Healthcare (SSH). (2014). *Certified healthcare simulation educator handbook.* Retrieved from http://ssih.org/certification/handbook

Steehler, M. K., Chu, E. E., Na, H., Pfisterer, M. J., Hesham, H. N., & Malekzadeh, S. (2013). Teaching and assessing endoscopic sinus surgery skills on a validated low-cost task trainer. *Laryngoscope, 123*(4), 841–844.

Steehler, M. K., Pfisterer, M. J., Na, H., Hesham, H. N., Pehlivanova, M., & Malekzadeh, S. (2012). Face, content, and construct validity of a low-cost sinus surgery task trainer. *Otolaryngology-Head & Neck Surgery, 146*(3), 504–509.

Zerth, H., Harwood, R., Tommaso, L., & Girzadas, D. V. (2012). An inexpensive, easily constructed, reusable task trainer for simulating ultrasound-guided pericardiocentesis. *Journal of Emergency Medicine, 43*(6), 1066–1069.

Interprofessional Simulation

SHARON GRISWOLD, KYMBERLEE MONTGOMERY, KATE MORSE,
AND GREGORY J. OWSIK

> *The status quo of educating health professionals*
> *in silos without preparing them for the current realities of*
> *everyday practice is no longer tenable.*
> —Frenk et al. (2010)

This chapter addresses Content Area 3: Educate and Assess
Learners Using Simulation (Society for Simulation in Healthcare
[SSH], 2014).

LEARNING OUTCOMES

- Discuss the history of interprofessional education (IPE) over the past century
- Define IPE principles that foster a climate of patient/population care that is safe, timely, effective, and equitable
  - Values and ethics (VE)
  - Roles and responsibilities (RR)
  - Interprofessional communication/Communication competency (IC/CC)
  - Teams and teamwork (TT)
- Discuss interprofessional communication techniques in simulation-based education (SBE) to translate an improved team approach to daily patient care
  - Application of closed-loop communication techniques in all professional interactions
  - Creation of a climate where providers apply a shared mental model
  - Support of learner understanding and respect of individual providers' roles and those of other professions to collaboratively address the healthcare needs of patients
- Discuss how IPE principles taught via SBE have begun to translate to patient care outcomes

HISTORY OF IPE

The newly recognized and often-used term "interprofessional education" has a variety of meanings and interpretations. The World Health Organization (WHO) defines IPE as a form of experiential learning whereby "students from two or more professions learn about, from, and with each other to enable effective collaboration and improve health outcomes" (WHO, 2010, p. 1). For many, learning through some type of active participation, experience, and reflection (experiential learning) provides a fresh lens in viewing the educational process (Kolb, 1984). To mimic real-life environments as the backdrop can be even more powerful. Thus, to practice together better, it is imperative that students have the opportunity to collaborate and learn together and from one another in a safe educational environment (Montgomery, Morse, Smith-Glasgow, Posmontier, & Follen, 2012).

BACKGROUND

The national recommendations to redesign the health education system to embrace the strengths of multidisciplinary skill sets are certainly not novel nor did they develop out of necessity to comply with the needs derived from healthcare reform. In fact, the origin of this challenge can be traced to the Flexner Report of 1910 (Flexner, 1910), and a call for healthcare educational transformations to include IPE initiatives has been a recurrent theme threaded through the following landmark reports of the Institute of Medicine (IOM) over the past half century (Table 14.1).

- *Educating for the Health Team* (IOM, 1972)
- *To Err Is Human: Building a Safer Health System* (Kohn, Corrigan, & Donaldson, 1999)
- *Crossing the Quality Chasm: A New Health System for the 21st Century* (IOM, 2001)

Unfortunately, although these reports provided the premise that IPE-based programs would decrease preventable medical errors though increased multidisciplinary team collaboration and communication and improved quality care delivery and patient safety outcomes, these challenges yielded slim results.

Years of escalating governmental spending, healthcare costs, numbers of uninsured and underinsured Americans, and fear of the individual's inability to afford basic healthcare spawned a unified consensus among governmental and private foundations to transform both the healthcare and health education system, strongly emphasizing the need for IPE in the United States (Montgomery et al., 2012; Montgomery, Griswold-Theodorson, Morse, Montgomery, & Farabaugh, 2012). Rethinking the IPE's call to action initiatives were postulated in three well-respected and nationally recognized sentinel reports.

1. *The Future of Nursing: Leading Change, Advancing Health* (IOM, 2010)
2. *Framework for Action on Interprofessional Education and Collaborative Practice* (WHO, 2010)
3. *Transforming Education to Strengthen Health Systems in an Interdependent World* (Frenk et al., 2010)

TABLE 14.1

Historical Landmark Reports That Have Made Recommendations Regarding the Integration of Interprofessional Education (IPE) to the Healthcare Environment

LANDMARK REPORTS	INTERPROFESSIONAL EDUCATION RECOMMENDATIONS
Flexner Report (1910)	Suggests a full redesign of medical school education systems
Educating for the Health Team (Institute of Medicine [IOM], 1972)	Challenges national healthcare educators and administrators to • Engage in interprofessional education • Develop clinical settings to begin interprofessional innovation • Lobby governmental and professional support of interprofessional education for healthcare delivery teams
To Err Is Human: Building a Safer Health System (IOM, 1999)	Encourages the reduction of preventable medical errors through • Provision of support to multidisciplinary teams of researchers, healthcare facilities, and organizations to determine the causes of medical errors • Development of new knowledge to assist in the creation of demonstration projects
Crossing the Quality Chasm: A New Health System for the 21st Century (IOM, 2001)	Provisions made to ensure licensing and accreditation organizations begin the evolution of our siloed educational processes through • Stressing evidence-based practice instruction • Providing opportunities for interprofessional training
Health Professions Education: Building a Bridge to Quality (IOM, 2003)	Reiterates the need for *all* healthcare professionals to be • Educated to deliver patient-centered care as members of an interprofessional team • Prepared to use evidence-based practice, quality-improvement approaches, and informatics

(continued)

TABLE 14.1
Historical Landmark Reports That Have Made Recommendations Regarding the Integration of Interprofessional Education (IPE) to the Healthcare Environment (*continued*)

LANDMARK REPORTS	INTERPROFESSIONAL EDUCATION RECOMMENDATIONS
The Future of Nursing: Leading Change, Advancing Health (IOM, 2010)	Recommends that nurses need to be an integral part of the healthcare team by • Practicing to the full extent of their education and training • Intertwining advanced competencies within higher levels of training and education • Becoming equal partners in redesigning and improving healthcare • Participating in workforce planning and policymaking initiatives
Framework for Action on Interprofessional Education and Collaborative Practice (World Health Organization [WHO], 2010)	Provides strategies to support global health workforce and • Identifies the necessity of IPE education and collaboration strategies to increase health profession work force • Defines IPE as the future of health education and in the delivery of quality patient care
Transforming Education to Strengthen Health Systems in an Interdependent World (Frenk; Harvard School of Public Health, 2010)	Suggests that health education reform should • Promote interprofessional and transprofessional education • Encourage nonhierarchical relationships in effective teams

After much time the initial IOM call to action for collaboration among healthcare professionals, six of the major national healthcare organizations convened an expert panel to produce documents containing the foundation of IPE (Montgomery, Morse, et al., 2012). *Team-Based Competencies: Building a Shared Foundation for Education and Clinical Practice* (2011) and *Core Competencies for Interprofessional Collaborative Practice* (2011) define four measurable core competency domains and 38 subcompetencies for curriculum foundation for IPE and practice in all healthcare realms.

1. VE for interprofessional practice
2. RR
3. IC/CC
4. TT

GENERAL IPE COMPETENCIES

The aforementioned competencies for IPE in health professions were developed by the Interprofessional Education Collaborative (IPEC), an expert panel including the American Association of Colleges of Nursing (AACN), the American Association of Colleges of Osteopathic Medicine, the American Association of Colleges of Pharmacy, the American Dental Education Association, the Association of American Medical Colleges, and the Association of Schools of Public Health. The overarching goal of this collaboration was to develop individual-level core interprofessional competencies. Originally developed with an authentic patient practice focus, these definitions are also foundational to IPE in simulated environments. IPEC defined interprofessional competencies in healthcare as "integrated enactment of knowledge, skills and values/attitudes that define working together across the professions, with other health care workers, and with patients, along with families and communities as appropriate to improve health outcomes in specific care contexts" (*Team-Based Competencies Building a Shared Foundation for Education and Clinical Practice*, 2011, p. 1).

The collaborative identified that core IPE competencies were needed in order to coordinate and direct the curricular revisions in health professions, including pedagogy and assessment strategies to promote success, to lay the foundation for a teaching curriculum in IPE that was connected to the development of student lifelong learning, to foster discussion regarding the divide between authentic patient care demands and IPE core competencies, to identify opportunities to integrate IPE content with current accreditation expectations, to provide a framework of common IPE competencies that would eventually link to a common set of accreditation standards, to provide licensing and credentialing bodies with potential testing content, and to promote the conduct of evaluation and research in this area to support outcomes (IPEC Expert Panel, 2011).

The competencies are based on a single, unifying concept, interprofessionality, which was originally defined as part of the work by Health Canada (D'Amour & Oandasan, 2005). It is not merely practicing in the same room or on the same team, but a deliberate practice of professionals to reflect and develop an integrated practice model focused on addressing the needs at the level of patient/family or population. The key elements include constant knowledge sharing between professionals and an emphasis on active patient participation. This is a paradigm shift from traditional care teams and educational models in most health professions. Thus, the development of core IPE competencies to describe the unique attributes of IPE practice was needed. The intent of the publication and competencies was to remain general in nature to provide for individual profession and institutional flexibility.

Exhibit 14.1 demonstrates IPE core competencies from the IPEC (Dieckmann, Molin Friis, Lippert, & Østergaard, 2009).

EXHIBIT 14.1

Core Competencies for Interprofessional Collaborative Practice From the Interprofessional Education Collaborative

1. Values and ethics: Work with individuals of other professions to maintain a climate of mutual respect and shared values.
2. Roles and responsibilities: Use the knowledge of one's own role and those of other professions to appropriately assess and address the healthcare needs of the patients and populations served.
3. Communication competency: Communicate with patients, families, communities, and other health professionals in a responsive and responsible manner that supports a team approach to the maintenance of health and the treatment of disease.
4. Teams and teamwork: Apply relationship-building values and the principles of team dynamics to perform effectively in different team roles to plan and deliver patient-/population-centered care that is safe, timely, efficient, effective, and equitable.

Each of the four core competencies or domains is further delineated into specific IPE competencies that are outlined here.

Detailed VE Competencies

This domain moves beyond the individual's professional ethics and focuses on the development of interprofessional ethics.

- VE 1: Place the interests of patients and populations at the center of the IPE health delivery
- VE 2: Respect the dignity and privacy of patients while maintaining confidentiality in the delivery of team-based care
- VE 3: Embrace the cultural diversity and individual differences that characterize patients, populations, and the healthcare team
- VE 4: Respect the unique cultures, values, roles/responsibilities, and expertise of other health professions

- VE 5: Work in cooperation with those who receive care, those who provide care, and those who contribute to or support the delivery of prevention and health services
- VE 6: Develop a trusting relationship with patients, families, and other team members
- VE 7: Demonstrate high standards of ethical conduct and quality of care in one's contribution to team-based care
- VE 8: Manage ethical dilemmas specific to interprofessional patient-/population-centered care situations
- VE 9: Act with honesty and integrity in relationships with patients, families, and other team members
- VE 10: Maintain competence in one's own profession appropriate to scope of practice

Detailed RR Competencies

The interaction between understanding your own roles and responsibilities and those of another within an interprofessional team while providing patient-centered or population-focused care are delineated in the roles and responsibilities-specific competencies. Each profession's roles and responsibilities are delineated within the legal scope of practice that may be significantly influenced by practice environment, region, or location. However, within the appropriate scope of practice, roles and responsibilities may also vary, depending on the particular situation. The specific RR (IPEC Expert Panel, 2011) competencies are

- RR 1: Communicate one's roles and responsibilities clearly to patients, families, and other professions
- RR 2: Recognize one's limitations in skills, knowledge, and abilities
- RR 3: Engage diverse healthcare professionals who complement one's own professional expertise, as well as associated resources, to develop strategies to meet specific patient care needs
- RR 4: Explain the roles and responsibilities of other care providers and how the team works together to provide care
- RR 5: Use the full scope of knowledge, skills, and abilities of available health professionals and healthcare workers to provide care that is timely, safe, effective, and equitable
- RR 6: Communicate with team members to clarify each member's responsibility in executing components of a treatment plan or public health intervention
- RR 7: Forge interdependent relationships with other professions to improve care and advance learning
- RR 8: Use unique and complementary abilities of all members of the team to optimize patient care

Detailed IC Competencies

This domain expounds on the critical nature of effective verbal, written, and health literacy communication to promote interprofessional collaboration. This includes using a shared language that is known to all team members, such as that suggested in *TeamSTEPPS®: National Implemenation* (Agency for Healthcare Research Quality; 2012).

- CC 1: Choose effective communication tools and techniques, including information systems and communication technologies, to facilitate discussions and interactions that enhance team function
- CC 2: Organize and communicate information with patients, families, and healthcare team members in a form that is understandable, avoiding discipline-specific terminology when possible
- CC 3: Express one's knowledge and opinions to team members involved in patient care with confidence, clarity, and respect, working to ensure common understanding of information and treatment and care decisions
- CC 4: Listen actively, and encourage ideas and opinions of other team members
- CC 5: Give timely, sensitive, instructive feedback to others about their performance on the team, responding respectfully as a team member to feedback from others
- CC 6: Use respectful language appropriate for a given difficult situation, crucial conversation, or interprofessional conflict
- CC 7: Recognize how one's own uniqueness, including experience level, expertise, culture, power, and hierarchy within the healthcare team, contributes to effective communication, conflict resolution, and positive interprofessional relationships (University of Toronto, 2008)

Detailed TT Competencies

The last domain addresses the concepts of effective team members and team behaviors that may influence, positively or negatively, the team's overall effectiveness.

- TT 1: Describe the process of team development and the roles and practices of effective teams
- TT 2: Develop consensus on the ethical principles to guide all aspects of patient care and team work
- TT 3: Engage other health professionals—appropriate to the specific care situation—in shared patient-centered problem solving
- TT 4: Integrate the knowledge and experience of other professions—appropriate to the specific care situation—to inform care decisions, while respecting patient and community values and priorities/preferences for care
- TT 5: Apply leadership practices that support collaborative practice and team effectiveness
- TT 6: Engage self and others to constructively manage disagreements about values, roles, goals, and actions that arise among healthcare professionals and with patients and families
- TT 7: Share accountability with other professions, patients, and communities for outcomes relevant to prevention and healthcare

- TT 8: Reflect on individual and team performance for individual as well as team performance improvement
- TT 9: Use process improvement strategies to increase the effectiveness of inter-professional teamwork and team-based care
- TT 10: Use available evidence to inform effective teamwork and team-based practices
- TT 11: Perform effectively on teams and, in different teams, perform roles in a variety of settings

---

Simulation Teaching Tip 14.1
Pearls and Pitfalls Implementing Interprofessional Simulation-Based Education

Pearls
Medical errors can often be traced back to common root causes: lack of team communication or provider knowledge or organizational transfer of knowledge to a relevant clinical encounter (*AHRQ's Patient Safety Initiative: Building Foundations, Reducing Risk*, 2003).

One of the greatest changes in the healthcare communication culture may be advanced by bringing multidisciplinary healthcare professionals together to practice improved situational awareness, a shared mental model, or "huddle" as defined by TeamSTEPPS (*TeamSTEPPS: National Implemenation*, Agency for Healthcare Research Quality, 2012). The TeamSTEPPS curriculum is a product developed jointly by the Department of Defense (DoD) and the Agency for Healthcare Research and Quality (AHRQ) in the United States to improve institutional collaboration and communication relating to patient safety. The cultural implications of any team member speaking up when concerned and open sharing of situational monitoring of the **S**tatus of the patient, **T**eam status, **E**nvironment, and the **P**rogress toward the goal (STEP) are best practiced in the simulation environment. The TeamSTEPPS educational materials are readily available in the public domain: teamstepps.ahrq.gov.

Pitfalls
The enormity of bringing healthcare providers together to practice without risk to patients and to improve patient care is systematically challenging. The practical issues of scheduling and time commitment may be some of the most significant barriers to successful implementation. Successful implementation requires a committed interprofessional team of educators.

EVIDENCE-BASED SIMULATION PRACTICE (EBSP) 14.1

Teamwork training, including IPE principles conducted using simulation and debriefing, has begun to translate to improved patient care process outcomes (Marr et al., 2012; Riley, Davis, Miller, Hansen, Sainfort, & Sweet, 2011). Although it is extremely difficult to understand the specific methodology used in each of these studies to definitively understand what, when, and how IPE principles practiced outside of the patient care environment lead to patient care improvements, the following studies are promising. In 2010, Capella

(continued)

EVIDENCE-BASED SIMULATION PRACTICE (EBSP) 14.1 (*continued*)

and colleagues studied trauma team performance after simulation-based TeamSTEPPS Training. In this study, the time to computed tomography (CT), time to tracheal intubation, and appropriateness of time to the operating room were all significantly improved after training. Another study by Marr and colleagues (2012) was able to demonstrate similar patient care process outcomes after multidisciplinary providers practiced high-stress clinical situations in a simulated environment.

Riley and colleagues (2011) demonstrated that a simulation-based intervention in addition to interprofessional team training resulted in a statistically significant 37% improvement in perinatal morbidity scores. The authors used the Weighted Adverse Outcome Score measure of perinatal morbidity and a culture-of-safety survey (safety attitudes questionnaire) before and after intervention to compare three hospital groups. The first group served as a control, and the second hospital received the US AHRQ-supported curriculum, the TeamSTEPPS didactic training program. The third hospital received both the TeamSTEPPS program and a series of in situ simulation training exercises. The authors found that a comprehensive interprofessional team training program using in situ simulation in addition to interprofessional educational team training in nontechnical skills improved perinatal safety in the hospital setting. They also reinforced the idea that didactic instruction alone without simulation was not effective in improving perinatal outcomes.

In 2013, Theilen and colleagues published a prospective cohort study of all deteriorating inpatients of a tertiary pediatric hospital requiring admission to a pediatric intensive care unit (PICU) the year before and after the introduction of a pediatric rapid-response medical emergency team (pMET) and concurrent team training. The article suggests improvements in patient outcomes specifically related to the in situ simulation training. Lessons learned by ward staff during regular training that brought physicians and nurses together for weekly, in situ team training led to significantly improved recognition and management of deteriorating inpatients with evolving critical illness.

It is imperative to understand the methodology of these recent studies and how IPE has contributed to each study's success and limitations. Table 14.2 outlines the EBSP described here and demonstrates evidence of patient care–related outcomes after interprofessional simulation practice.

CASE STUDY 14.1

A Certified Healthcare Simulation Educator™ (CHSE™) is arranging an interprofessional simulation experience with multiple disciplines in a teaching hospital laboratory. All the healthcare professionals are licensed and needed for the simulation experience of a prolapsed cord on a laboring patient. It is imperative that nursing, medicine, the obstetrical operating room (OR) team, respiratory, and neonatology disciplines respond. The simulation experience is scheduled three separate times, and all three times, one of the participants cancels due to "being busy in the labor and delivery suites." What pitfall is the CHSE falling into and how can this be overcome?

TABLE 14.2
Teamwork and Interprofessional Education Principles and Clinical Outcomes

ARTICLE TITLE	COMPARISON	OUTCOMES MEASURED	PARTICIPANTS	CONCLUSIONS
Theilen et al. (2013; Tertiary Hospital, UK), *Resuscitation*				
"Regular In Situ Simulation Training of Pediatric Medical Emergency Team Improves Hospital Response to Deteriorating Patients"	Pediatric medical emergency team (pMET) Rotating team training	Prospective study of all deteriorating inpatients requiring admission to PICU	Key ward staff and on-call staff	Statistically significant faster recognition and management of deteriorating inpatients
Marr et al. (2012; Level I Trauma Center, US), *Journal of Surgical Education*				
"Team Play in Surgical Education: A Simulation-Based Study"	Performance in videotaped trauma cases, pre- and postsimulation	# of HCWs in resuscitation % HCW in role Time to intubation Time to intubation from paralysis Time to first imaging Time to leave to CT/OR Spinal stabilization	NY state level 1 trauma center staff	High-stress situations simulated in a low-stress environment can improve team interaction and competencies
Riley et al. (2011; Community Hospital, US), *Joint Commission Journal on Quality and Patient Safety*				
"Didactic and Simulation Nontechnical Skills Team Training to Improve Perinatal Patient Outcomes in a Community Hospital"	Compared curriculum of three hospitals: control, TeamSTEPPS alone, and TeamSTEPPS with simulation training	WAOS score—summary metric of adverse event score per delivery	Labor and delivery staff	Improvement in WAOS score

(continued)

TABLE 14.2
Teamwork and IPE Principles and Clinical Outcomes (continued)

ARTICLE TITLE	COMPARISON	OUTCOMES MEASURED	PARTICIPANTS	CONCLUSIONS
Capella et al. (2010: Tertiary Teaching Hospital, US), *Journal of Surgical Education*				
"Teamwork Training Improves the Clinical Care of Trauma Patients"	Score sheet and clinical trauma registry data pre- and postteam training	Team performance time to computed tomography, OR, and endotracheal tube Percentage survival at discharge	Trauma team consisting of residents, faculty, and nurses	Significantly improved communication, leadership, mutual support, and situational monitoring scores after SBT Significant improvement in clinical process outcomes such as time to computed tomography, OR, and endotracheal tube and no significant change in survival

HCW, healthcare worker; OR, operating room; NY, New York; PICU, pediatric intensive care unit; pMET, pediatric medical emergency team; SBT, simulation-based training; UK, United Kingdom; US, United States; WAOS, Weighted Adverse Outcome Score.

PRACTICE QUESTIONS

1. Which of the following best describes the WHO definition of IPE?

   A. A form of testing in which different disciplines write questions for each other
   B. A form of didactic learning in which students learn about different professions
   C. A form of experiential learning in which students spend time observing other professions
   D. A form of experiential learning in which students from two or more professions learn about, from, and with each other

2. Which of the following are the four core competency domains identified for IPE?

   A. VE, RR, IC, and TT
   B. VE, individual scope of practice, team communication, and leadership
   C. RR, evidence-based guidelines for care, IC, and TT
   D. Professional ethics, team leadership, scope of practice, and teamwork

3. Which of the following is an example of a simulation-based IPE program?

   A. Nurse practitioner students and undergraduate nursing students participating in rapid-response scenarios
   B. Nurse practitioner students, medical residents, and respiratory therapy students participating in complex simulation scenarios
   C. Undergraduate nursing students and medical students participating in individual standardized patient scenarios
   D. Medical residents learning how to place central lines on a simulator

4. Which of the following is a *primary goal* for the development of IPE competencies?

   A. For healthcare professions to understand each other's roles
   B. To improve health outcomes in authentic patient care
   C. To increase the use of simulation to promote IPE
   D. To help the patient understand the healthcare team

5. Which of the following has been identified as a barrier in developing and promoting simulation-based IPE?

   A. Persistent separation of healthcare disciplines
   B. Accreditation lagging behind practice
   C. Students not interested in learning together
   D. The reduction in tuition costs that would occur based on combining programs

6. For an individual faculty member, which of the following activities would promote the development of simulation-based IPE experiences?

   A. Designing a simulation-based curriculum and then inviting students to participate
   B. Inviting an interprofessional team of faculty to evaluate current curriculum and identify opportunities to design IPE experiences
   C. Collaborating with one other discipline to design simulation-based IPE experiences to evaluate the two student groups at the end of their curriculum
   D. Publishing a review of IPE articles in your own profession only

7. The simulation educator overhears a particpant of the IPE experience barking orders at another member. The simulation educator understands that one of the main reasons this occurs is a violation of which of the following principles?

   A. VE
   B. RR
   C. CC
   D. TT

8. The simulation educator overhears a particpant of the IPE experience barking orders at another member. The simulation educator would best handle this situation initially by

   A. Dealing with the behavior of the inappropriate participant at the end of the scenario
   B. Developing a learning plan for the inappropriate participant
   C. Asking the team to restart the scenario and provide additional patient background data
   D. Stopping the scenario, discussing the actions with the team, and then restarting

9. The simulation educator overhears a particpant of the IPE experience continuously asking an English-as-a-second-language (ESL) learner to speak up because he cannot be heard. The simulation educator understands that one of the main reasons this occurs is a violation of which of the following principles?

   A. VE
   B. RR
   C. CC
   D. TT

10. The simulation educator overhears a particpant of the IPE experience continuously asking an ESL learner to speak up because he cannot be heard. The simulation educator would best deal with this situation by

    A. Dealing with the behavior at the end of the scenario
    B. Developing a learning plan for the inappropriate participant
    C. Asking the team to restart the scenario and asking the person to speak up
    D. Stopping the scenario, discussing the actions with the team, and then restarting

REFERENCES

Agency for Healthcare and Research Quality (AHRQ). (2012). *TeamSTEPPS: National implemenation*. Retrieved February 13, 2014, from http://teamstepps.ahrq.gov

AHRQ's Patient Safety Initiative: Building Foundations, Reducing Risk. (2003). *Efforts to reduce medical errors: AHRQ's response to Senate Committee on Appropriations questions*. Retrieved February 13, 2014, from http://www.ahrq.gov/research/findings/final-reports/pscongrpt/psini2.html

Capella, J., Smith, S., Philp, A., Putnam, T., Gilbert, C., Fry, W., . . . Remine, S. (2010). Teamwork training improves the clinical care of trauma patients. *J Surg Educ, 67*(6), 439–443. doi: 10.1016/j.jsurg.2010.06.006

D'Amour, D., & Oandasan, I. (2005). Interprofessionality as the field of interprofessional practice and interprofessional education: An emerging concept. *Journal of Interprofesssional Care, 19*(Suppl. 1), 8–20. doi:10.1080/13561820500081604

Dieckmann, P., Molin Friis, S., Lippert, A., & Østergaard, D. (2009). The art and science of debriefing in simulation: Ideal and practice. *Medical Teacher, 31*(7), e287–e294.

Flexner, A. (1910). *Medical education in the United States and Canada: A report to the Carnegie Foundation for the Advancement of Teaching.* New York, NY: The Carnegie Foundation for the Advancement of Teaching.

Frenk, J., Chen, L., Bhutta, Z. A., Cohen, J., Crisp, N., Evans, T., . . . Zurayk, H. (2010). Health professionals for a new century: Transforming education to strengthen health systems in an interdependent world. *Lancet, 376*(9756), 1923–1958. doi:10.1016/s0140-6736(10)61854-5

Institute of Medicine (IOM). (1972). *Educating for the health team.* Washington, DC: Institute of Medicine of the National Academies.

Institute of Medicine (IOM). (1999). *To err is human: Building a safer health system.* Retrieved from https://www.iom.edu

Institute of Medicine (IOM). (2003). Health professions education: A bridge to quality. Institute of Medicine of the National Academies. Retrieved February 13, 2014, from http://www.iom.edu/Reports/2003/Health-Professions-Education-A-Bridge-to-Quality.aspx

Institute of Medicine (IOM). (2010). The Future of Nursing Leading Change, Advancing Health. Institute of Medicine of the National Academies. Retrieved February 13, 2014, from http://www.iom.edu/Reports/2010/The-Future-of-Nursing-Leading-Change-Advancing-Health.aspx

Institute of Medicine of the National Academies (IOM). (2001). *Crossing the quality chasm: A new health system for the 21st century.* Retrieved February 13, 2014, from http://iom.edu/Reports/2001/Crossing-the-Quality-Chasm-A-New-Health-System-for-the-21st-Century.aspx

Interprofessional Education Collaborative Expert Panel. (2011). *Core competencies for interprofessional collaborative practice: Report of an expert panel.* Washington, DC: Interprofessional Education Collaborative.

Kohn, L. T., Corrigan, J. M., & Donaldson, M. S. (Eds.). (1999). *To err is human: Building a safer health system.* Washington, DC: National Academies Press.

Kolb, D. A. (1984). *Experiential learning: Experience as the source of learning and development* (Vol. 1). Englewood Cliffs, NJ: Prentice-Hall.

Marr, M., Hemmert, K., Nguyen, A. H., Combs, R., Annamalai, A., Miller, G., . . . Cohen, S. M. (2012). Team play in surgical education: A simulation-based study. *Journal of Surgical Education, 69*(1), 63–69. doi:http://dx.doi.org/10.1016/j.jsurg.2011.07.002

Montgomery, K., Griswold-Theodorson, S., Morse, K., Montgomery, O., & Farabaugh, D. (2012). Transdisciplinary simulation: Learning and practicing together. *Nursing Clinics of North America, 47*(4), 493–502.

Montgomery, K., Morse, C., Smith-Glasgow, M. E., Posmontier, B., & Follen, M. (2012). Promoting quality and safety in women's health through the use of transdisciplinary clinical simulation educational modules: Methodology and a pilot trial. *Gender Medicine, 9*(1, Suppl.), S48–S54. doi:http://dx.doi.org/10.1016/j.genm.2011.11.001

Riley, W., Davis, S., Miller, K., Hansen, H., Sainfort, F., & Sweet, R. (2011). Didactic and simulation nontechnical skills team training to improve perinatal patient outcomes in a community hospital. *Joint Commission Journal on Quality and Patient Safety, 37*(8), 357–364.

Society for Simulation in Healthcare (SSH). (2014). *Certified healthcare simulation educator handbook.* Retrieved from http://ssih.org/certification/handbook

Team-Based Competencies Building a Shared Foundation for Education and Clinical Practice. (2011). *Health Resources Service Administration.* Retrieved February 13, 2014, from http://www.aacn.nche.edu/leading-initiatives/IPECProceedings.pdf

Theilen, U., Leonard, P., Jones, P., Ardill, R., Weitz, J., Agrawal, D., & Simpson, D. (2013). Regular in situ simulation training of paediatric medical emergency team improves hospital response to deteriorating patients. *Resuscitation, 84*(2), 218–222. doi:http://dx.doi.org/10.1016/j.resuscitation.2012.06.027

World Health Organization (WHO Framework for Action on Interprofessional Education & Collaborative Practice). (2010). In D. Hopkins (Ed.), *World Health Organization*. Retrieved February 13, 2014, from http://www.who.int/hrh/resources/framework_action/en

Debriefing

RUTH A. WITTMANN-PRICE, LELAND J. (ROCKY) ROCKSTRAW, AND TERRY KIRK

Sometimes, you have to look back in order to understand the things that lie ahead.
—Yvonne Woon

This chapter addresses Content Area 2: Demonstrate Knowledge of Simulation Principles, Practice, and Methodology (Society for Simulation in Healthcare [SSH], 2014).

LEARNING OUTCOMES

- Discuss the importance of simulation debriefing in the learning process
- Discuss the principles of simulation debriefing
- Describe a variety of simulation debriefing methodologies

When using simulation as a learning tool, debriefing is an essential component of the learning process (Cantrell, 2008). Most simulation experts concur that the debriefing process of learners, which takes place after the simulation experience, is in effect the most important element of the learners' experience. Cant and Cooper (2009) describe debriefing as one of the "core components" of simulation learning. Alinier (2011) describes debriefing by stating, "Experiential learning experience must then be reinforced and analyzed with the participants through a debriefing process that is as, if not more, important than the experience itself as it helps them to reflect about what happened and understand and assimilate the learning objectives" (p. 14). The ultimate goal of the learning process that takes place during debriefing is to foster clinical decision making (Dreifuerst, 2009).

Dewey (1933, p. 9) suggests that reflection is a process and requires a process; he describes reflection as "active, persistent and careful consideration"; furthermore, Dewey believed that reflection could be caused by "a state of doubt, hesitation, [or] perplexity" (p. 12). This active approach to reflection requires that the learner recognize actions or events and enter a state of questioning of held beliefs and learned behaviors to identify issues and begin to problem solve.

BACKGROUND

Debriefing was originally used in the military in order for personnel to describe what happened during a mission. Debriefing accomplished two objectives for the military. First, it assisted them with operational understanding and strategic planning and, second, it helped to reduce the psychological impact of a traumatic event on the participant. Reconstructing the event through narrative was therapeutic for the participant. By conducting debriefing in groups, participants received several different perspectives (Fanning & Gaba, 2007).

THE DEBRIEFING PROCESS

Learning is facilitated during the debriefing process of simulation (Dieckmann, Lippert, Glavin, & Rall, 2010). Debriefing is a process that commonly involves face-to-face discussion between a group of learners and an educator after a simulation scenario has taken place. Debriefing is often distinguished as a separate process from feedback, which can occur using different modalities (face to face, written, or electronic), and normally occurs between one learner and an educator after a simulation experience (Archer, 2010). When standardized (simulated) patients (SPs) are used in simulation experiences, they are often included in the feedback process to provide insights to the learner, but they are not usually participants in debriefing processes (Barrows, 1993).

The debriefing process is normally facilitated retrospectively after simulation with the simulation participants as soon as possible after the experience is completed (Cantrell, 2008), and it includes all the learners actively involved in the entire experience (Alinier, 2011). Timing of the debriefing process is important, and it is beneficial to provide debriefing as close to the simulation experience as possible (Cantrell, 2008).

Some simulation experts refer to the process of debriefing as *team debriefing*, which highlights the aspect that it is a group activity (Alinier, 2011). Debriefing should be facilitated by a certified educator who has observed the entire simulation learning experience and has taken physical or mental notes about the details of the experience (Alinier, 2011). Recording of the simulation experience is important to the debriefing process and can also effectively include videotaping of the experience. Videotaping may assist learners to analyze their performance and provide structure to the debriefing process. At times, depending on the complexity of a scenario, learning is facilitated by having a second certified educator observing the simulation scenario and participating in the debriefing process in order to note all the details of a simulation experience (Alinier, 2011).

Debriefing sessions are often approximately 20 to 30 minutes in length, and researchers have noted that 10-minute debriefing sessions are inadequate to facilitate the learning process (Cantrell, 2008). Therefore, as a critical component of simulation learning, adequate time must be assigned to the debriefing process.

Another type of debriefing is called *in-simulation* debriefing. This debriefing technique is done by suspending the scenario to discuss a specific incident or aspect of learning (Van Heukelom, Begaz, & Treat, 2010).

EVIDENCE-BASED SIMULATION PRACTICE (EBSP) 15.1

Matthews and Viens (1998) found that videotaping a simulation experience and having learners critically critique the experience during debriefing decreased learner anxiety.

Lederman (1984) describes the essential, structural elements of debriefing as having the following seven components.

1. Debriefer or simulation educator
2. Participants or learners to debrief
3. A simulation experience
4. The impact of the simulation experience
5. Recollection of the simulation experience
6. Report about the simulation experience
7. Time required for debriefing (Lederman, 1984)

DEBRIEFING AND THE LEARNING PROCESS

Using simulation experiences provides learners an opportunity to practice and acquire knowledge and clinical skills in a safe environment (McGaghie, Issenberg, Petrusa, & Scalese, 2010). Much of the knowledge acquisition is facilitated during the debriefing process because it is a teaching strategy (Cantrell, 2008).

Debriefing as a teaching strategy supports a constructivist theory of education, which is fully explained in Chapters 6 and 17. Some of the learning processes that take place during debriefing include

- Promoting communication skills
- Appropriately integrating emotions into the learning process
- Reinforcing skill acquisition (Cantrell, 2008)

Debriefing is a learning process that ties in all three domains of learning:

1. Psychomotor—during debriefing, skills are analyzed
2. Affective—feelings and emotions are discussed
3. Cognitive—learning takes place by having events deconstructed (Cantrell, 2008)

Warrick, Hunsaker, Cook, and Altman (1979) defined the objectives of debriefing as

1. Identification of the different perceptions and attitudes that have occurred
2. Linking the exercise to specific theory or content and skill-building techniques
3. Development of a common set of experiences for further thought

4. Opportunity to receive feedback on the nature of one's involvement, behavior, and decision making

5. Reestablishment of the desired classroom climate, such as regaining trust, comfort, and purposefulness

DEFINING ATTRIBUTES OF DEBRIEFING

Dreifuerst (2009) describes the following defining attributes of debriefing in a concept analysis.

- Reflection
- Emotion
- Reception
- Integration
- Assimilation

Each attribute is described in the following text.

Reflection

An important aspect of the debriefing process as pointed out by Dieckmann, Gaba, and Marcus (2007) is that no one has the "correct view." Debriefing comprises perceptions of educator(s) and learners of what took place in the simulation experience. Different views assist learners with understanding different elements of the scenario, and in that way, it mimics clinical situations. Debriefing discussions should begin with asking participants about their view of the situation just experienced and initiate the reflective learning process (Dieckmann, Gaba, & Marcus, 2007).

Fanning and Gaba (2007) call reflection "the cornerstone" of both experiential learning and lifelong learning. The following text lists different ways to conceptualize reflection and some important points about using reflection as a learning activity.

- In 1983, Schön published his landmark book, *The Reflective Practitioner: How Professionals Think in Action*, and called on educators to develop themselves as reflective practitioners in order to gain competence in their individual practices.
- Boud, Keogh, and Walker (1985) defined "reflection" as "an important human activity in which people recapture their experience, think about it, mull it over, and evaluate it" (p. 19).
- Reflection is a technique that encourages critical thought, either with oneself (self-dialogue) or another individual or group (dialogue; Shor, 1992).
- Reflection is a thoughtful and self-regulating process (Kaakinen & Arwood, 2009).

Reflection can be facilitated in different ways.

- Many certified healthcare educators use the technique after an experience in a free-flow attempt to assist learners to uncover what affective behaviors they can identify as assets and to highlight those behaviors that may be deficits.

- Others pose reflective questions to learners, such as "What was the one thing (incident or patient) that affected you most?" or "What was the best thing that happened to you during the experience?"
- Usually, questions like these are followed up with questions such as, "What one thing would you do differently if you were in that situation again?"

> **Simulation Teaching Tip 15.1**
> Several issues must be considered when asking learners to reflect.
>
> - Reflection is a self-disclosing process that can elicit sensitive information.
> - What one does with information revealed during reflective sessions may become an ethical issue.

Having learners reflect facilitates finding deeper meanings and thinking critically about experiences, especially critical incidents (Montagna, Benaglio, & Zannini, 2010).

Scanlon and Chernomas (1997) identified three stages of reflection.

1. Awareness
2. Critical analysis
3. New perspective

Riley-Doucet and Wilson (1997) describe a three-step process for reflection:

1. *Critical appraisal* is done by a learner in free form to drill down to the meaning of the experience.
2. *Peer group discussions* share questions that the learners might have become aware of during the experience.
3. *Self-awareness* or *self-evaluation* is the last step and relates the learning outcomes for evaluative purposes.

Montagna, Benaglio, and Zannini (2010) also recommend that educator feedback to learners be done with care and be certain that resources are available if needed.

Emotions

Debriefing provides the learner the opportunity to reexamine the experience and deal with emotions, thereby providing an emotional release as well as a thinking process (Dreifuerst, 2009).

Reception

Reception has to do with how "open" the learner is to accepting the information provided or revealed during debriefing. The simulation educator needs to establish an environment that facilitates positive reception by

- Presenting learners' strengths and challenges in a nonthreatening manner
- Maintaining learner–facilitator respect at all times
- Providing confidentiality as appropriate (Dreifuerst, 2009)

FIGURE 15.1 Attributes of learning in debriefing as defined by Dreifurest (2009).

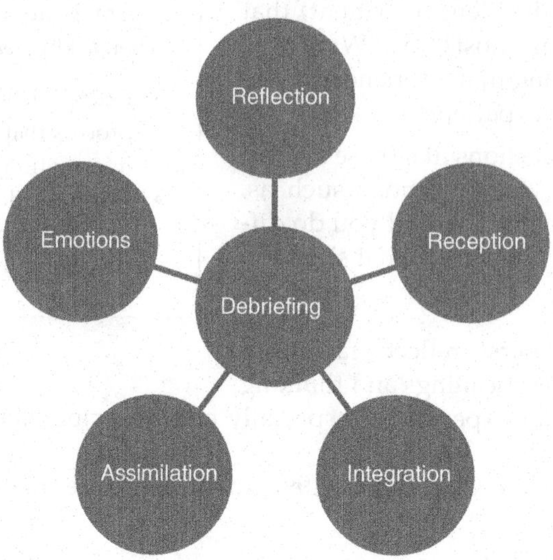

Integration

Using a conceptual framework that is familiar to the learners in their discipline and integrating the context of the simulation scenario fosters learning. Integration links knowledge gained from the simulation experience to knowledge already familiar to the learning. By facilitating integration, the simulation educator is promoting deep learning (refer to Chapter 6 for an explanation of deep, surface, and strategic learning; Dreifuerst, 2009).

Assimilation

Assimilation has to do with the ultimate goal of simulation, which is the transfer of knowledge from the experience to actual clinical practice. Further assimilation studies are needed, but assimilation may be encouraged by techniques used by the facilitator, such as the Socratic dialogue. Dreifurest (2009) reminds simulation educators that all attributes defined as elements of debriefing work together to promote learning as shown in Figure 15.1.

ORAL (SOCRATIC) QUESTIONING

Oral questioning or Socratic dialogue can promote the learners' critical thinking and prompt them to reflect. Questions that involve synthesizing concepts rather that questions that can be answered with a "yes" or "no" or regurgitating facts are the most beneficial. Promoting thinking through questioning can be accomplished by using "what if" questions and changing the situation to encourage learners to think beyond the experience (Dreifuerst, 2009).

EXHIBIT 15.1

Benefits of Questioning

- Increases motivation and participation
- Helps monitor the learners' acquisition of knowledge and understanding
- Promotes higher cognition
- Assesses learners' progress
- Facilitates environmental management
- Encourages learners to ask and to answer questions
- Promotes dialogue/interaction/debate between and among educators and learners (Ralph, 2000)

DEBRIEFING AS AN ASSESSMENT PROCESS

Debriefing, which usually involves a group of learners, is most often used as a formative evaluative mechanism. Summative evaluations of learner performance are most commonly done on an individual basis using feedback (McGaghie, Issenberg, Petrusa, & Scalese, 2010). A method of using debriefing as an evaluation has been outlined by Rudolph, Simon, Raemer, and Eppich (2008); it is a four-step process, which is shown diagrammatically in Figure 15.2.

FACILITATOR ROLE IN THE DEBRIEFING PROCESS

Fanning and Gaba (2007) describe facilitator involvement in debriefing as high to low. Table 15.1 demonstrates the differences in involvement.

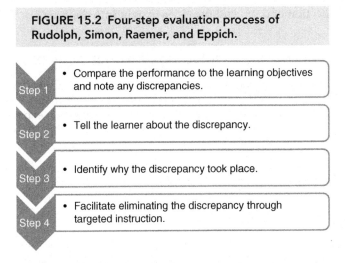

FIGURE 15.2 Four-step evaluation process of Rudolph, Simon, Raemer, and Eppich.

Step 1
- Compare the performance to the learning objectives and note any discrepancies.

Step 2
- Tell the learner about the discrepancy.

Step 3
- Identify why the discrepancy took place.

Step 4
- Facilitate eliminating the discrepancy through targeted instruction.

Adapted from Rudolph, Simon, Raemer, and Eppich (2008).

TABLE 15.1 Involvement of Facilitator in Debriefing	
High-level facilitation	The facilitator outlines the debriefing process Facilitator guides the discussion when necessary Facilitator has low-level involvement Learners are highly involved
Low-level facilitation	Facilitation takes on an involved role Learners are less involved and have less initiative Facilitators use a direct debriefing process Simulation educator may overinstruct

Source: Fanning and Gaba (2007).

TYPES OF DEBRIEFING METHODS

Structured Debriefing

Debriefing sessions often begin with establishing group rules in order to focus the learners on the meaning of the scenario rather than have them focus on the fidelity of the scenario (Dieckmann, Gaba, & Marcus, 2007). Cantrell (2008) used a structured debriefing process in her study with nursing learners and used guiding questions that were developed by Ham and O'Rouke (2004)

- What were the patient's goals for this episode of care?
- Were these goals met by your nursing behaviors?
- How did you prioritize the patient's needs?
- What would you do differently if actually caring for him or her and the family in an acute care setting? (Cantrell, 2008, p. e20)

Structured debriefing provides guidance in the learning process, facilitates the collection of data, and provides insight into the learners' thinking processes.

> **EVIDENCE-BASED SIMULATION PRACTICE (EBSP) 15.2**
>
> Birch and colleagues (2007) used debriefing in the simulation education of learners using a scenario about postpartum hemorrhage. The study found that those learners who participated in the simulation experience and were debriefed had increased knowledge immediately after the scenario and at 3 months after the scenario.

Case Study Analysis Debriefing

One of the most common methods of debriefing is review of a case study. One method to accomplish this has been outlined in 12 steps by Salas and colleagues (2008) and includes the following

1. Use debriefing to diagnose the case
2. Provide a supportive environment
3. Always note teamwork, which is critical to patient safety
4. Team leaders should be educated in debriefing
5. Members should not be threatened during a debriefing session
6. Focus on critical incidents during the scenario
7. Describe the interactions of the team
8. Use objective data when possible
9. Provide process feedback before outcome feedback
10. Provide both individual and team feedback appropriately
11. Provide feedback as soon as possible
12. Record outcomes of the debriefing to use in the future

Advocacy–Inquiry

A nonjudgmental approach to debriefing uses the simulation educator as a patient advocate by asking questions using "I" and referring to the patient (advocacy). The simulation educator then requests the learner to describe the thought process used, and this is the inquiry process (Rudolph, Simon, Rivard, Dufresne, & Raemer, 2007).

An example is provided in Exhibit 15.2.

EXHIBIT 15.2
An Example of Advocacy–Inquiry

Simulation educator:	"Karen, during the simulation I noticed you giving the wrong dose of pitocin to the patient. That concerns me because it is important to give the correct dose because an incorrect dose could produce tectonic contractions. Can you tell me what you were thinking at that time?"
Learner:	"I was trying to figure out the dosage but it is a complicated formula and I remember that micro units is a small amount so when I arrived at the dose I thought it was correct."
Simulation educator:	"That is true, it is a small amount because of its potency. I observed you looking for a paper to write on and then writing something on the alcohol swab before programming the intravenous pump. That concerns me because the pump can be programmed to ensure the correct dose calculation. Can you tell me what you were thinking at that time"?

Adapted from Rudolph, Simon, Rivard, Dufresne, and Raemer (2007).

There are many methods used to debrief simulation learners. Table 15.2 describes techniques currently used.

TABLE 15.2
Debriefing Techniques

TECHNIQUE	DESCRIPTION OF THE TECHNIQUE
Funneling	Learners are guided during debriefing, but the debriefer does not comment (Fanning & Gaba, 2007).
Framing	A technique used during debriefing to present the simulation experience to the participants in a relevant way (Fanning & Gaba, 2007).
Frontloading	Providing specific questions before the debriefing to guide the direction of the debriefing (Fanning & Gaba, 2007).
Plus–delta	Developing a two-column tool in which the participants list positive and negative aspects of the simulation experience (Fanning & Gaba, 2007).
Good cop–bad cop	Technique used if there is more than one debriefer. This technique provides opposing sides to an issue (Fanning & Gaba, 2007).
Advocacy–inquiry (debriefing with good judgment)	A nonjudgmental approach to debriefing that uses the simulation educator as a patient advocate by asking questions using "I" and referring to the patient (**advocacy**). The simulation educator then requests the learner to describe the thought process, and this is the **inquiry** process (Rudolph, Simon, Rivard, Dufresne, & Raemer, 2007).
Case review	An organized review of the patient condition starting with diagnosis and then a review of systems.

Adapted from Fanning and Gaba (2007).

THE DEBRIEFING ENVIRONMENT

The environment in which debriefing is conducted is also important. Besides having an appropriate amount of time set aside for debriefing, there should to be enough room for the members being debriefed. Rooms for debriefing should be large, private, and comfortable. Large groups of learners pose special challenges to debriefing, and two methods used to overcome group learning that may exclude individuals are

Simulation Teaching Tip 15.3
Dieckmann, Gaba, and Marcus (2007) discuss the importance of simulation educators paying attention to the semantical sense that learners develop during the analysis of a scenario during debriefing. The use of words and language in descriptions of the scenario can provide insight into how learners phenomenally experienced the scenario.

1. Separate groups—Have more than one debriefer, and separate the large group into smaller groups.

2. Use the fishbowl method—Have an inner circle of learners and an outer circle. Debrief the learners in the inner circle and then have learners switch to the outer circle and outer-circle learners move in for debriefing (Fanning & Gaba, 2007).

> **Simulation Teaching Tip 15.4**
> Steinwachs (1992) describes using a process of seating that avoids "energy gaps." In order to facilitate this concept, learners must sit next to each other, and there should be no empty spaces. Decker (2007) suggests a circular design for seating that allows spherical movement while questioning the learners as discussion is promoted.

An additional consideration for establishing an environment that feels safe for debriefing includes a space away from where the simulation was conducted, a comfortable and private area (Decker, 2007).

DEBRIEFING DIFFICULTIES

Debriefing sessions are goal oriented, but at times difficulties can occur when learners interpret debriefings differently than what was intended in the learning outcomes. In this case, extra time is often needed to explain what was supposed to occur as opposed to what did occur. Many simulation educators then re-enact the scenario to accomplish the intended learning outcomes (Dieckmann, Lippert, Glavin, & Rall, 2010).

CASE STUDY 15.1

Women's Health – Healthy Delivery (Cultural)

PATIENT NAME: Isha Smith (and husband John Smith)

DATE OF BIRTH: Use own

DIAGNOSIS: Pregnant 32-year-old (38-weeks gestation/G3P2) with early labor

VITAL SIGNS: Use own

CHANGE IN VITAL SIGNS: None

SETTING: Clinic, office, or inpatient hospital

TIME:
- For scenario: 20–30 minutes
- For debriefing: 40–60 minutes
- Time of day of scenario: As offered

PATIENT CONDITION:
- Clothing: Causal, loose fitting, may become soiled (dirty)
- Props (for mannequin, i.e., glasses, etc.): NONE
- Moulage (makeup): NONE
- Abdomen vest, pregnancy/birthing simulator

(continued)

CASE STUDY 15.1 (*continued*)

EQUIPMENT LIST:
- Typical medical clinical

MEDICATIONS: None

OBJECTIVES FOR STUDENTS:
- Provide safe patient care
- Correctly assess and treat common women's health pregnancy conditions
- Relate therapeutic communication skills to care of the intrapartum woman and her significant other(s)
- Identify nursing priorities when assisting the woman to give birth

Provide oral handoff (report) to senior nurse or physician

SCENARIO OBJECTIVES (with evaluation outcomes):
- Conduct mother and fetus assessment
  - Provide admitting assessment
  - Provide continued focused assessment
  - Correctly identify active labor, prepare, and deliver healthy newborn
- Establish a therapeutic relationship with patient and significant other
  - Make them feel welcome
  - Determine expectations about birth
  - Convey confidence
  - Use touch for comfort
- Respect cultural values of patent and significant other
  - Ask mother and significant other about cultural beliefs and practices
  - Offer support to mother and significant other
  - Ask for clarification of cultural beliefs and practices

REPORT TO STUDENTS: You are working in a clinic and are asked to provide assessment and basic care for the local community members. Due to a flu outbreak, most of the primary nursing staff and doctors are home, sick. The administration of the clinic has a physician who will try to make daily visits to the clinic. Should any critically ill patients present, do call a local hospital for advice. You have typical medical supplies, oral medications, and comfort measures.

REPORT TO ACTORS: (Patient and husband): Isha Smith, 32-year-old Indian woman pregnant for the third time; she is traveling with John Smith, her husband of 12 years; they are visiting her parents who live in (your town); today, she is preparing to travel home to Philadelphia, PA, via train. The excitement of travel seems to have precipitated active labor. Isha is concerned about the safety of her child being born away from her doctor in Philadelphia. Both Isha and John want John to remain at Isha's side during labor and delivery of the child. They also are asking that the medical staff provide medication to stop the labor for a day or so to allow for travel back to Philadelphia.

ROLES FOR ACTORS (FACULTY):

Patient: Grunting sounds, bearing down, sitting on one buttock, attentive to nurses, polite but determined to have husband stay at side and is requesting to have labor stopped.

Husband: Quiet, polite, but determined to stay at wife's side and is requesting to have labor stopped for travel.

CASE STUDY 15.1 (*continued*)

ROLES FOR STUDENTS:

Primary provider:

Secondary provider:

Resource (gathers equipment):

Recorder:

DEBRIEFING QUESTIONS:

1. What went well? What did not go well?
2. If you were to experience the same occurrence, what might you do differently? What might you ask your patient and/or family member?
3. Whose direction should the nurse follow when providing respect for cultural value(s) for the patient? Why?
4. Explore cultural differences and comfort of student/local culture versus other country
5. Therapeutic relationship
   a. Introduces self
   b. Asks woman how she wants to be addressed, father too
   c. Asks woman to communicate when contractions occur (pauses interview during contractions)
   d. Demonstrates sensitivity

6. Assessment
   a. Mother
      i. Prenatal healthcare/screening
      ii. Estimated date of delivery (2 weeks from today's date)
      iii. Gravidity, parity, abortions
      iv. Pregnancy history
      v. Labor status, contractions, membrane status
      vi. Food intake, recent illness, mediations, tobacco or alcohol use, birth plans

   b. Fetal
      i. Fetal heart rate

   c. Physical examination
      i. Appearance
      ii. Vital signs
      iii. Heart and lungs
      iv. Breasts
      v. Abdomen
      vi. Deep tendon reflexes
      vii. Midstream urine specimen

7. Cultural respect
   a. Special plans? What do you want to avoid?
   b. Special cultural practices

PRACTICE QUESTIONS

1. The simulation educator requests a group of learners to gather in an auditorium-style room to debrief. In order to encourage active learning, the simulation educator may

   A. Request a spokesperson for the group
   B. Ask a question of each learner individually
   C. Bring in chairs, so half the learners can face the front row
   D. Use an audience response system to question about the scenario

2. One of two debriefers for a group of learners states that the learner team was slow to respond to the simulated patient's deterioration. The second debriefer says that even though the learner team used time, they executed the resuscitation well. This type of debriefing can be described as

   A. Good cop–bad cop
   B. Advocacy–inquiry
   C. Funneling
   D. Plus–delta

3. A novice simulation educator requires additional mentoring when he states

   A. "I will place the learners in a circle to debrief."
   B. "I will provide adequate time for the learners to discuss the experience."
   C. "I will ask the learners to return tomorrow for the debriefing."
   D. "I think the learners would benefit from high-intensity debriefing."

4. The simulation educator asks the learners to take 5 minutes at the start of the debriefing session and write down what went well and what needs improvement in the performance of the team. This method of debriefing is known as

   A. Good cop–bad cop
   B. Advocacy–inquiry
   C. Funneling
   D. Plus–delta

5. The simulation educator understands that in the advocacy–inquiry debriefing technique, the goal of advocacy is

   A. Safe student learner space
   B. Simulation educator's instruction
   C. Patient safety
   D. Teamwork development

6. The simulation educator understands that when using the advocacy–inquiry technique, the goal is to

   A. Explain to the learners what needs improvement
   B. Understand the patient's perception
   C. Provide a nonjudgmental environment
   D. Have the learner decide on the corrections

7. A useful tool when using case study analysis is to provide the learners with

    A. Past stories of the experience with other learners
    B. The patient outcome first, then the process
    C. The actual written scenario that was used
    D. Objective data from observation or videotape

8. A novice simulation educator is asking questions during a debriefing that facilitate "yes" and "no" answers from the learners. This may be interpreted as a case in which the instructor is

    A. Overinstructing
    B. Using plus–delta
    C. Encouraging reflection
    D. Oversimplifying

9. Which of the following examples is a Socratic question?

    A. "Did you remember to turn the oxygen on when you placed the face mask on the patient?"
    B. "How did you feel about the family crying?"
    C. "Was patient safety your first thought?"
    D. "After the oxygen level was adequate, what was your next priority and why?"

10. The simulation educator is viewing a scenario with a group of learners performing a sterile technique. The simulation educator observes two learners breaking the sterile technique and calls through the microphone to "freeze the action." This type of debriefing is known as

    A. Plus–delta
    B. Advocacy–inquiry
    C. In simulation
    D. Spontaneous learning

REFERENCES

Alinier, G. (2011). Developing high-fidelity health care simulation scenarios: A guide for educators and professionals. *Simulation and Gaming, 42*(1), 9–26.

Archer, J. C. (2010). State of the science in health professional education: Effective feedback. *Medical Education, 44,* 101–108.

Barrows, H. S. (1993). An overview of the uses of standardized (simulated) patients for teaching and evaluating clinical skills. *Academic Medicine, 68*(6), 443–451.

Birch, L., Jones, N., Doyle, P. M., Green, P., McLaughlin, A., Champney C., Williams, D., . . . Taylor, K. (2007). Obstetric skills drills: Evaluation of teaching methods. *Nurse Education Today, 27*(8), 915–922.

Boud, R. K., & Walker, D. (Eds.). (1985). *Reflection: Turning experience into learning* (pp. 7–8), London, UK: Kogan.

Cant, R. P., & Cooper, S. J. (2009). Simulation-based learning in nursing education: Systematic review. *Journal of Advanced Nursing, 66*(1), 3–15.

Cantrell, M. A. (2008). The importance of debriefing in clinical simulation. *Clinical Simulation in Nursing, 4,* e19–e23.

Decker, S. (2007). Integrating guided reflection into simulated learning experiences In P. R. Jeffries (Ed.), *Simulation in nursing education: From conceptualization to evaluation* (pp. 73–85). New York, NY: National League for Nursing.

Dewey, J. (1933). *How we think: A restatement of the relation of reflective thinking to the educative process*. Lexington, KY: D. C. Health.

Dieckmann, P., Gaba, D., & Marcus, R. (2007). Deepening the theoretical foundations of patient simulation as social practice. *Simulation in Healthcare, 2*(3), 183–193.

Dieckmann, P., Lippert, A., Glavin, R., & Rall, M. (2010). When things do not go as expected: Scenario life savers. *Simulation in Healthcare, 5*, 219–225.

Dreifuerst, K. T. (2009). The essentials of debriefing in simulated learning: A concept analysis. *Nursing Education Perspectives, 30*(2), 109–114.

Fanning, R. M., & Gaba, D. M. (2007). The role of debriefing in simulation-based learning, *Simulation in Healthcare, 2*(2), 115–125.

Ham, K., & O'Rourke, E. (2004). Clinical strategies. Clinical preparation for beginning nursing students: An experiential learning activity. *Nurse Educator, 29*(4), 139–141.

Kaakinen, J., & Arwood, E. (2009). Systematic review of nursing simulation literature for use of learning theory. *International Journal of Nursing Education Scholarship, 6*(1), 1–20. doi: 10.2202/1548-923X.1688

Lederman. L. (1984). Debriefing: A critical reexamination of the post experience analytic process with implications for its effective use. *Simulation Games, 15*, 415–431.

Matthews, R., & Viens, D. C. (1988). Evaluating basic nursing skills through group video testing. *Journal of Nursing Education, 27*(1), 44–46.

McGaghie, W. C., Issenberg, S. B., Petrusa, E. R., & Scalese, R. J. (2010). A critical review of simulation-based medical education research: 2003–2009. *Medical Education, 44*, 50–63.

Montagna, L., Benaglio, C., & Zannini, L. (2010). Reflective writing in nursing education: Background, experiences and methods. *Assistenza Infermieristica e Ricerca, 29*(3), 140–152.

Ralph, E. (2000). Oral-questioning skills of novice teachers: Any questions? *Journal of Instructional Psychology, 26*(4), 286–296.

Riley-Doucet, C., & Wilson, S. (1997). A three-step method of self-reflection using reflective journal writing. *Journal of Advanced Nursing, 25*, 964–968.

Rudolph, J. W., Simon, R., Raemer, D. B., & Eppich, W. J. (2008). Debriefing as formative assessment: Closing performance gaps in medical education. *Academic Emergency. Medicine, 15*, 1010–1016.

Rudolph, J. W., Simon, R., Rivard, P., Dufresne, R. L., & Raemer, D. B. (2007). Debriefing with good judgment: Combining rigorous feedback with genuine inquiry. *Anesthesiology Clinics, 25*, 361–376.

Salas, E., Klein, C., King, H., Salisbury, M., Augenstein, J. S., Birnbach, D. J., . . . Upshaw, C. (2008). Debriefing medical teams: 12 evidence-based best practices and tips. *Joint Commission Journal on Quality and Patient Safety, 34*, 518–527.

Scanlon, J. M., & Chernomas, W. M. (1997). Developing the reflective teacher. *Journal of Advanced Nursing, 25*(6), 1138–1143.

Schön, D. A. (1983). *The reflective practitioner: How professionals think in action*. New York, NY: Basic Books.

Shor, I. (1992). *Empowering education: Critical teaching for social change*. Chicago, IL: University of Chicago Press.

Society for Simulation in Healthcare (SSH). (2014). *Certified healthcare simulation educator handbook*. Retrieved from http://ssih.org/certification/handbook

Steinwachs, B. (1992). How to facilitate a debrief. *Simulation Gaming, 23*, 186–195.

Van Heukelom, J. N., Begaz, T., & Treat, R. (2010). Comparison of postsimulation debriefing versus in-simulation debriefing in medical simulation. *Simulation in Healthcare, 5*, 91–97.

Warrick, D. D., Hunsaker, P. L., Cook, C. W., & Altman, S. (1979). Debriefing experiential learning exercises. *Journal of Experiential Learning and Simulation, 1*, 91–96.

Standardized Patient Debriefing

and Feedback

ANTHONY ERRICHETTI

Thinking is easy, acting is difficult, and to put one's
thoughts into action is the most difficult thing in the world.
—Johann Wolfgang von Goethe

> This chapter addresses Content Area 2: Demonstrate Knowledge of
> Simulation Principles, Practice, and Methodology (Society for
> Simulation in Healthcare [SSH], 2014).

LEARNING OUTCOMES

- Discuss debriefing as a self-reflective learning process
- Describe how debriefing and feedback are necessary components in the patient simulation learning process, requiring learners to reflect on their work
- Compare the different roles the clinical educators and standardized patients (SPs) have in the debriefing process
- Discuss SP selection and training for the debriefing–feedback process

SPs have been used for more than 50 years to teach and assess clinical skills (Barrows, 1993). Originally used to facilitate medical student training through simulated patient encounters, SPs are now used in high-stake licensure examinations (Dillon, Boulet, Hawkins, & Swanson, 2004). Their full potential, however, is realized when used in formative assessment exercises where skills assessment and debriefing are part of an educational plan. Selection of appropriate SPs and preparation for the debriefing and feedback process are required. This chapter presents an overview of how SPs can be selected and prepared for debriefing with suggestions for basic to advanced debriefing approaches.

DEBRIEFING FOUNDATIONS

Debriefing, as we know it today, has roots in the military and in adult and experiential learning theories and practices. The military "after-action review"(AAR) is a professional discussion of an event that enables soldiers and units to discover for themselves what happened and develop a strategy for improvement (Bartone & Adler, 1995).

"An AAR is not a critique. No one, regardless of rank, position, or strength of personality, has all of the information or answers. After-action reviews maximize training benefits by allowing soldiers, regardless of rank, to learn from each other" (Department of the Army, 1993, p. 1).

Simulation learning is experiential learning, that is, learning through direct experience (Itin, 1999). American educator John Dewey noted, however, that experience alone does not guarantee learning, but that learning occurs when experience is reflected on or "reconstructed" (Dewey, 1933). Experiential learning therefore requires the learners to reflect on their actions (Kolb, 1984) and, in the context of simulation learning, actions taken during SP and other simulation exercises. It integrates personal experience with academic learning, structures opportunities for reflection, is inquiry based, and facilitates face-to-face communication (Hatcher, 1997).

Debriefing is a process that facilitates learner self-reflection. It is a "rigorous reflection process" that focuses on clinical (e.g., critical thinking and actions) and behavioral (e.g., interpersonal communication) issues raised by a simulation exercise (Rudolph, Simon, Rivard, Dufresne, & Raemer, 2007). Feedback, a tool of debriefing, is information given to the learners about their performance intended to be used to promote positive and desirable development (Archer, 2010). For feedback to be effective, the debriefer must be aware of the needs of the learner and be able to judge whether or not the learner is ready accept it.

Adult learners, the focus of simulation education, have life experience, opinions, emotions, and assumptions ("frames"), well-developed personalities, and relationship patterns that drive their behaviors (Rudolph, Simon, Rivard, Dufresne, & Raemer, 2007). They expect learning to be goal directed, relevant, and applicable. Simulation learning, the antithesis of teacher-led classroom learning, is learning through experience and interaction with experts who understand adult learners' mind-set. Vygotsky's (1978) "zone of proximal development" describes the stage at which we find many adult learners who are, for example, students of healthcare science, that is, between unsupervised and supervised practice. This transition occurs with expert guidance (Vygotsky, 1978), the type of guidance that could come from a debriefing encounter.

SP CORE COMPETENCIES

SPs are professionals trained to accurately simulate medical problems and conditions, document and assess skills, and provide feedback (Boulet & Errichetti, 2008). They must continually demonstrate a number of "core competencies" to remain effective. The following is a list of those competencies, from the basic/foundational to the advanced, all of which are directly or indirectly related to mastering the debriefing process (Exhibit 16.1).

Foundational Competencies

Professional Conduct

SPs are required to demonstrate professional behaviors that guide their actions. These include

- **Reliability:** Being on time and carrying out scheduled activities as planned
- **Emotional intelligence:** The ability to be aware of and monitor one's own emotions as well as others' (Mayer & Salovey, 1997)
- **Social intelligence:** The awareness of how one interacts in social situations (Goleman, 2006; Thorndike, 1920)
- **Lifelong learning:** The willingness and ability to learn new things (e.g., medical problems and conditions) in new ways (e.g., through experiential and web-based learning)

Acting/Simulating

SPs have the ability to learn patient roles and credibly simulate or imitate a patient's condition, including physical symptoms, believably enough to convince learners that they are in an authentic clinical encounter. It requires SPs to play a role while simultaneously observing the learner for postencounter assessment and debriefing. Overidentifying with a role (e.g., when portraying an illness one actually has) or getting too deeply into it (e.g., through "method acting") undermines the learner assessment and debriefing. SPs must come out of the character immediately and prepare for postencounter activities.

Professionalism and credible acting may be all that are needed for clinical simulations that do not require the following advanced competencies.

Advanced Competencies

Documentation

When history-taking and physical examination skills are used, SPs must be able to memorize the checklist items, observe the learner during the encounter, and then document on the checklists what the learner accomplished.

Communication Assessment

SPs are in the best position to assess the interaction and communication skills of the learner. They are in close proximity to the leaner in the exam room during the encounter and are observing such skills as rapport building, empathic responses, nonverbal communication, eliciting information, active listening, information exchange, and physical examination quality.

Debriefing and Feedback

These are arguably the most difficult skills for SPs to master. It requires SPs to come out of the character immediately, assess the learner, and quickly formulate a debriefing agenda. SPs, using their social and emotional intelligence, engage the learner for a short, productive review of the encounter. They must be prepared to work with learners whose responses to the SP exercise can range from apathy to engagement. And most important, SPs must create a climate of psychological safety in which learners disclose and discuss needed areas of improvement (Schön, 1983). Indeed, empathy and compassion for the learner are key debriefing requirements.

EXHIBIT 16.1

Standardized Patient Core Competencies

FOUNDATIONAL SKILLS
Professional conduct
Acting/simulating

ADVANCED SKILLS
Documenting skills (checklists)
Assessing communication
Debriefing–feedback

SELECTING SPs FOR DEBRIEFING—SCREENING PROCESS

Not every SP is appropriate for debriefing and feedback activities. These are tasks requiring maturity, psychological awareness, and discernment. Before SPs can be used for this purpose, they must be rigorously screened to determine whether they have the potential to demonstrate the communication assessment and debriefing core competencies. They must be literate, have the ability and willingness to learn, and demonstrate the goodwill toward learners that is critically important to debriefing (Adamo, 2003), and they must have a modicum of acting skills. A robust screening process will determine whether SP candidates can be trained to engage learners in debriefing. The following are suggested steps to SP selection.

Prescreening SP Candidates

The following activities evaluate SP capabilities.

- Candidates submit a curriculum vitae (CV) and complete an electronic application (to determine a candidate's comfort level with technology).
- Candidates are provided with an "SP Program Information Sheet," listing job skills, activities, and requirements to review before the first interview.
- A phone or video (e.g., Skype) interview with the SP recruiter is required to evaluate motivation (e.g., the candidate's impression of the medical healthcare field, why she or he wants to do this work, etc.), work history, understanding of SP work, and comfort level with educational technology.

SP Information Meeting

If candidates are appropriate, they are invited to an unpaid "information meeting," an extended group interview and exercise that provides a didactic and experiential overview of the work. The goal of the meeting is to get an impression of the candidates' abilities to demonstrate and master the SP core competencies.

Group Interview and Introduction

- Candidates introduce themselves.
- Group question: "What draws you to this work?"
- SP trainer provides an overview of SP work through, for example, videos.
- Candidates are asked to give their opinion about the quality of the work demonstrated by the student on the videos.
- "Veteran" SPs discuss their experience.

This process allows candidates to present themselves as they might be when functioning as SPs and reveals their potential to provide debriefing. For example, some candidates will demonstrate respect and consideration for other candidates, will listen and respond appropriately, and ask questions. The process may also reveal candidates who lack emotional and social intelligence, for example, by "grandstanding" or making themselves the center of attention. Or candidates may appear to be overly reticent to speak, ask questions, or render an opinion. By reviewing videos, you can access if candidates view learners' abilities in a positive light. A "red flag" would be raised when candidates are overly judgmental in their opinion of a learner (Exhibit 16.2).

Experiential SP Exercise

Candidates learn a short sample SP case in order to assess reading ability and memory. They are then asked to voluntarily play the case as an SP several times and provide feedback to a simulated "student" played by an SP. Feedback given could include how the student communicated and interacted with the SP. This exercise provides candidates the opportunity to "try out" different components of SP work and for the trainer to determine candidate capabilities.

SP Candidate Debriefing

Following this exercise, the candidates are debriefed about the SP information meeting. "What was the meeting like for you?" "What did you learn about SP work? "What did you learn about yourselves?" "Any suggestions about how to improve this process?" It is important that the SP trainer conducting the meeting understands and demonstrates an empathic debriefing approach as a prelude to preparing new SPs for debriefing training.

EXHIBIT 16.2

Standardized Patient Selection Process: Steps

1. Prescreening
   - Submit CV and application
   - Phone/video interview

2. SP information meeting
   - Group interview
   - SP exercise
   - Candidate debriefing

PREPARING SPs FOR DEBRIEFING AND FEEDBACK

After it has been determined whether SPs have the potential ability to provide debriefing and feedback, they are trained for the process. Although there is considerable variability among SP programs regarding how debriefing and feedback are conducted, the following learning points are general guidelines for all programs.

Debriefing Concepts for SPs

- *Understand the difference between debriefing and feedback.* If debriefing is a process used to reflect on work, feedback is a tool of debriefing that clearly articulates "positive feedback" (what was done well) and "constructive feedback" (what could be improved upon with continued practice).

- *Debriefing is conducted in an empathic but straightforward way* that models the ideal healthcare encounter SPs expect from learners. It creates a climate of "psychological safety" in which learners can disclose without shame or humiliation.

- *Feedback and inquiry are linked.* The debriefer seeks to understand the learner through *empathic inquiry* (Rudolph, Simon, Rivard, Dufresne, & Raemer, 2007).

- *SP debriefing is focused on interpersonal and communication skills.* Because debriefing potentially has a medical/healthcare component (e.g., reviewing how a differential diagnosis was determined, critical thinking and problem solving, patient management, etc.) and an interpersonal and communication component, an experienced clinician would perform the former and SPs the latter.

- *Understand the goals and objectives of the exercise.* SPs are briefed on what the learners are expected to accomplish during a given exercise.

- *Understand the learner's level of training and expertise.* SPs are instructed, for example, to not expect expertise in novice learners and to avoid comparing student learners to their ideal healthcare provider.

Small-Group Debriefing and Feedback Exercises

Moving from concepts to practice, the following small-group training methods help SPs understand how they will follow a debriefing plan.

- *Review and discuss* the debriefing–feedback model used.

- *View videos depicting "gold standard" debriefing examples.* These can come from actual encounters or simulated encounters.

- *View SP–student encounter videos and rate communication* as a group, compare ratings, and discuss: "What positive and constructive feedback would you give this student?"

- *Role-play and discuss.* SPs greatly benefit from small-group practice and receiving immediate feedback. Role-play option: Pair SPs, one playing the student, the other playing the SP who will give feedback. The SP as student can be coached to portray a common student issue, for example, a nervous student who has difficulty making eye contact.

- *Use side coaching*: The trainer sits close to the SP and quietly gives instructions or redirects actions during role-play training.

- *Use earbud coaching*: A variation of side coaching, the SP in training wears an earbud during debriefing and receives instructions or redirections from the trainer.

> **Simulation Teaching Tip 16.1**
> Watch a prerecorded actual student–SP encounter, make notes on student communication issues to be addressed, and then have one SP portray the student and the other assume the role of the SP who gives feedback.

DEBRIEFING AND FEEDBACK MODELS

Models of debriefing range from the basic (giving positive and constructive feedback) to the reflective/exploratory (encouraging learner self-reflection and exploring learner "frames of reference"). All models require giving specific feedback on observable behavior. Also, the SP debriefer must prepare by reviewing learner communication ratings and/or exercise objectives and identify areas to review.

The following are several examples of feedback and debriefing for SP encounters.

Basic Feedback Approach

The *feedback sandwich* (Chowdhury & Kalu, 2004) softens constructive feedback by *sandwiching* it between two examples of positive performance (Exhibit 16.3).

- Advantages: Easy to teach to SPs and satisfactory to students who want specific feedback: "Tell me what I did well, and what I could have done better."

- Disadvantages: Prescriptive, formulaic; reinforces passivity on the part of the learner; more a report than a reflection on work done.

EXHIBIT 16.3
FEEDBACK SANDWICH
Positive feedback: "This is what I thought you did well." **Constructive feedback:** "When you did X, I would have preferred Y." **Positive feedback:** "This is another example of what I thought you did well."

Pendleton's Rules

Pendleton's Rules (Exhibit 16.4) structures feedback so that positive feedback is highlighted first, followed by a discussion of "what could have been done differently" (Pendleton, Schofield, Tate, & Havelock, 1984).

EXHIBIT 16.4
PENDLETON'S RULES—STEPS
Learners Self-assess performance List two things done well and two things the learner could improve on with more practice **SPs** Assess learner List two things done well and two things the learner could improve on with more practice **SP and Learner** Compare notes, discussing areas of agreement and disagreement, and actions that could improve performance

- Advantages: Learners actively prepare themselves for debriefing by identifying strengths and areas to improve. SPs can address and focus on areas to improve identified by the student.

- Disadvantages: By rigidly focusing on the positives first, valuable debriefing time may be lost that could have been spent discussing more relevant issues.

Reflective Debriefing Model

Based on the work of Rudolph and colleagues (Rudolph, Simon, Rivard, Dufresne, & Raemer, 2006, 2007) this approach promotes reflection on the work between learner and SP in which the SP encourages self-reflection, provides concrete and specific feedback, and most important attempts to understand the learners' "frame of reference" or assumptions about why she did what she did (Exhibit 16.5). In this approach, the SP debriefer raises issues of concern (e.g., why the learner did not demonstrate empathy during a "giving bad news" exercise), but tries to understand the learner's point of view. The SP models empathy and the desire to understand the other, a fundamental stance of patient-centered treatment. This, like other feedback and debriefing models, requires the debriefing facilitator to create a climate of psychological safety in which the learner will feel comfortable discussing and critiquing his or her work. The SP is a learner in this process as well because the learner's frame of reference is inferred and not always evident through his or her actions. Therefore, the learners' rationale for his or her actions may either be accepted ("Now I understand, that makes sense") or challenged ("Now I understand what you were doing, but let's explore another option").

EXHIBIT 16.5

STANDARDIZED PATIENT REFLECTIVE DEBRIEFING STEPS

SP

- Encourage learner self-reflection by first taking the *emotional pulse* of the learner
  "How are you? How did you feel during the encounter?"
  (A focus on the learner's affect)
- Encourage the learner to self-reflect on *positive actions*
  "What do you think went well?"
- Encourage the learner to self-reflect on *future actions*
  "With enough practice, what do you think could be improved?"
  When done well, the learner's concerns and questions are the primary focus of attention.

When feedback is given:

- Positive, specific feedback is given when appropriate
- Constructive feedback (areas of questions or concerns) is given, but the learner's frame of reference is explored
  "Here is some feedback....help me to understand why you did X."
- Empathically explore the learner's thinking and be prepared to change your mind about your own assumptions or make rational challenges.

- Advantages: Promotes mutual understanding of the learner's frame of reference, models empathy, and promotes true experiential learning.
- Disadvantages: Requires a high level of training, maturity, and psychological sophistication on the part of the SP learner.

Debriefing the Physical Examination

If the physical examination was technically correct but of poor quality, or if done with thoroughness and care but technically incorrect, SPs are encouraged to have the learners retry the exam in question and correct the technique.

STARTING DEBRIEFING

The following is a suggested opening appropriate for all types of debriefing and feedback.

Set the Stage

- Debriefing dress: Wear a robe, gym pants, and so on, over the exam gown if wearing one.
- Welcome the learner: Open the door, invite the learner in, and make the individual feel comfortable: "Please come in and have a seat."

Set the Collaborative Agenda

"We have X minutes to discuss your work. We're going to focus on your communication and our patient–clinician relationship. I will not be reviewing your clinical reasoning, the questions you asked, and so forth. This is a dialogue so please ask me any questions. How does this sound?"

ADDITIONAL APPROACHES TO ENSURE DEBRIEFING QUALITY

- To ensure debriefing and feedback quality, SP encounters should be video recorded and those videos reviewed on a regular basis. A debriefing quality-assurance checklist can be used to note SP behaviors.
- Prepare learners for debriefing. If learners are to get the most from the debriefing–feedback process, they can be instructed on how the process works, what they should expect from the SP, and how they should prepare themselves for the debriefing.

SUMMARY

Debriefing and feedback are sophisticated skills, arguably among the most difficult to master. SPs must be screened for appropriateness. Although there are no formal screening exams to determine skill and psychological readiness, the experienced SP trainer can determine through experiential exercises and communication assessment training the most appropriate candidates. SPs must have a high degree of emotional and social intelligence, and have the ability to distinguish between low- and high-quality performance appropriate for the level of learner. They must practice, receive feedback, and be debriefed in such a way that closely approximates the model of debriefing used. Indeed, debriefing trainers must model debriefing and feedback's best practices.

CASE STUDY 16.1

You are interviewing three SPs and ask them to role-play a patient with active appendicitis. The first one doubles over and moans continuously while you are trying to examine him. The second SP states that he has a pain level of 3 on a scale of 0 to 10 and is sitting on the table smiling. The third one asks several questions about the condition and asks if he can "read up" on it first on his electronic device. Assess all three SPs for their appropriateness to provide SP service and feedback to learners.

PRACTICE QUESTIONS

1. One of the most beneficial uses of SPs is

   A. Summative evaluation
   B. Group enhancement
   C. Promotion of critical thinking
   D. Formative feedback

2. Experiential learning is a learning methodology that combines

    A. Deep learning with hands-on experience
    B. Personal experience with academic learning
    C. Academic learning and critical thinking
    D. Reflective learning and lecturing

3. An experienced debriefer understands that the learner who is not ready to accept feedback may say

    A. "I understand that I was slow to react because I was overthinking the procedure."
    B. "I never thought that watching myself would be so revealing."
    C. "This is not like it is in the hospital, so I am not concerned about being slow."
    D. "This experience made me look at things differently."

4. Adult learners may not respond to the debriefer's explanation about the simulation experience's

    A. Relevance
    B. Use
    C. Theoretical background
    D. Applicability

5. An SP is portraying symptoms of respiratory distress, and while the learners are doing lung assessments, continues to cough uncontrollably. This type of situation is referred to as

    A. A symptomatic SP
    B. Overidentifying
    C. Intentional obstruction
    D. Overacting

6. Foundational competencies for an SP include all of the following except

    A. Emotional intelligence
    B. Reliability
    C. Healthcare background
    D. Lifelong learning

7. Advanced competencies for SPs include all of the following except

    A. The ability to understand the learning theory
    B. The ability to effectively communicate
    C. Documentation skills
    D. Evaluation skills

8. It is important to carefully screen SPs because they should

    A. Be award-winning actors or actresses
    B. Be able to provide negative feedback
    C. Fit the physical role of the patient being portrayed
    D. Care about the learning process

9. During a group interview of four SPs, one actor keeps dominating the conversation by describing his many roles while name-dropping about famous people he has worked with. This may be a red flag because it can be interpreted as
   A. Narcissism
   B. Emotional liability
   C. Grandstanding
   D. Ineffective communication

10. The following interaction describes sandwich-style feedback
    A. "I think you did a good job with the sterile technique initially, but then contaminated the field."
    B. "I watched you contaminate the field and this concerns me. Can you tell me what you were thinking?"
    C. "Contaminating the field is serious and can cause a patient to get infected; do you understand how necessary it is to be more careful?"
    D. "You did a good job putting on sterile gloves, you reached over the corner of the field, but then you changed the contaminated sheet, which was good."

REFERENCES

Adamo, G. (2003). Simulated and standardized patients in OSCEs: Achievements and challenges 1992–2003. *Medical Teacher, 25*(3), 262–270.

Archer, J. C. (2010). State of the science in health professional education: Effective feedback. *Medical Education, 4*(1), 101–108.

Barrows, H. S. (1993). An overview of the uses of standardized patients for teaching and evaluating clinical skills. *AAMC Academic Medicine, 68*(6), 443–451.

Bartone, P. T., & Adler, A. B. (1995). Event-oriented debriefing following military operations: What every leader should know. *US Army Pamphlet, 95*(2), 1–12.

Boulet, J. R., & Errichetti, A. (2008). Training and assessment with standardized patients. In R. H. Riley (Ed.), *Manual of simulation in healthcare.* New York, NY: Oxford University Press.

Chowdhury, R. R., & Kalu, G. (2004). Learning to give feedback in medical education. *Obstetrician and Gynecologist, 6,* 242–247.

Department of the Army. (1993). A leader's guide to after action reviews. *Training circular* (pp. 25–20). Washington, DC.

Dewey, J. (1933). *How we think: A restatement of the relation of reflective thinking to the educative process.* Boston, MA: D.C. Heath.

Dillon, G. F., Boulet, J. R., Hawkins, R. E., & Swanson, D. B. (2004). Simulations in the United States Medical Licensing Examination (USMLE). *Quality & Safe Health Care, 13* (Suppl. 1), i41–i45.

Goleman, D. (2006). *Social intelligence: The new science of human relationships.* New York, NY: Bantam Dell.

Hatcher, J. A. (1997). The moral dimensions of John Dewey's philosophy: Implications for undergraduate education. *Michigan Journal of Community Service Learning, 4*(1), 22–29.

Itin, C. M. (1999). Reasserting the philosophy of experiential education as a vehicle for change in the 21st century. *Journal of Experiential Education, 22*(2), 91–98.

Kolb, D. A. (1984). *Experiential leaning theory: Experience as the source of learning and development.* Englewood Cliffs, NJ: Prentice-Hall.

Mayer, J. D., & Salovey, P. (1997). What is emotional intelligence? In P. Salovey & D. Sluyter (Eds.), *Emotional development and emotional intelligence: Implications for educators* (pp. 3–31). New York, NY: Basic Books.

Pendleton, D., Schofield, T., Tate, P., & Havelock, P. (1984). *The consultation: An approach to teaching and learning.* Oxford, MS: Oxford University Press.

Rudolph, J. W., Simon, R., Rivard, P., Dufresne, R. L., & Raemer, D. B. (2006). There's no such thing as non-judgmental debriefing: A theory and method of debriefing with good judgment. *Simulation in Healthcare, 1*(1), 49–55.

Rudolph, J. W., Simon, R., Rivard, P., Dufresne, R. L., & Raemer, D. B. (2007). Debriefing with good judgment. *Anesthesiology Clinics, 15*, 361–376.

Schön, D. (1983). *The reflective practitioner.* New York, NY: Basic Books.

Society for Simulation in Healthcare (SSH). (2014). *Certified healthcare simulation educator handbook.* Retrieved from http://ssih.org/certification/handbook

Thorndike, E. L. (1920). Intelligence and its use. *Harper's Magazine, 140*, 227–235.

Vygotsky, L. (1978). Interaction between learning and development. *Mind in society.* (pp. 79–91). Cambridge, MA: Harvard University Press.

Virtual Reality

ROSEMARY FLISZAR

Unless you try to do something beyond what you have already mastered, you will never grow.
—Ralph Waldo Emerson

This chapter addresses Content Area 3: Educate and Assess Learners Using Simulation (Society for Simulation in Healthcare [SSH], 2014).

LEARNING OUTCOMES

- Discuss the basic components of virtual reality (VR)
- Identify ways in which VR can be used to facilitate learning
- Discuss the platforms used to design virtual learning (VL) activities
- Discuss the feasibility of using VL and virtual simulation in designing classroom and clinical activities

The healthcare environment of today is fast paced and with the advancement of technology is moving rapidly in the provision of patient care and learning environments. There is a large demand for clinical sites within the nursing field alone, and acute care facilities are not able to accommodate the large numbers of students seeking clinical placements. There has also been a proliferation of distance education programs, which traditionally have been delivered in a two-dimensional environment with limited interaction between the learners and faculty member. Additionally, the complexity of healthcare in today's world is moving toward interprofessional collaboration among healthcare providers, increased teamwork, enhanced critical thinking skills and clinical judgment, and time for skill practice. Changes are needed in the way learners are educated to meet the demands of complex healthcare settings.

Virtual worlds (VWs) are evolving as strategies to meet the demands of this changing environment, thereby changing the way nursing education is delivered (Billings, 2009; Farra, Miller, & Hodgson, in press; Kilmon, Brown, Gnosh,

& Mikitiuk, 2010; Phillips, Shaw, Sullivan, & Johnson, 2010; Walsh & van Soeren, 2012). This chapter begins with a description of VL environments. The components of VL worlds are discussed, as well as the three-dimensional (3-D) platforms used to create these worlds. Advantages and disadvantages are presented with regard to VWs. Examples of application of VR to areas of practice are presented. The chapter concludes with a case study and review questions.

VIRTUAL LEARNING

Several terms are used to describe VL, including virtual reality simulation (VRS), VR, VWs, and virtual patients (VPs). VR is a broad term that encompasses a wide range of technology. However, the common definition of VR is that learners immerse themselves in a multimedia, computer-generated, 3-D simulated environment that simulates reality and allows learners to interact, practice skills, learn teamwork and collaboration, and manipulate medical equipment (Billings, 2009; Billings & Halstead, 2012; Farra, Miller, & Hodgson, in press). Sensory stimulation is presented to the user, and the VR environment is designed to prevent users from perceiving influences from the real world (Kilmon, Brown, Ghosh, & Mikitiuk, 2010).

Key features of the VR environment include

- 3-D imaging
- The ability to interact with the virtual environment
- Visual and auditory feedback (Kilmon, Brown, Ghosh, & Mikitiuk, 2010)

A VW is a 3-D computer-based simulated healthcare environment. The environment, or "world," provides an interactive experience based on teacher-designed case scenarios (Bai, Duncan, Horowitz, Graffeo, Glodstein, & Lavin, 2012). Other benefits of VWs are they

- Provide dynamic feedback
- Allow for learner experimentation
- Allow for creativity
- Provide opportunities for social networking and social interaction
- Facilitate collaboration among participants
- Lower learner anxiety
- Provide opportunities to bridge education and experience (Jarmon, Traphagan, Mayrath, & Trivedi, 2009)

The faculty and learners enter the VW, otherwise known as being "in world," by creating an avatar. An avatar is a digitized person created in 3-D, which represents the individual participating in the VW and is created by that person (Second Life, n.d.). The participant creates the characteristics of the avatar, including eye and hair color, clothing, age, race, ethnicity, and gender. However, it is highly recommended that the learners create an avatar that mimics their own features and appearance (Phillips et al., 2010). Avatars interact with each other through online chat by typing messages or talking using a headset with a microphone and Internet or telephone connection (Billings, 2009). The avatar can function in the world, move around, perform skills, role-play, and participate in meetings and communicate with other avatars in the world, such as patients, doctors, or nurses. The VW provides the learner the opportunity to simulate real-life experiences either synchronously or asynchronously and can be used in various settings in the learning environment. The virtual environment allows options for the development of social and professional relationships, especially in areas of distance learning. It also allows the learner to practice and demonstrate skills and knowledge without the fear of harming a live patient, and can be used as an evaluative tool to determine whether learning has occurred. Examples of areas in which VWs have been created include

- Classrooms
- Distance education
- Clinical agency
- Staff orientation
- Operating room (Baker, 2009; Patel, Aggarwal, Cohen, Taylor, & Darzi, 2013)
- Community settings
- Disaster training (Farra & Miller, 2013)
- Pediatric primary care clinic (Cook, 2012)
- Mental health education (Guise, Chambers, & Valimaki, 2012)

> **Simulation Teaching Tip 17.1**
> Avatars represent the individuals creating them and should be as realistic as possible.

VIRTUAL PATIENTS

A VP is an interactive computer-based simulation of a real-life clinical case scenario. Learners assume the role of the healthcare professional as an avatar, such as a nurse or doctor, and make judgments and clinical decisions based on the assessments made of the VP (Guise, Chambers, & Valimaki, 2012; Patel, Aggarwal, Cohen, Taylor, & Darzi, 2013). Participants learn the role of the professional they represent with regard to assessment, clinical diagnosis, treatment and care of the patient, just as they would if interacting with a real-life patient. VP simulations are case-based educational computer games in which the user progresses through various steps and applies clinical knowledge and critical thinking skills in making judgments about the care and treatment of the VP (Guise, Chambers, & Valimaki, 2012). The pathway for clinical decision making may be preprogrammed or may have a branching structure, which allows for several alternative pathways depending on each action taken by the learner.

SERIOUS GAMES

The term *serious games* has loosely been defined in several contexts, including technology for professional use, interactive video simulation, avatars, and watching videos (Baker, 2009; dit Dariel, Raby, Ravuat, & Rothan-Tondeur, 2013). The serious game has as its primary purpose educational and professional goals and not entertainment (Hogan, Kapralos, Cristancho, Finney, & Dubrowski, 2011; Skiba, 2008). Zyda (2005, p. 26) defines a serious game as "a mental contest, played with a computer in accordance with specific rules, that uses entertainment to further government or corporate training, education, health, public policy, and strategic communication objectives."

Serious games allow for experiential learning, problem-based learning, and a more learner-centered approach, as the student is immersed in the virtual environment and becomes engaged in the learning process (dit Dariel et al., 2013; Hogan et al., 2011). Students enter the VW on a computer and can interact in a realistic environment to practice skills and develop different competencies. The learner-centered approach is used as the player controls the learning through interactivity (Hogan et al., 2011). The game can be designed so that as the student makes a choice, with regard to an action or intervention, it leads to another step based on the previous decision. This design fits nicely with Kolb's (1984) experiential learning theory.

The design of a serious game should be based on several key components (Billings & Halstead, 2012).

- Identify the content of the lesson
- Identify the information the learner is to receive
- Base the game on objectives and outcomes

Several platforms have been identified for the serious games' simulation environment, also known as multi-user virtual environments (MUVEs) (Jarmon et al., 2009; Wang & Braman, 2009).

- Second Life
- mSTREET (modular Synthetic Training, Research, Evaluation, and Extrapolation Tool)
- Task trainers
- vSim by Laerdal
- Active Worlds
- Twinity

Second Life and mSTREET are serious game 3-D software platforms, or frameworks, which deliver computerized virtual training and research environments (mSTREET, 2010; Skiba, 2009). Scenarios can be constructed by faculty to design simulations in which the student may practice skills, make decisions, try new ideas, and learn from mistakes in a safe and controlled environment. The creation of a serious game is more complex than a case study or laboratory simulation designed for a classroom. The serious game is not linear in nature, but rather is a dynamic experience in which the player participates in the unfolding of a sequence of problems, and the interaction with the game influences the outcomes (dit Dariel et al., 2013). Serious games can be designed so that rules may be broken or the scenario changed based on the decisions made and actions of the learner (Charsky, 2010). Serious games may be designed as a means of summative evaluation based on specific outcomes or provide a means for formative evaluation to determine whether learning is occurring.

VL PLATFORMS

The Second Life platform allows faculty and students to perform some of the following activities (Second Life, n.d.).

- Build an avatar designed by the participant
- Join or create groups
- Develop one's own online community
- Attend or organize events
- Participate in forums
- Use 3-D voice chats, gestures, language, and so on

The mSTREET platform comprises "specialty modules" in a supported field, such as nursing. Scenarios can be constructed by educators in the fields, which can be played in real time in a safe, controlled 3-D environment using several approaches (mSTREET, 2010).

- Structured scripts—require adherence to time- or sequence-sensitive action protocols
- Unstructured—require satisfactory real-time response to emerging events and information
- Student responses can take several forms:
  - Direct-action response, also called emergency or protocol-based response, can occur in real time and be measured through expected response behaviors, trigger events, and sequencing. An example of this in nursing would be critical care nursing in which adherence to strict protocols is required for the situation.
  - Investigative response—recommendations for further action are made after studying the situation.

Task trainers are specific tools that are used to train the professional for a specific purpose. These may include

- Intravenous (IV) arm for venipuncture
- Airway trainers
- Blood pressure skills
- Femoral artery access
- Intubation trainers
- Chest tube insertion
- Neonatal procedures

> **Simulation Teaching Tip 17.2**
> The simulation or scenario must be appropriate for the level of the learner.

THEORETICAL FRAMEWORKS

Serious games should be designed based on the objectives for the game, outcomes to be met by students, and processes that have a theoretical basis. Three main theoretical approaches include constructivist theory, Kolb's experiential learning theory, and Knowles's adult learning theory.

The constructivist learning theory states that learners construct knowledge based on their experiences in relation to an event (Keating, 2011). The constructivist theory supports the movement of the learner from the novice to advanced beginner level, and recognizes that actions by the learner may be determined by previous exposure to a situation as well as the knowledge base of the learner.

According to Woolfolk (2010, p. 315), there are five conditions for learning that are integral to the constructivist theory.

* The learning environment should provide a realistic and relevant learning experience
* Social interactions and peer collaboration are essential to the learning process
* Multiple perspectives of the experience are important to support, especially as the learner gains more knowledge and moves through more complex situations
* Learners must be aware of their own beliefs and knowledge that shapes their learning and assumptions, which allows them to respect that others may have a different perspective of the scenario
* Learners must assume ownership of learning and use multiple resources to enhance learning

When designing a serious game using the constructivist theory, it is important to formulate objectives and outcomes prior to the development of the scenario for the game. The level of the learner must also be taken into consideration; for example, a scenario designed for a beginning nursing student may require the instructor to be more actively involved in the game based on limited knowledge of the learner. As the student moves through the curriculum, there is less involvement by the instructor, and eventually the student assumes total control of the decision making for the scenario. This type of design is termed *instructional scaffolding* (Keating, 2011).

Kolb's (1984) experiential learning theory provides a solid platform for the design of VL activities. Kolb described learning "as the process whereby knowledge is created through transformation of experience" (p. 41). Kolb suggests that a person learns through a concrete experience, which provides a basis for observation and reflection on the experience in the virtual simulated environment, and discovers new knowledge (Rogers, 2011). Kolb further proposes that reflections are then assimilated into abstract concepts and can be applied to a new experience. This in turn suggests that learning, which has occurred from a simulation in a virtual environment, can be applied to situations encountered in the real world (Rogers, 2011).

Knowles's adult learning theory (1978) can also be applied to the VR environment and development of serious games. Knowles proposed that adults learn differently from children, and their learning is dependent on autonomy, life experiences, personal goals, and relevance of the experience. He termed this "andragogy." This theory is applicable to the VR environment as the learners can apply theoretical principles to the situation and receive immediate

> **Simulation Teaching Tip 17.3**
> The development of a serious game should be based on sound theoretical principles and designed around the purpose, objectives, and outcomes of the learning exercise.

> **Simulation Teaching Tip 17.4**
> The learning outcomes that result from using technology cannot be educationally effective unless the design of the learning activities are made based on the evidence and concepts presented from cognitive science (Rogers, 2011).

feedback on their decisions and actions. Virtual environments can stimulate adult learners to apply their knowledge and experiences to concrete situations in a controlled environment, then consider the consequences of their actions and make changes to future choices. The learner is actively engaged in the learning process through simulated activities and can apply what is learned to real-life situations.

ADVANTAGES AND DISADVANTAGES OF VR LEARNING

The integration of VR learning is important in the learning environment in order to allow the learners an opportunity to immerse themselves in environments where they can practice skills, interact and collaborate with peers or other professionals, make decisions related to care and interventions, and manipulate equipment without fear of harming an individual. VL simulations can be used in any area of clinical practice, but is especially useful in environments where limited access to the experience is available, such as disaster or perioperative nursing. Some benefits and limitations are described in Table 17.1.

ENTERING AND DESIGNING A VIRTUAL SIMULATION

There are several issues that need to be considered in order to develop a simulation in the VW using a platform, such as Second Life, in order to enhance teamwork and problem solving for the simulated experience. In order to participate in the VW, the individual

- Must be able to access the Internet through a high-speed connection
- Creates an avatar the first time the platform is accessed
- Participates in the simulation community through one of two ways
  - Types messages as done in texting or online chats
  - Communicates using a headset with a microphone or Internet telephone connection
- Participates either synchronously (in real time) or asynchronously (virtual time; Billings, 2009) (Table 17.2)

Once the participant enters the simulation or serious game, the participant is able to interact in the environment created in the VW. This may include role-playing, practicing skills, decision making, or participating in conferences or classroom activities.

Several steps should be taken in designing the MUVE (Rogers, 2011, p. 612).

- Briefing stage
  - Learners create their avatar and familiarize themselves with the platform interface
  - Learners view the VW videos for an introduction to the scenario and how to interact with and view objects in the scenario and how to communicate with peers or others in the virtual environment for the scenario

TABLE 17.1
Advantages and Disadvantages of Virtual Learning Environments

ADVANTAGES/BENEFITS	DISADVANTAGES/CHALLENGES
Provide learning experiences in a safe environment to enhance experiential learning (Herold, 2012)	Virtual reality (VR) learning environments, such as serious games, are expensive to produce
Virtual worlds (VWs) are highly interactive and provide dynamic feedback (Jarmon et al., 2009)	Educators and learners must be oriented on how to use the virtual game or task trainer
Simulate clinical experiences, have a student-centered approach, and promote active learning (Rogers, 2011)	Time must be allotted for development of the scenario and creation of avatars (Billings, 2009)
Provide opportunities for learning, which are not readily available in clinical practice or situations that may be dangerous (Kilmon et al., 2010)	Technological support must be available to users and designers
Foster collaboration with peers and users from other disciplines, both locally and globally	Scenario must be relevant for the learning community for which it is designed, and globally relevant if used in a multidisciplinary context (Hogan et al., 2011)
Engage students in role-playing in a more natural environment	Educators and learners must keep an open mind and be willing to learn how to function within the virtual environment
Manipulate equipment and perform procedures in a safe environment (Billings & Halstead, 2012)	Lacks a comprehensive theoretical framework to support and guide the use of simulation in nursing (Guise, Chambers, & Valimaki, 2012)
Incorporate a variety of problems and information the learner can use as part of the assessment phase and test solutions (Hogan et al., 2011)	Lack of empirical evidence on impact of virtual learning (VL)

ADVANTAGES/BENEFITS	DISADVANTAGES/CHALLENGES
Reflect on outcomes related to learner actions and propose new strategies or interventions for the situation	Computer requirements for VL environments may not be available on entry-level computers (Billings & Halstead, 2012)
Evaluate student performance to determine whether learning outcomes have been met	
Standardize scenarios and reuse them with a variety of learners (Billings, 2009)	
Present information to allow learners to learn from each other and enrich the learning experience (Billings, 2009)	
Achieve technology and informatics competencies (Baker, 2009, p. 174)	
Expose learners to a diversity of worldviews through development of virtual social relationships (Jarmon et al., 2009, p. 171)	
Communicate effectively across disciplines	
Useful in a multitude of disciplines and environments, such as community health nursing, disaster preparedness, and perioperative areas (Kaplan et al., 2011; Patel et al., 2013)	

- Action phase
  - Learners enter the VW scenario created for them
  - Learners are given the scenario for the VL experience
  - Learners interact in the environment based on the design of the simulation, which may be acting alone or working in teams and collaborating with others
- Debriefing stage (Billings & Halstead, 2012, p. 361)
  - A key feature in designing VWs and should be done after each VL experience
  - Educators facilitate the reflection (reflective observation) of learners' experiences during the simulation
  - Meaning (abstract conceptualization) is derived from the experience
  - Further application of the meaning may be initiated

EVIDENCE-BASED SIMULATION PRACTICE (EBSP) 17.1

Perceptions and experiences of nursing students using a virtual game (Chia, 2013)

Purpose: To examine the perception and experiences of nursing students using a virtual game prior to the related simulation-based activity in the simulation laboratory.

Design: The game was designed to reinforce knowledge about chronic obstructive pulmonary disease (COPD) and to teach students how to apply this knowledge in the simulated clinical setting.

Method: One hundred sixty-one second-year diploma students participated in the study. Ten students were absent for the virtual game, thereby yielding a response rate of 94.8%. A self-developed questionnaire was used to ask students about their perception and experiences of using the virtual game to collect data. The game was available to the students for 1 week prior to the simulation-based learning (SBL) session. Feedback through a questionnaire was obtained from the participants and included whether or not they felt the virtual game prepared them for the simulated learning experience.

Results: Overall, the participants felt that the game did prepare them for the SBL activity in the laboratory and that it was relevant. A total of 91% of participants felt that their knowledge base on patient management was enhanced in managing the care of patients with COPD.

Conclusion: The results of the study provided useful data to use in Phase 2 of the design of the game. The next phase will incorporate constructivist learning theory resulting in more challenging segments in patient assessment and history.

EVIDENCE-BASED SIMULATION PRACTICE (EBSP) 17.2

Design of a virtual pediatric primary care clinic in Second Life (Cook, 2012)

Purpose: To present an example of an educational strategy to design and evaluate a VW simulation for family nurse practitioner (FNP) students.

Design and Development: The virtual pediatric primary care clinic was created by a team of instructional designers, instructional technologists, and FNP faculty. The FNP faculty created the case studies and questions for the clinic. The instructional technologists developed the interactive display and provided illustrations of the characters in the simulation. The instructional designer integrated the pedagogy, learner, context, and representation for the learning experience. The simulation was based on constructivist learning and experiential learning theories.

Results: VW simulations have the potential to provide a safe environment for FNP students to practice in a pediatric clinic and interact with pediatric patients. However, several areas for improvement were noted, including the development of faculty to create a virtual environment and support students using the technology. Student skills in using the technology need to be investigated before designing the VL activities. Students felt the virtual simulation enhanced their learning of pediatric cases, but that it needed to be presented earlier in their learning experiences. It also provided an opportunity to interact with more pediatric cases.

TABLE 17.2
Virtual Learning Websites

WEBSITE ADDRESS	PURPOSE
Active Worlds https://www.active worlds.com/worlds.html	To create a virtual world using 3-D technology; real-time, interactive 3-D content over the web; create avatars
Second Life www.secondlife.com	Serious game platform using 3-D technology to create avatars
mSTREET http://www.tubettiworld.com/mstreet/info.php	Serious game platform using 3-D technology
mSTREET Critical Care Nursing www.tubettiworld.com/mSTREET/CCN.php	Serious game platform designed for critical care nursing
vSim from Laerdal www.nln.org/newsreleases/laerdal_021214.htm	News release from the National League for Nursing (NLN) about Laerdal V simulations
Twinity www.twinity.com	Free virtual 3-D world and 3-D community chats can be created using avatars

CONCLUSION

This chapter has discussed VL modalities, including VR, VPs, VRS, MUVEs, and serious games, and has looked at the design of these modalities and their effectiveness in the learning environment. Second Life and mSTREET were two examples of serious game platforms discussed, including factors that need to be considered when designing a game for educational purposes. There are concrete advantages to using VL environments, which include promoting interprofessional collaboration and providing experiences that mimic real-life situations and are easily transferred to the clinical practice setting. Disadvantages of VL include the cost and extensive faculty development required to design the scenario. The learner must also be oriented to the VL platform in order to be successful in maneuvering within the scenario to enhance the learning experience. VL and VRSs can be used in both prelicensure and postlicensure education when there is a great demand for clinical placement and, at the same time, fewer resources available, both time and space, for learning. The uses of VL and their outcomes are in the infancy stages of development and show much promise in enhancing the learning environment.

CASE STUDY 17.1

Students in their last semester of nursing at the local university are enrolled in the community health nursing course. The course has been designed within the context of public health nursing. Disaster preparedness is one of the topics taught in the course. The faculty member has collaborated with faculty in other disciplines, including medical students, physician-assistant students, and emergency management services (EMS) as well as paramedic students, to plan a VR learning experience in the management of disasters. Faculty members are developing the scenario, but are not sure how to design the simulation using Second Life as the VL platform. How should they begin the process to design the simulation so that it is a meaningful learning experience?

Discussion: A major factor to consider is the cost of designing the virtual simulation. Does the university support the learning platform, and are they willing to provide funds for the project? An initial action to be considered when designing the virtual serious game is the determination of the purpose of the activity. The scenario should be designed based on the objectives and outcomes of the exercise. That is the key factor in developing a VL situation. It is advisable to base the VW on a sound learning theory, which then influences the activities that are constructed within the activity. Faculty should receive some professional development on how to design the simulation using the Second Life platform. What computer requirements are needed for the learner to interact in the VW? Instructional technology services at the university need to be available to support both faculty and students through the process. Faculty should conduct an assessment of the students' abilities and/or needs to interact with technology and plan orientation based on the data obtained. The value of professional collaboration across disciplines, especially in disaster preparedness, should be emphasized prior to the start of the VL simulation so that learners from all of the disciplines are actively involved in the game.

PRACTICE QUESTIONS

1. When choosing an avatar, the most important consideration is
   A. Design the avatar with as much humor as possible
   B. Design the avatar as realistically as possible for the scenario
   C. The design doesn't matter and can be anything the participant chooses
   D. To allow the learning platform to choose the avatar

2. When designing a VL platform using the constructivist theory, the designer bases the scenario on which principle of learning?
   A. Constructivist theory is experiential in nature
   B. Constructivist theory is based on adult learning principles
   C. Actions are based on building upon previously learned principles
   D. Maslow's hierarchy of needs should be considered as part of the design

3. A major reason for choosing VL is which of the following?
   A. Self-learning is important when interacting in VWs
   B. VWs provide a safe environment for the learner to practice new skills
   C. Designers show off their creativity in designing a serious game
   D. Outcomes of the activity are not important when interacting in VWs

4. An avatar is best described as
   A. A 3-D digitized person that best represents the participant
   B. A passive figure created to mimic the nurse
   C. A computer-generated representation of a person
   D. A person who can only move in one direction based on input of the designer

5. A major advantage or benefit of VL is that
   A. It does not require much work to complete the exercise
   B. It is a cost-effective method of learning
   C. It requires minimal preparation on the part of the designer
   D. It allows interprofessional collaboration on best practices

6. When designing MUVEs, the briefing stage should be initiated. During this stage, which of the following occurs?
   A. Learners enter the VW to begin the simulation
   B. Learners make sense of the experience and build new knowledge
   C. Faculty holds sessions with the learner to allow for reflection on the experience
   D. Students watch videos before entering the VW as part of orientation

7. Instructional scaffolding means that the VL environment
   A. Can be applied to any level of the learner
   B. Builds on previous knowledge and experiences of the participant
   C. There is only one correct action or answer allowed in the scenario
   D. The scenario is linear in nature

8. Kolb's theory espouses which of the following principles?

A. Reflections are assimilated into abstract concepts and applied to a new experience

B. Adults learn best when the material can be immediately applied

C. Andragogy is key to this theory

D. Learning is linear and is based on effective faculty teaching

9. During the debriefing stage, which of the following occurs?

A. Learners enter the VW using their avatar

B. Learners create an avatar for the virtual simulation

C. Faculty develop outcomes for the VL experience

D. Educators facilitate learner reflection on the experience

10. A limitation of incorporating MUVEs in the learning environment is

A. Participants view it as a game with no value in the learning process

B. VL does not provide opportunities for interaction with others

C. The cost of developing an MUVE may be prohibitive

D. It does not allow the transfer of knowledge to the real world

REFERENCES

Bai, X., Duncan, R. O., Horowitz, B. P., Graffeo, J. M., Glodstein, S. L., & Lavin, J. (2012). The added value of 3D simulations in healthcare education. *International Journal of Nursing Education, 4*(2), 67–72.

Baker, J. D. (2009). Serious Games and perioperative nursing. *AORN, 90*, 173–174.

Billings, D. M. (2009). Teaching and learning in virtual worlds. *Journal of Continuing Education in Nursing, 40*, 489–490.

Billings, D. M., & Halstead, J. M. (2012). *Teaching in nursing* (4th ed.). St. Louis, MO: Elsevier.

Charsky, D. (2010). From entertainment to serious games: A change in the use of game characteristics. *Games and Cultures, 5*, 177–198.

Chia, P. (2013). Using a virtual game to enhance simulation based learning in nursing education. *Singapore Nursing Journal, 40*(3), 21–26.

Cook, M. J. (2012). Design and initial evaluation of a virtual pediatric primary care clinic in Second Life. *Journal of the American Academy of Nurse Practitioners, 24*, 521–527.

dit Dariel, O. J., Raby, T., Ravaut, F., & Rothan-Tondeur, M. (2013). Developing the serious games potential in nursing education. *Nurse Education Today, 12*, 1569–1575.

Farra, S. L., & Miller, E. T. (2013). Integrative review: Virtual disaster training. *Journal of Nursing Education and Practice, 3*, 93–101.

Farra, S. L., Miller, E. T., & Hodgson, E. (in press). Virtual reality disaster training: Translation to practice. *Nurse Eduction in Practice*. Retrieved from http://dx.doi.org/10.1016/j.nepr.2013.08.017

Guise, V., Chambers, M., & Valimaki, M. (2012). What can virtual patient simulation offer mental health nursing education? *Journal of Psychiatric and Mental Health Nursing, 19*, 410–418.

Herold, D. K. (2012). Second Life and academia—Reframing the debate between supporters and critics. *Journal of Virtual Worlds Research, 5*, 1–22.

Hogan, M., Kapralos, B., Cristancho, S., Finney, K., & Dubrowski, A. (2011). Bringing community health nursing education to life with Serious Games. *International Journal of Nursing Education Scholarship, 8*, 1–13.

Jarmon, L., Traphagan, T., Mayrath, M., & Trivedi, A. (2009). Virtual world teaching, experiential learning, and assessment: An interdisciplinary communication course in Second Life. *Computers & Education, 53*, 169–182.

Kaplan, B. G., Holmes, L., Mott, M., & Atallah, H. (2011). Design and implementation of an interdisciplinary pediatric mock code for undergraduate and graduate nursing students. *CIN: Computers, Informatics, Nursing, 29*(9): 531–538.

Keating, S. B. (2011). *Curriculum development and evaluation in nursing* (2nd ed.). New York, NY: Springer Publishing Company.

Kilmon, C. A., Brown, L., Ghosh, S., & Mikitiuk, A. (2010). Immersive virtual reality simulations in nursing education. *Nursing Education Perspectives, 31*, 314–317.

Knowles, M. S. (1978). *The adult learner: A neglected species* (2nd ed.). Houston, TX: Gulf.

Kolb, D. A. (1984). *Experiential learning: Experience as the source of learning and development.* Englewood Cliffs, NJ: Prentice-Hall.

mSTREET (2010). *Modular synthetic, training, research, evaluation and extrapolation tool.* TubettiWorld Games, Inc. Retrieved from http://www.tubettiworld.com/mstreet/info.php

Patel, V., Aggarwal, R., Cohen, D., Taylor, D., & Darzi, A. (2013). Implementation of an interactive virtual-world simulation for structured surgeon assessment of clinical scenarios. *Journal of American College of surgeons, 217*, 270–279. http://dx.doi.org/10.1016/j.jamcollsurg.2013.03.023

Phillips, B., Shaw, R. J., Sullivan, D. T., & Johnson, C. (2010). Using virtual environments to enhance nursing distance education. *Creative Nursing, 16*, 132–135.

Rogers, L. (2011). Developing simulations in multi-user virtual environments to enhance healthcare education. *British Journal of Educational Technology, 42*, 608–615. doi:10.1111/j.1467-8535.2010.01057.x

Second Life. (n.d.). *Retrieved from Second Life.* Retrieved from http://secondlife.com

Skiba, D. J. (2008). Nursing education 2.0: Games as pedagogical platforms. *Nursing Education Perspectives, 29*, 174–175.

Skiba, D. J. (2009). Nursing education 2.0: A second look at Second Life. *Nursing Education Perspectives, 30*, 129–131.

Society for Simulation in Healthcare (SSH). (2014). *Certified healthcare simulation educator handbook.* Retrieved from http://ssih.org/certification/handbook

Walsh, M., & van Soeren, M. (2012). Interprofessional learning and virtual communities: An opportunity for the future. *Journal of Interprofessional Care, 26*, 43–48.

Wang, Y., & Braman, J. (2009). Extending the classroom through Second Life. *Journal of Information Systems Education, 20*, 235–247.

Woolfolk, A. (2010). *Educational psychology* (11th ed.). Upper Saddle River, NJ: Merrill.

Zyda, M. (2005). From virtual simulation to virtual reality to games. *Computer, 38*(9), 25–32.

Planning Simulation Activities

KAREN K. GITTINGS

It takes as much energy to wish as it does to plan.
—Eleanor Roosevelt

This chapter addresses Content Area 3: Educate and Assess
Learners Using Simulation (Society for Simulation in Healthcare
[SSH], 2014).

LEARNING OUTCOMES

- Discuss the importance of developing goals and objectives for simulation activities that are relevant to student learning outcomes
- Describe formative and summative methods that can be used to evaluate learning outcomes for simulation activities
- Design a simulation day or simulation activities to promote learning

Simulation activities are a valuable adjunct for student learning and evaluation if linked appropriately to student learning outcomes. Planning ahead is vitally important for the overall success and effectiveness of simulation activities. The process begins with an assessment of learner needs, after which goals for the simulation activities and measurable learning objectives must be identified. The educator must then decide on whether the evaluation should be formative or summative and what methods of evaluation would be most appropriate. After these initial steps are completed, the simulation activities are designed with consideration to resources needed and those that are available. A well-planned simulation activity will minimize problems in the implementation phase. The focus of this chapter is to discuss the planning process for simulation activities; a sample simulation day is reviewed to illustrate each step in the process.

NEEDS ASSESSMENT

The first step in the planning process for simulation activities is to identify the needs of the learners. This can be accomplished through several methods. In some instances, it may be helpful to administer a formal needs assessment at the onset of the planning process; this allows learners to self-identify their educational needs. The needs assessment can also be done informally by the educator who is responsible for the simulation activities and has the most knowledge of the context in which the simulation is being used and how it links to student learning outcomes. Both methods will serve to provide a starting point for the planning process and further guide the development of goals and objectives.

Case Study

Karen, a nurse educator, is planning a simulation day for her learners. To begin the process, she reviews the student learning outcomes of her Adult Health II course. The learners are first-semester seniors (third-semester nursing students) in a baccalaureate nursing program. Karen identifies areas of new content and skills that will be introduced to learners this semester, and from those, determines what knowledge and skills would be best taught through simulation activities. It is decided that learners will be taught intravenous (IV) insertion and principles of IV therapy during the simulation day.

In further assessing her learners' needs, Karen recognizes that they gain little clinical experience in working with

- Nasogastric (NG) tubes
- Small-bore feeding tubes
- Tube feeding
- Administration of medications through enteral feeding tubes

Even though learners are introduced to these skills in the Fundamentals of Nursing course, they may not have the opportunity to use them again because of their clinical placement. It was therefore decided to include these skills as part of the simulation day for review and re-education.

GOAL DEFINITION

Once learner needs have been assessed, it is important to set achievable goals for the day. The words *goals* and *objectives* are often erroneously used interchangeably. Goals are usually statements that serve as a long-term target; they describe the expected outcome at the end of the teaching–learning process. Goals can be used to broadly identify the purpose and final outcomes of the day and lead to the development of more specific objectives (Bastable, 2014).

Case Study, Continued

With an understanding of learner needs, Karen is able to develop goals for the simulation day. It is important to keep student learning outcomes for the course in mind to ensure that the goals are relevant and support learning within the course. Goals include

1. The simulation day will enable learners to develop an understanding of IV insertion and principles of IV therapy.
2. The simulation day will enable learners to review knowledge and skills related to feeding tube insertion, tube feedings, and enteral medication administration.

LEARNING OBJECTIVES

Learning objectives are specific actions that are measurable, tangible, and designed to support attainment of the goals. Written to be short term, objectives are a statement about a single behavior that is to be accomplished after a teaching session or within a short period of time. Objectives are often used to describe a behavior or performance that the learner must accomplish before being considered competent (Bastable, 2014).

The number of learning objectives depends on the number of simulation activities and time involved, but generally vary from one to four. In addition to being relevant, the learning objectives should also be at the appropriate level for the learner; for example, the learning objectives for a simulation activity should be different if the learner is a student nurse compared to an experienced practitioner. When running the simulation activities, it is important to always keep the learning objectives in mind. Avoid having learning objectives overshadowed by allowing learners to become too focused on the completion of skills, unless that is the original intent (Alinier, 2010).

Case Study, Continued

After setting her goals for the simulation day, Karen develops measurable objectives that will be used to evaluate the effectiveness of the simulation activities. Objectives include the following:

At the completion of the simulation day, learners will

1. Demonstrate correct technique in IV insertion using the IV simulator
2. Demonstrate the correct steps for hanging a secondary IV and programming the smart pump
3. Assess and perform nursing interventions for a simulated patient having abdominal pain
4. Demonstrate the correct technique for NG insertion and enteral administration of medications

TYPES OF EVALUATION

Evaluation of simulation activities can be formative or summative. Formative evaluation is done during the learning activity, allowing the educator to assess learners' progress toward achieving learning objectives. In this manner, the learning activity is used to facilitate learning and identify student learning deficits; the activity can also be evaluated and improved upon (Billings & Halstead, 2012).

Summative evaluation is completed at the conclusion of a learning activity, course, or program. The focus is generally on evaluating the extent to which objectives or outcomes were met, leading to a grade assignment. Because summative evaluation occurs at the end, the biggest disadvantage is that nothing can be done to alter the results (Billings & Halstead, 2012).

Case Study, Continued

In deciding whether to use formative or summative evaluation, Karen considers her goals for the day. Because the simulation day is designed to introduce new skills related to IV therapy and reinforce knowledge related to NG tubes and enteral medication administration, Karen decides to use this day as a teaching opportunity with formative evaluation to assess learners' progress. At each learning station, students will be required to return demonstrate their new skills. Faculty members are responsible for facilitating the learning of new skills and correction of identified learning deficits.

As learners will only attend one simulation day associated with the Adult Health II course, a summative evaluation will be completed by learners and faculty. This evaluation will be used to determine whether the learning activities were effective in meeting the planned goals and objectives.

> **Simulation Teaching Tip 18.1**
> Let learners know up front that they will be evaluating the day and provide them with the criteria so that, as they move through the day, they have an idea of what aspects they should be paying particular attention to in order to complete the appraisal.

EVALUATION METHODS

After determining the type of evaluation to be used, different methods of evaluation must be considered. Debriefing is considered an integral part of the teaching–learning process that occurs with high-fidelity simulation. This follow-up discussion provides learners the opportunity to process what they have learned. Debriefing sessions also provide learners with constructive critique for improvement, as well as an opportunity for self-reflection (Cantrell, 2008).

When other low-fidelity simulations are used, observation and feedback may be a more appropriate means of evaluation. Observation is the direct visualization of learner performance of a task or behavior. This is a useful method for evaluating skills competence. Faculty members observing learner performance are able to provide immediate feedback; additionally, learners have the opportunity to remediate and improve on skills. An objective tool to be used with observation is important to avoid bias and accurately record information (Billings & Halstead, 2012).

Feedback is defined by van de Ridder, Stokking, McGaghie, and ten Cate (2008) as information that is provided, after comparing the learner's performance against a standard, in order for improvement to occur. In order to provide appropriate feedback, observation must have occurred. The person providing feedback must also know the standard against which the learner is being compared; for this reason, it is important that the person providing feedback has expertise in the content area.

To evaluate the effectiveness of the simulation day, a survey with a rating scale can be used to elicit learners' and faculty's feedback on the extent to which the day's objectives were met. Objectivity of the evaluation process is increased by using a rating scale (Billings & Halstead, 2012). Information from the survey can identify issues with the learning activities and lead to improvement for future simulation day activities.

EVIDENCE-BASED SIMULATION PRACTICE (EBSP) 18.1

Handley and Dodge (2013) found that evaluation of simulation as a teaching mode for healthcare professionals is overwhelmingly positive in the literature. Less studied is how to best incorporate simulation into curricula. Further outcomes studies are needed to demonstrate the effectiveness of simulation on clinical competency.

Case Study, Continued

For the purposes of formative evaluation, Karen elects to use debriefing, observation, and feedback. Debriefing will follow the high-fidelity simulation of the patient with abdominal pain. Each simulation will run 15 to 20 minutes followed by a 30-minute debriefing. The simulation coordinator will lead the debriefing because of her expertise and advanced training in this skill.

Faculty members will use observation and feedback at the three other low-fidelity simulation stations. Skills' checklists or other tools will be used to objectively document learner performance. Learners will be provided feedback during their performance to assist with process improvement.

Learners and faculty will be asked to complete a brief survey at the conclusion of the simulation day. This tool will be developed with the assistance of the simulation coordinator. Information will be collected anonymously and used to determine whether learning objectives were met. Suggestions for further improvement will also be solicited.

EVALUATION TOOLS

Measurements of learner performance can range from self-reporting surveys to external reviewers using validated assessment tools. Many educators use self-reports of satisfaction and confidence to evaluate learning objectives and outcomes. For those educators unskilled in tool development, self-reporting provides a means of evaluation that is easily obtained, although not necessarily a valid measure of simulation effectiveness (Kardong-Edgren, Adamson, & Fitzgerald, 2010). The objective structured clinical examinations (OSCEs) are well known as valid assessment tools used in medical schools for evaluation, but they can also be used to objectively evaluate clinical nursing skills (Cant & Cooper, 2009). Several evaluation tools that use checklists or evaluation scales are documented in the literature, but many have not been evaluated for reliability or validity (Kardong-Edgren et al., 2010).

Case Study, Continued

Because the simulation day is designed to provide opportunities for learners to acquire new knowledge and skills, Karen elects to use skills' checklists at the IV therapy and NG tube stations to evaluate learner performance. At the conclusion of the day, learners will be asked to complete a survey that is a self-report of their satisfaction with the simulation day activities, and their confidence in meeting the learning objectives. In the future, when simulation activities are used to document competency, a more valid and reliable evaluation tool will need to be used.

DESIGNING THE SIMULATION ACTIVITY

Planning and organization of the simulation activities are vital to a successful simulation day. Decisions must be made about the time frame for the learning activities. For example, will the simulations be run during class or clinical time? If simulation activities occur on a clinical day, what will the learners do if simulation activities are completed in less time than their designated clinical hours?

Simulation activities must be planned that are consistent with student learning outcomes for the course. What simulation activities would reinforce student learning and promote achievement of student learning outcomes? How many simulation activities would be appropriate?

Consideration must also be given to the number of learners enrolled in the course. Simulation activities are most effective when learners are placed in smaller groups. Even when using low-fidelity simulations, smaller numbers of learners allow for more time for interaction with faculty members and hands-on practice. This leads to questions about how to schedule the learners in smaller numbers and still fit into the simulation laboratory schedule.

Case Study, Continued

In the nursing department where Karen teaches, course coordinators are given the opportunity to schedule a week for simulation activities for their course. Karen elects to schedule her simulation week early in the semester so learners will have the opportunity to learn new skills (IV therapy) and review old skills (NG tubes) prior to starting back to clinical in the hospital setting. She further decides to have four simulation stations that will support the identified learning objectives. The first station will be an IV station where learners will learn proper technique for IV insertion. The second station will be an IV station where learners will learn principles of IV therapy, including hanging a secondary medication and programming the smart pump. At the third station, learners will be required to assess and intervene in a simulated patient having abdominal pain. Last, learners will review procedures for inserting NG tubes and administering enteral medications. These simulation activities will be scheduled over a period of 7.5 hours. In order to keep the number of learners low, only two clinical groups (16 learners) will be scheduled per day. Learners will be divided into four groups of four. For a class of 50 learners, 3 to 4 days will be necessary to rotate all learners in the Adult Health II course through the simulation activities. A sample schedule for the simulation day is noted in Table 18.1.

TABLE 18.1
Sample Schedule for Simulation Day

TIMES	STATION 1 IV SIM	STATION 2 IV PUMP	STATION 3 SIMULATOR	STATION 4 NG/MEDS
8:30–9:45 a.m.	Orientation	Orientation	Orientation	Orientation
9:50–10:40 a.m.	Blue Team	Green Team	Purple Team	Red Team
10:45–11:35 a.m.	Red Team	Blue Team	Green Team	Purple Team
11:35–12:35 p.m.	Lunch	Lunch	Lunch	Lunch
12:40–1:30 p.m.	Purple Team	Red Team	Blue Team	Green Team
1:45–2:35 p.m.	Green Team	Purple Team	Red Team	Blue Team
2:40–3:00 p.m.	Evaluations	Evaluations	Evaluations	Evaluations
3:00–4:00 p.m.	Math Work	Math Work	Math Work	Math Work

IV, intravenous; med, medication; NG, nasogastric; sim, simulator.

SELECTING THE SIMULATION MODALITY

After designing the simulation day and activities, careful consideration must be given to selection of the modalities that will best support learning objectives. Simulation modalities are referred to as high fidelity and low fidelity, but with continued technological advances, even the simplest trainers are becoming more realistic. High fidelity generally refers to the use of software-controlled, full-body mannequins, whereas low fidelity refers to the traditional task trainers that are used for procedural training. When used in an interactive environment, low-fidelity task trainers can become a high-fidelity experience (Wang, 2011).

Case Study, Continued

Karen continues planning for the simulation day by identifying the simulation modalities that will be used at each station. In the first station, learners will work with the screen-based IV computer simulator to learn correct technique for IV insertion; because this program provides feedback at the conclusion of each scenario, learners will be provided with an objective evaluation of their technique.

At the second station, learners will have the opportunity to work with IV equipment and practice priming IV lines, hanging secondary IVs, and programming the smart pump. This simulation activity involves the use of a task trainer (smart pump) in which learners have the opportunity to practice IV therapy skills.

Learners will work with a high-fidelity mannequin at the third station where they will be required to assess and intervene with a patient having abdominal pain. Learners will be observed during the simulation activity and feedback will be provided as part of the debriefing process.

The fourth and final station will use low-fidelity simulation to allow learners to practice the technique of NG tube insertion and administration of enteral medications. A task trainer that is a model of a human's head and upper torso will be used to practice NG tube insertion. Enteral medication administration can be practiced with a very simple setup of an NG tube inserted into an empty jug. Evaluation will be through observation and feedback.

RESOURCE IDENTIFICATION

Once the simulation day has been planned, it is important to identify the resources that will be needed, as well as those that are available. First to consider is the location. Although many nursing/medical schools have simulation laboratories, the size and room availability may be limited. Scheduling and reserving space are an early priority.

Equipment needs should also be identified. This should include a detailed list of everything that is needed at each simulation station. If resources permit, it may be helpful to create prop boxes that can be used to store equipment needed for each simulation activity (Alinier, 2010). This simplifies the preparation that occurs each time a simulation is run.

It is also important to identify the content experts/educators and their availability for the simulation activities. Although some low-fidelity simulation activities can be designated as self-directed, generally, a monitor is needed at each station to orient learners to the activity and keep them on target. For simulation done in nursing/medical schools, learners who are at a higher class level could be used to monitor some of the low-fidelity stations. For activities that involve high-fidelity or more complex learning activities, an adjunct clinical instructor or a graduate-level learner would be able to function as the content expert in instructing and assisting learners to meet learning objectives. Some schools have dedicated laboratory personnel or technicians whose responsibilities include simulation and management of laboratory activities.

Simulation activities that are carried out in healthcare organizations are usually developed and organized by the staff of the education department. The educators have the primary responsibility of providing and managing the simulation activities, but other resources are often available. Nurses and medical personnel within the organization have unique knowledge and skills that make them valuable resources in assisting with simulation activities. Additionally, healthcare organizations that have collaborative relationships with nursing/medical schools can invite faculty to participate in simulation activities.

Case Study, Continued

In order to plan for simulation and schedule laboratory space each semester, the simulation coordinator requests that course coordinators sign up for their simulation week at the end of the preceding semester. A master schedule is then generated so that all faculty are aware of their simulation week, as well as other courses using the laboratory. Prior to her assigned week, Karen notifies the simulation coordinator of her planned learning activities and space needs so that rooms/space in the laboratory can be designated in advance.

After carefully considering each simulation activity, Karen identifies potential personnel for each station. At the IV simulator station, a full-time faculty or trained adjunct faculty will need to run and demonstrate the IV simulator. The second station with IV therapy can be led by an adjunct clinical faculty member. As the third station involves the high-fidelity mannequin, the simulation coordinator will lead the simulation and debriefing because of her advanced knowledge and skill in this area. The NG tube and enteral medication administration station has previously been designated as a self-directed station, but feedback from previous learners has led to this station also being directed by a content expert. This is a simulation activity that could be led by an adjunct clinical faculty or graduate learner.

SIMULATION TEAM

Once the resources have been identified, it is important to organize the simulation team. Educators/content experts must be recruited to participate in simulation day activities. In the academic setting, if other faculty are to be used, consideration must be given to their workload and responsibilities. If the simulation activities are to be conducted on the learners' clinical days, the adjunct clinical instructors can be requested to assist with leading the simulation activities on the day their learners are in the laboratory setting. Adjunct clinical instructors may be recruited to assist with other days, but it must be clear whether additional pay is expected and whether departmental or laboratory budgets can support this. Graduate learners can also be recruited, as an example, from the nurse educator students; simulation hours may be used to fulfill hour requirements in a practicum course.

In the healthcare organizational setting, educators who are recruiting assistance from other agency personnel must often request release of the employees from their primary department. Arrangements need to be made as early as possible to prevent scheduling conflicts. This is also true when collaborating with faculty from nursing/medical schools.

If standardized (simulated) patients are used, actors must be also be recruited. In collaboration with the drama department in academic settings, drama learners may portray patients as part of an assignment. Other educators or faculty may also be used. Volunteers may be recruited as well. Professional actors skilled in playing standardized (simulated) patients are also available for hire, although costs can be prohibitive.

Once the members of the simulation team have been recruited and confirmed, arrangements must be made to orient and train them for their roles. It can be challenging to schedule extra time for team members to train, especially when they have other jobs and responsibilities. This becomes less of an issue when the same content experts, whether clinical professionals, educators, or adjunct clinical instructors, are used frequently and simulation activities are done repetitively. Standardized (simulated) patients may require a more in-depth orientation and training depending on the role to be played.

Case Study, Continued

In order to have enough content experts to lead each simulation station, Karen needs to recruit at least four additional members to the simulation team. The simulation coordinator is the first person recruited to run the high-fidelity simulation. Three clinical faculty will also be used.

1. The first is an adjunct clinical faculty member who has worked in this adult health course for several years and participated in multiple simulation exercises; as her expertise is IV therapy, she has been asked to lead this station.
2. The second clinical faculty is actually a full-time faculty member with experience on the IV simulator, so she was asked to lead this particular station.
3. The final clinical faculty member is new to this adult health course and simulation. Because her clinical experience is in acute care surgical nursing, she is very comfortable with NG tubes and has agreed to lead this station.

As the course coordinator, Karen is also in the simulation laboratory with her learners to troubleshoot any problems that may occur.

In order to orient her team members to the simulation activities, Karen sends out, in advance, an agenda with the day's schedule of activities. Learning objectives are shared, and the simulation activities at each station are listed in detail. The goal of the simulation experience and the course coordinator's expectations for the day are made clear to all members. To accommodate everyone's schedule, training is held 1 hour prior to the learners' arrival. As three of the team members have participated in this simulation day previously, only a brief review is necessary. More time is spent with the new adjunct clinical faculty to familiarize her with the equipment and learning objectives for the station she is assigned. Because she is an experienced nurse, she has no difficulty grasping the activities of this station.

PREPARATIONS

Prior to the simulation day, multiple tasks must be accomplished in preparation for the learners and simulation team. A week in advance, learners and team members should be sent an agenda with a schedule of the day's activities. Learners should additionally be provided information about

- Dress requirements
- Equipment required (e.g., stethoscope)
- Any preplanning work/assignment (Table 18.2)

The laboratory must also be prepared with all equipment set up and ready for use. If the laboratory is heavily used, it may not be possible to set up until late in the preceding week. The laboratory setting should be fully prepared and functional so that simulation can be started and kept on schedule. When learners are required to stand around and wait because of lack of planning on the part of the coordinator, it reflects poorly on the simulation day, overall. Learners appreciate well-run, organized learning activities.

It may be advisable to pilot a new simulation before conducting it with learners. This can be done in the form of a run-through or field test and can be as

TABLE 18.2
Learner Instructions for Simulation Day
Please bring the following items on your simulation day. 1. Clinical uniform 2. Stethoscope 3. Simulation-day agenda 4. Class notes on nasogastric tubes 5. Medical–surgical nursing textbook 6. Nursing skills book 7. Medications reference

simple as the course coordinator and simulation coordinator running the simulation scenario through with various unfolding events or endings. This process assists in identifying potential issues and problems that may occur during the simulation; additionally, this is an opportunity to ensure nothing has been forgotten, all necessary resources are available, and every simulation activity is running seamlessly (Alinier, 2010).

Case Study, Continued

Using the university's online learning platform, Karen created a folder within her course's site with information pertaining to simulation day activities. Learners were also encouraged to visit the simulation site to meet their simulated patient and review his past medical–surgical history. This provides learners with additional information about the high-fidelity simulation activity in an attempt to reduce anxiety and fear of the unknown.

As the simulation laboratory is in use at least 3 days a week, Karen and the simulation coordinator prepare the simulation rooms the Friday before simulation activities are scheduled to begin for her adult health course. Handouts are prepared and copied for use at some stations. All equipment and supplies are laid out and organized; computerized simulators are calibrated as necessary. A final walk-through of the stations is conducted early Monday morning before the learners arrive. Because these four simulation activities have been used previously with success, no prior run-through was needed.

SUMMARY

Simulation days are very valuable to learners and can provide clinical skill practice that will be needed in the clinical area. Being true to the goals and objectives of the experience is of utmost importance. Deciding on the logistics of how stations will be set up and what type of evaluation of skills will be accomplished is needed. It is also important to organize the day beforehand by setting up the laboratory, notifying people, and providing the learners with expectations.

PRACTICE QUESTIONS

1. A simulation educator is explaining to a novice the reason for completing a needs assessment prior to planning simulation activities. The best explanation is
   A. "This allows the student to choose what she really wants to learn."
   B. "This is a starting point for assessing learner needs before the planning begins."
   C. "This is nice to do, but not always needed when planning for simulation."
   D. "This is a requirement for accreditation and must be done."

2. A simulation educator is teaching a class on planning for simulation activities. She determines that the instruction is effective when one of the learners states
   A. "A goal should be short term and easily accomplished with simple activities."
   B. "Goals are very complex and may require several simulation activities to accomplish."
   C. "Goals are broadly defined to identify the purpose and final outcomes of the simulation activity."
   D. "Goals and objectives are the same and the terms can be used interchangeably."

3. The simulation coordinator is assisting one of the hospital educators to develop objectives for a simulation experience for new nursing hires. The hospital educator demonstrates understanding when she states
   A. "Objectives must be a measurable statement of a single behavior."
   B. "Objectives are broad statements of what is to be attained."
   C. "There is no need for objectives unless they are to be used for continuing education credit."
   D. "There should only be one objective per simulation activity."

4. Evaluating student learning during the simulation activity to facilitate further instruction and identify deficits is an example of
   A. Summative evaluation
   B. Debriefing
   C. Outcome evaluation
   D. Formative evaluation

5. In discussing the debriefing process with a novice educator, the simulation coordinator's best explanation is that debriefing is
   A. "Ideally done after each simulation, but can be eliminated if time runs short."
   B. "An opportunity for learners to reflect and derive meaning from the experience."
   C. "The time to critique the learners' experience and point out all faults."
   D. "An activity that should be done on the following day after learners have had a time to reflect."

6. In planning for a simulation activity, the simulation educator elects to use a simple pelvic model for learners to practice insertion of indwelling urinary catheters. This is an example of what type of simulation modality?

   A. High-fidelity simulator
   B. Standardized patient
   C. Task trainer
   D. Virtual reality

7. The simulation coordinator is working with a graduate learner to plan a simulation activity. The learner correctly identifies that resources do not include

   A. Learners
   B. Location
   C. Content experts
   D. Laboratory technicians

8. The clinical nurse educator and simulation coordinator are working together to organize a simulation team for a code II simulation activity. The first step is to

   A. Orient team members
   B. Develop a training schedule
   C. Recruit content experts
   D. Advertise the event

9. While planning a simulation activity, a novice educator asks why an agenda needs to be prepared and sent out to learners ahead of time. The simulation coordinator's best response is

   A. "It is expected to always have an agenda for an educational event."
   B. "If there are any typos, we can correct them ahead of time."
   C. "This is required for hospital employees to request time off to attend."
   D. "This helps learners to know what to expect and identifies any preplanning needs."

10. A content expert who has agreed to participate in a new simulation activity asks the coordinator why he needs to pilot the simulation ahead of time. The best response is

    A. "This is a good way to identify problems or issues before running a first-time simulation activity."
    B. "This is something that should be done before every simulation activity."
    C. "Piloting a simulation allows the planner to determine whether the content experts are appropriate for the simulation activity."
    D. "This is the only way to make sure the equipment is all working."

REFERENCES

Alinier, G. (2010). Developing high-fidelity health care simulation scenarios: A guide for educators and professionals. *Simulation & Gaming, 42*(1), 9–26. doi:10.1177/1046878109355683

Bastable, S. B. (2014). *Nurse as educator: Principles of teaching and learning for nursing practice* (4th ed.). Burlington, MA: Jones & Bartlett Learning.

Billings, D. M., & Halstead, J. A. (2012). *Teaching in nursing: A guide for faculty* (4th ed.). St. Louis, MO: Saunders.

Cant, R. P., & Cooper, S. J. (2009). Simulation-based learning in nurse education: Systematic review. *Journal of Advanced Nursing, 66*(1), 3–15. doi: 10.1111/j.1365-2648.2009.05240.x

Cantrell, M. A. (2008). The importance of debriefing in clinical simulations. *Clinical Simulation in Nursing, 4*(2), e19–e23. doi:10.1016/j.ecns.2008.06.006

Handley, R., & Dodge, N. (2013). Can simulated practice learning improve clinical competence? *British Journal of Nursing, 22*(9), 529–535.

Kardong-Edgren, S., Adamson, K. A., & Fitzgerald, C. (2010). A review of currently published evaluation instruments for human patient simulation. *Clinical Simulation in Nursing, 6*(1), e25–e35. doi:10.1016/j.ecns.2009.08.004

Society for Simulation in Healthcare (SSH). (2014). *Certified healthcare simulation educator handbook.* Retrieved from http://ssih.org/certification/handbook

van de Ridder, J. M. M., Stokking, K. M., McGaghie, W. C., & ten Cate, O. T. J. (2008). What is feedback in clinical education. *Medical Education, 42*, 189–197. doi: 10.1111/j.1365-2923.2007.02973.x

Wang, E. E. (2011). Simulation and adult learning. *Disease-a-Month, 57*(11), 664–678.

Evaluation of Simulation Activities

MELANIE LEIGH CASON AND FRANCES WICKHAM LEE

*One of the great mistakes is to judge policies and programs
by their intentions rather than their results.*
—Milton Friedman

> **This chapter addresses Content Area 3: Educate and Assess
> Learners Using Simulation (Society for Simulation in Healthcare
> [SSH], 2014).**

LEARNING OUTCOMES

- Discuss the basic components of performance and activity evaluation
- Discuss the importance of evaluation of simulation activities
- Identify current practices for individual learner evaluation, team evaluation, and activity evaluation in simulation-based training (SBT)
- Discuss the future of evaluation in SBT

The healthcare world continues to evolve at an amazing speed with increasing individual and organizational accountability at the forefront. Experts agree that simulation is a valuable tool for healthcare education learning and for determining clinical competency (Cant & Cooper, 2010; Chappell & Koithan, 2012; Wilhaus, Burleson, Palaganas, & Jeffries, 2014). However, the question remains: How does one determine the effectiveness of simulation at the individual, team, organizational, and system levels? Assessing learner outcomes, whether for students or practicing healthcare professionals, individually or in teams, requires valid and reliable tools to ensure that instructional goals are achieved (Boulet, Jeffries, Hatala, Korndorffer, Feinstein, & Roche, 2011). Although a variety of SBT and simulation-based team training (SBTT) evaluation tools exist, there continues to be a need for establishing the validity and reliability of both the simulator and the tools (Adamson & Kardong-Edgren, 2012; Eppich, Howard, Vozenilek, & Curran, 2011; Rosen et al., 2008; Schaefer, Vanderbilt, Cason, Bauman, Glavin, Lee, & Navedo, 2011).

In addition to accurately evaluating learners, outcome data are needed to determine the overall effectiveness of SBT, including demonstration of translation to practice within organizations and the overall healthcare system.

This chapter begins with a brief discussion of evaluation and its importance in SBT, both today and in the future. Next, the chapter focuses on evaluation of the individual learner, including the differences between formative and summative evaluation and a discussion of self and peer evaluation, followed by an overview of the evaluation of team members during SBTT. A summary of selected SBT and SBTT evaluation instruments is presented. The chapter concludes with a discussion of methods and current tools available for evaluating the simulation activity itself.

EVALUATION IN SBT

Rosen and colleagues (2008) offer an overview of three key concepts for understanding evaluation in SBT: "issues of purpose (i.e., why evaluate?), content (i.e., what to evaluate?), and method (i.e., how to evaluate?)" (p. 353). There are multiple reasons for evaluating SBT, including providing formative and summative feedback to learners, defining key outcomes, validating the usefulness of the training, and demonstrating translation to practice. What to evaluate is often challenging. High-quality simulation design begins with a clear understanding of the learning objectives. These objectives focus on what is to be evaluated. For example, is the focus on individual performance or overall effectiveness or impact on the organization? Performance refers to the "actual behaviors" demonstrated, whereas effectiveness addresses the results of the performance (Rosen et al. 2008). Actual behaviors within SBT are often divided into knowledge, skills, and attitudes (KSAs). These relate to the recognized learning domains, that is, cognitive (knowledge), affective (attitude), and psychomotor (skills). The "how to evaluate" must be determined by the "why" and the "what." Clearly, the tools used to evaluate straight performance versus effectiveness or translation would be quite different. The instrument chosen for assessment or evaluation should reflect the appropriate domain in which the learning has occurred or an integration of all three if appropriate (Kardong-Edgren, Adamson, & Fitzgerald, 2010).

There has been a great deal of attention given to developing evaluation methods and tools to demonstrate that SBT "translates to practice" (Eppich et al., 2011; Rosen et al., 2008; Schaefer et al., 2011). In other words, if the learner performs in a competent manner in the SBT, will this translate into actual clinical practice? Eppich and colleagues (2011) discuss a need to examine SBT and SBTT as "interrelated conceptual" levels of training the individual, team, organization, and system. Translation to practice occurs at the organizational and system levels. Although the current state of evaluation for SBT and SBTT has not reached the level of demonstrating translation, any discussion of evaluation should include it as an ultimate goal. To date, the majority of work related to SBT evaluation has been at the individual learner and team levels, with some work targeting the evaluation of effective simulation design and implementation. We examine these three areas in more detail in the subsequent sections of this chapter.

INDIVIDUAL LEARNER SBT EVALUATION

SBT learner evaluation focuses primarily on the individual's performance and outcomes. There are existing evaluation tools developed for this purpose. In evaluating learners, it is important to determine desired specific learning outcomes, maintain consistency, and apply standardization in order to be fair and objective with feedback (Motola, Devine, Chung, Sullivan, & Issenberg, 2013). All evaluations of learners begin with the development of clear, measurable objectives for the SBT. Evaluation should always be tightly aligned with the learning objectives. The appropriate choice of the evaluation tool is specific to the measurement of learning outcomes, whether the activity is an individual or group activity. The outcome of the evaluation may be formative or summative, and this will be a large determinant of the tool selected. A few of the more well-known SBT evaluation tools are listed in Table 19.1 with brief descriptions.

> **Simulation Teaching Tip 19.1**
> Remember to determine what you are evaluating and make sure it is appropriate for the level of the student. Approaches will depend on formative or summative activities. If summative, then you should not give students unfair advantages by cueing or assisting in any way. Are you *evaluating* clinical judgment, competency, psychomotor skills, or critical thinking or *teaching* them? Scenarios in simulation cannot encompass all aspects of a case study, so it is important to define the desired learning outcomes or assessment measures clearly before you begin.

FRAMEWORKS FOR EVALUATION STRATEGIES

There are several applicable frameworks that support the evaluative process in SBT. These include Kirkpatrick's levels of evaluation, translational science research (TSR) phases, and Miller's pyramid (Adamson, Kardong-Edgren, & Willhaus, 2012; Downing & Yudkowsky, 2009; McGaghie, Draycott, Dunn, Lopez, & Stefanidis, 2011).

Kirkpatrick's Levels of Evaluation

- Level 1 is **reaction**. How satisfied are the learners with the activity, how did they like it? As the lowest level of evaluation, it is usually reflected by self-reporting on surveys, observations, or verbal feedback: "It was fun" or "I didn't like it."

- Level 2 is **learning**. How much did they learn? This level reflects a change in attitudes, skills, or knowledge.

- Level 3 is **behavior**. How has the learner's behavior changed as a result of this activity? Level III relates to a change in behavior and application of what he or she has learned.

- Level 4 is **results**. This relates to a change in practice based on the learning that benefits clients (patients) and/or contributes to a change in the organization with improved outcomes (Adamson, 2014; Downing & Yudkowsky, 2009; Kirkpatrick, 1998; McGaghie, Issenberg, Petrusa, & Scalese, 2010).

TSR Phases

The evaluation of the transfer of the KSAs learned with simulation to patient care and outcomes is appropriate for translational research (Adamson et al., 2012). TSR provides three levels of evaluation.

1. T-1 is the lowest level in relation to simulation activities. It consists of learning in the simulation lab.
2. T-2 is the carryover to patient care.
3. T-3 is that the results of the simulation activity improve patient outcomes. As the name implies, evidence is required to prove the translation to practice, and this requires measurable outcomes at every level. Research design and data collection for the highest level of TSR continue to be a challenge in simulation education (McGaghie et al., 2011).

Miller's Pyramid

Miller's pyramid provides a visual model with "Knows" as the base of the pyramid, followed by "Knows how" and "Shows how." "Does" is the top level of the pyramid (Figure 19.1). The "Shows how" level relates to a demonstration of learning, for example, in objective simulated clinical examinations (OSCEs) or with simulations. The highest level "Does" again relates to transfer to practice in the workplace (Miller, 1990).

A comparison of the levels, phases, and features of these frameworks confirms that the lowest level of learner evaluation relates to obtaining information and assessing learner reactions. The highest level involves translation to practice and health outcomes. The "in between" levels or phases contain the observation of the learned behavior, that is, performance. Most learner evaluation during SBT, whether formative or summative, is recognized as falling into these "in between" levels (see Figure 19.2).

FIGURE 19.1 Miller's pyramid.

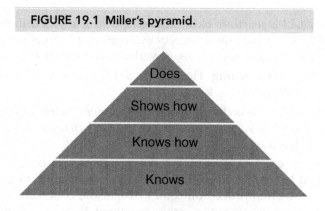

Adapted from Miller (1990).

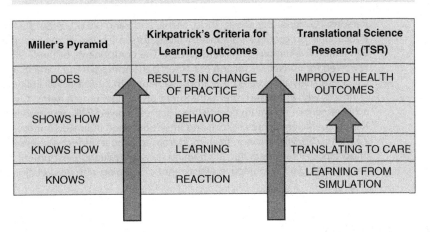

FIGURE 19.2 Selected frameworks for evaluation strategies.

FORMATIVE EVALUATION

Formative evaluation involves the learning process and occurs during or within instruction (Downing & Yudkowsky, 2009). Generally, formative evaluation does not result in a recorded grade or assessment score. Rather, it provides the learners with important feedback to guide them in obtaining appropriate KSAs relative to the study topic. Active learning with simulation promotes an opportunity for formative feedback, particularly regarding the higher level KSAs that encompass critical thinking and competencies (Glynn, 2012; Jeffries, 2012; Tanner, 2006). Tools, such as performance tests, checklists, and pre- and post-learning assessments are valuable in formative evaluation, enabling deliberate practice toward mastery (Downing & Yudkowsky, 2009; Sando et al., 2013).

SUMMATIVE EVALUATION

Summative evaluation measures the achievement of learning objectives by "summing up" the results of the formative experiences (Downing & Yudkowsky, 2009; Sando et al., 2013). Summative evaluation generally results in a recorded grade, score, or certification of competence or proficiency. A "high-stakes" simulation activity refers to a simulation designed as an assessment tool with an outcome that affects a grade, certification, and has consequences attached to the final rating (Rizzolo, 2014; Sando et al., 2013). There is increasing interest in using simulation not only for training, but also as the basis for learner evaluation. For summative assessment with high stakes, clear objectives and standard, informed measures are critical. In addition, facilitators should never cue the participants or provide information that would affect the evaluation (Wilhaus et al., 2014). According to McGaghie and Issenberg (2009), a major component in developing a simulation-based evaluation is to standardize the "test conditions," that is, the simulation activity, so that the *only* variable in the experience is the learner.

> **EVIDENCE-BASED SIMULATION PRACTICE (EBSP) 19.1**
>
> Parsons, Hawkins, Hercinger, Todd, Manz, and Fang (2012) created a formal educational program to train faculty facilitators in the use of the Creighton Simulation Evaluation Instrument (C-SEI). The components of the C-SEI were reviewed for consensus for the expected behaviors from the participants prior to use. Data analysis revealed that improvement with interrater reliability occurred as noted, with increased rater agreement on the instrument items. Overall achievement of minimum competency scores showed 94% agreement by faculty. Kappa coefficient scores before and after education indicated improvement from 27.7% to 75% with a range from moderate to almost perfect agreement. The importance of facilitator/faculty training for any evaluation instrument is critical for implementing a fair, objective assessment of learning with a simulation activity.

SELF-EVALUATION

Self-evaluation commonly occurs in debriefing after SBT. It can also occur during SBT in which structured feedback is provided. Effective debriefing provides the opportunity to reflect and is a valuable learning experience for the learner. Learning occurs individually during the experience of the simulation and during debriefing (Dreifuerst, 2009). Self-evaluation may be enhanced with recording the simulation activities. Previous self-efficacy studies with nursing students and physicians indicate that abilities may be overrated (Davis, Mazmanian, Fordis, Harrison, Thorpe, & Perrier, 2006; Shinnick & Woo, 2013; Watts, Rush, & Wright, 2009).

PEER EVALUATION

Removing the facilitator from the evaluative process and allowing the participants to evaluate each other has certain benefits. Participants working collaboratively learn from each other and develop the ability to make judgments and give and receive constructive criticism. The success in peer evaluation depends on how the activity is structured to prevent erroneous information, bias, and subjectivity (Rush, Firth, Burke, & Marks-Maran, 2012). Cooperative Learning with Simulation-Based Skills Training (CLSST)™ is one method of pairing students with a standardized programmed event menu for peer assessment with scoring. This method alleviates the need for a paper checklist and provides immediate feedback to the participants (Lee, Schaefer, Houck, Walker, & Cason, 2014).

EVALUATION IN SBTT

There are significant challenges in evaluating both the performance and the effectiveness of SBTT. Healthcare teams are complex entities, often comprising ever-changing members in a high-stress environment. The Agency for Healthcare Research and Quality (AHRQ, 2005) defines a team as

- Consisting of two or more individuals
- Having specific roles, performing specific tasks, and interacting to achieve a common goal or outcome
- Making decisions

- Possessing specialized knowledge and skill and often functioning under conditions of high workload
- Differing from small groups in that teams embody a collective action arising out of task interdependence

One of the most significant challenges in SBTT evaluation is the need to assess the KSAs of the team members within the context of the team. The team performance and effectiveness must also be considered. If individual team members do not have the KSAs needed to perform the tasks associated with their respective roles, the effectiveness of the team may be impacted. Most of the existing SBTT evaluation tools are observational checklists that focus primarily on the "soft skills" and overall team characteristics rather than outcomes. For example, one of the most used team frameworks is TeamSTEPPS™, developed by the AHRQ. (Although, not an evaluation tool, per se, TeamSTEPPS has been used as the foundation for many SBTT evaluation tools.) The four key skills emphasized in TeamSTEPPS are

1. Leadership
2. Communication
3. Situational monitoring
4. Mutual support

A few of the more well-known SBTT tools are listed in Table 19.1 with brief descriptions.

Rosen and colleagues (2008) have recently suggested the event-based training and assessment (EBTA) technique to address the complexities of rating team and other complex simulation training. EBTA is designed to facilitate the evaluation, not only of the team skills, but also the events that impact patient outcomes. EBTA is built on a specifically designed scenario that focuses on a subset of teamwork competencies. Diagnostic measurement tools are developed for each scenario.

CURRENT EVALUATION INSTRUMENTS

Instruments for evaluating individual and team SBT performance continue to be developed and tested. Appropriate feedback and evaluation require valid and reliable tools to avoid subjectivity, bias, and incorrect interpretation of the simulation experience (Motola, Devine, Chung, Sullivan, & Issenberg, 2013). Many instruments have been developed without established or reported reliability and validity data (Kardong-Edgren, Adamson, & Fitzgerald, 2010).

- *Validity* relates to the degree that the instrument or tool measures what it is intended to measure, for example, communication skills.
- *Reliability* is the consistency and dependability of the measurement of a particular attribute by the instrument or tool (Polit & Beck, 2012).

More multisite studies are needed to establish validity and reliability of many tools, and choosing a tool that is already developed supports this initiative (Adamson & Kardong-Edgren, 2012). Additionally, the importance of facilitator education regarding the appropriate use of an evaluative tool has been established (Parsons et al., 2012; Patton, 2012).

Simulation evaluation instruments vary in design and levels of measurement. As noted in Table 19.1, these may include Likert scales with rankings from

TABLE 19.1
Characteristics of Simulation-Based Team Training Evaluation Instruments

SELECTED CITATIONS	NAME OF INSTRUMENT	CHARACTERISTICS	REQUIREMENTS	MEASURES	OTHER
Fletcher, Flin, McGeorge, Glavin, Maran, and Patey (2004)	Anesthetists' Non-Technical Skills (ANTS)	Observational checklist for team performance	Evaluator rates four categories on a 4-point scale; Good 4, Acceptable 3, Marginal 2, Poor 1, Not Observed 0	Task management Team working Situation awareness Decision making	
Thomas, Sexton, and Helmreich (2004)	University of Texas Behavioral Marker Audit Form (UTBMAF)	One-page behavioral rating scale designed for team performance in neonatal resuscitation	Each behavior is rated on observability and frequency	10 behavior markers: information sharing, inquiry, assertion, intentions shared, teaching, evaluation of plans, workload management, vigilance/environmental awareness, teamwork overall, and leadership	Derived from methodologies used in aviation: Line Operations Safety Audit (LOSA)
Healey, Undre, and Vincent (2004)	Observational Teamwork Assessment of Surgery (OTAS)	Clinical checklist by surgical expert; teamwork behaviors by expert researcher	Clinical checklist is Yes or No; behaviors are rated on 7-point Likert scale	Task work and teamwork in three stages: preoperative, intraoperative, and postoperative; teamwork behaviors include communication, leadership, coordination, monitoring, and cooperation	Developed for use in the operating room (OR), not specifically simulation

SELECTED CITATIONS	NAME OF INSTRUMENT	CHARACTERISTICS	REQUIREMENTS	MEASURES	OTHER
Todd, Manz, Hawkins, Parsons, and Hercinger (2008); Kardong-Edgren et al. (2010); Adamson, Kardong-Edgren, and Willhaus (2012)	Creighton Simulation Evaluation Instrument (2008; C-SEI)	A rating tool designed for evaluation of nursing students using simulation	Evaluator scores either a 0 or 1 for 22 specific criteria; example: "Responds to abnormal findings appropriately"	Assessment Communication Critical thinking Technical skills	Modified for use in the NLN high-stakes assessment and NCSBN Simulation Research Study
Lasater (2007); Tanner (2006)	Lasater Clinical Judgment Rubric (2007; LCJR)	A rubric based on a clinical judgment model by Tanner (2006)	Evaluator rates participant as exemplary, accomplished, developing, or beginning with detailed rubric criteria	Effective noticing Effective interpreting Effective responding Effective reflecting	Has been modified for numeric grading (Ashcraft, Opton, Bridges, Caballero, Veesart, & Weaver, 2013)
Mikasa, Cicero, and Adamson (2012)	Seattle University Evaluation Tool (2008)	A tool based on curricular objectives and the American Association of Colleges of Nursing (AACN) baccalaureate competencies	Evaluator circles observed behaviors that relate to a score from the range of "Below expectations" to "Exceeds expectations"	Assessment Intervention Evaluation Critical thinking/clinical decision making Direct patient care/communication/collaboration Professional behaviors	

NCSBN, National Council of State Boards of Nursing; NLN, National League for Nursing.

0 to 5, scoring rubrics outlining expected behaviors linked to a score, or dichotomous scales of 0 to 1 (did not meet or met). In deciding the tool most appropriate to use, the most recently reported reliability and validity should be considered in addition to the objective of the evaluation (Adamson & Kardong-Edgren, 2012).

EVALUATING THE SIMULATION ACTIVITY

Another topic within the simulation community involves evaluating the simulation activity itself and the facilitator conducting the SBT. Questions, such as does the activity meet the objectives for which it was designed or is the facilitator effective, are important for improving activities and insuring quality. There are many ways to evaluate simulation activities, from direct observation by peers or formal to informal surveys and questionnaires. As with other evaluation tools, the surveys and questionnaires used to evaluate the simulation activities should be valid and reliable (Boulet et al., 2011; Jeffries, 2012). There are a handful of SBT assessment tools that address facilitator and activity effectiveness. The Simulation Design Scale (SDS) allows the participant not only to self-assess participation, but also to assess the effectiveness of the simulation activity. Another tool, the Educational Practices in Simulation Scale (EPSS), contains elements that assess for best practices in SBT, including active learning, high expectations, diversity in learning, and collaboration (Jeffries, 2012). Debriefing Assessment for Simulation in Healthcare© (DASH©; 2014) is a tool aimed at the evaluation of the debriefing experience following simulation (Center for Medical Simulation, 2014).

SUMMARY

This chapter has explored concepts and tools for evaluating performance and effectiveness of SBT at the individual and team levels, with some discussion related to the need to move to the higher levels of organizational and system impact. Although a variety of SBT, SBTT, and simulation activity evaluation tools exist, there continues to be a need for developing and establishing valid and reliable instruments, particularly those that will measure organizational impact and translation to practice (Eppich et al. 2011; Rosen et al., 2008; Schaefer et al., 2011). Outcomes data are needed to determine the overall effectiveness of the SBT, including demonstration of translation to practice within organizations and the overall healthcare system.

CASE STUDY 19.1

An academic medical university is planning an interdisciplinary professional education simulation activity involving medical students, nursing students, physician assistant students, and pharmacology students. The simulation will consist of teams of four, with one from each discipline. The scenarios are designed for specific behaviors, such as effective communication, teamwork and collaboration, procedural skill, and critical thinking. Evaluations consist of facilitator input at debriefing and self-assessment of performance and the activity with an online questionnaire. Results are positive, but the facilitators are determined to improve the evaluative results with peer evaluation and measurement of the achievement of the learning outcomes of effective communication, teamwork and collaboration, procedural skill, and critical thinking.

CASE STUDY DISCUSSION

There are several ways that the facilitators can evaluate the students' performance more effectively. The choice of a rubric could be time-intensive and involves an expert from each discipline observing the simulation either in real time, remotely or by video. Establishing interrater reliability by requiring another faculty member to review the simulation independently is desirable, especially if this type of activity may be used for high-stakes or summative assessments in the future. Programmed menu items allow for assessment while running the simulation and can be assimilated with data retrieval to evaluate the learning for the course overall, to identify knowledge gaps, and to inform curriculum development. Although it is important to evaluate how participants feel about an activity, simulation offers opportunities to evaluate learning in the cognitive, affective, and psychomotor domains.

PRACTICE QUESTIONS

1. A new faculty member wants to create and run a simulation "on the fly" to access the competency levels of the students for a pass/fail in clinical. The best response to this request is

   A. "We can try it, but I'm not sure this is the best way."
   B. "No, I don't think you should do that."
   C. "Best practices call for established objectives and learning outcomes."
   D. "Summative evaluation requires a valid and reliable assessment."

2. A simulation activity involves the use of deliberate practice to learn and perfect a skill. Students are given immediate feedback as to the correct and incorrect steps taken throughout the simulation to enhance their learning. This is an example of a

   A. Formative evaluation
   B. Summative evaluation
   C. Self-assessment
   D. Peer evaluation

3. The simulated patient has a terminal illness and is dying. The participant is evaluated on how professionally he communicates with the patient. This is an example of evaluating

   A. Attitude
   B. Skill
   C. Psychomotor ability
   D. Emotion

4. An evaluative instrument has criteria with possible scores from 0 to 5 in each category. This type of tool is best known as a

   A. Checklist
   B. Matrix
   C. Rubric
   D. Likert scale

5. Standardization of the evaluative process and evaluator training promotes which of the following?

   A. Increased reliability
   B. Improved validity
   C. Reduced bias potential
   D. Evidence-based practice

6. Following a simulation experience, students complete an anonymous online survey regarding their performance. This is an example of

   A. Self-evaluation
   B. Debriefing
   C. Peer assessment
   D. Formative assessment

7. A department head has mandated that faculty use a certain evaluation tool for summative evaluation with simulation. It is most important for faculty to

   A. Keep the evaluations hidden from the students.
   B. Be educated in the appropriate use of the tool.
   C. Use the tool as much as possible.
   D. Modify the tool as needed to meet the objectives of the course.

8. A hospital quality-assurance committee is analyzing patient satisfaction data related to communication between physicians and nurses following intensive team training with simulation. The results could support the achievement of which of the following?

   A. Kirkpatrick's Level 4
   B. TSR Phase 1
   C. Miller's pyramid base of "Knows"
   D. Kirkpatrick's Level 2

9. The hospital rapid-response team participates in SBT. At the conclusion of the training, the teams' adherence to protocol is evaluated using a valid and reliable tool to determine the impact of the SBT on actual team performance. This evaluation is aimed at

   A. Miller's "Does" and Kirkpatrick's Level 4
   B. Translating to practice and Kirkpatrick's Level 4
   C. Miller's "Shows how" and Kirkpatrick's Level 3
   D. Translating to practice and Kirkpatrick's Level 3

10. One of the most significant challenges in evaluating healthcare team performance is

    A. Understanding TeamSTEPPS as it relates to different types of healthcare teams
    B. Recognizing individual team member roles, as the healthcare teams are not static
    C. Evaluating the impact of team members on the overall team performance
    D. Evaluating communication strategies among team members

REFERENCES

Adamson, K. A. (2014). Evaluation tools and metrics for simulations. In P. R. Jeffries (Ed.), *Clinical simulations in nursing education: Advanced concepts, trends, and opportunities* (pp. 145–163). Philadelphia, PA: Wolters Kluwer, Lippincott Williams & Wilkins.

Adamson, K. A., & Kardong-Edgren, S. (2012). A method and resources for assessing the reliability of simulation evaluation instruments. *Nursing Education Perspectives, 33,* 334–339.

Adamson, K. A., Kardong-Edgren, S., & Willhaus, J. (2012). An updated review of published simulation evaluation instruments. *Clinical Simulation in Nursing,* e1–e13. http://dx.doi.org/10.1016/j.ecns.2012.09.004

AHRQ. (2005). *Chapter 2. Training teams medical teamwork and patient safety: The evidence-based relation.* Retrieved from http://www.ahrq.gov/research/findings/final-reports/medteam/chapter2.html

AHRQ. (2013). Introduction. In *TeamSTEPPS instructor guide.* Rockville, MD: Agency for Healthcare Research and Quality.

Ashcraft, A. S., Opton, L., Bridges, R. A., Caballero, S., Veesart, A., & Weaver, C. (2013). Simulation evaluation using a modified Lasater clinical judgment rubric. *Nursing Education Perspectives, 34*(2), 22–26.

Boulet, J. R., Jeffries, P. R., Hatala, R. A., Korndorffer, J. R., Feinstein, D. M., & Roche, J. P. (2011). Research regarding methods of assessing learning outcomes. *Simulation in Healthcare, 6,* S48–S51.

Cant, R. P., & Cooper, S. J. (2010). Simulation-based learning in nurse education: Systematic review. *Journal of Advanced Nursing, 66*(1), 3–15. http://dx.doi.org/10.1111/j.1365-2648.2009.05240.x

Center for Medical Simulation. (2014). *Debriefing Assessment for Simulation in Healthcare (DASH).* Retrieved from https://harvardmedsim.org

Chappell, K., & Koithan, M. (2012). Validating clinical competence. *Journal of Continuing Education in Nursing, 43,* 293–294. doi:10.3928/00220124-20120621-02

Davis, D. A., Mazmanian, P. E., Fordis, M., Harrison, R. V., Thorpe, K. E., & Perrier, L. (2006). Accuracy of physician self-assessment compared with observed measures of competence: A systematic review. *Journal of American Medical Association, 9,* 1094–1102.

Downing, S. M., & Yudkowsky, R. (2009). *Assessment in health professions education.* New York, NY: Routledge.

Dreifuerst, K. (2009). The essentials of debriefing in simulation earning: A concept analysis. *Nursing Education Perspectives, 10*(2), 109–114.

Eppich, W., Howard, V., Vozenilek, J., & Curran, I. (2011). Simulation based training in healthcare [Supplemental material]. *Simulation in Healthcare, 6*(7), S14–S19. http://dx.doi.org/10.1097/SIH.0b013e318229f550

Fletcher, G., Flin, R., McGeorge, P., Glavin, R., Maran, N., & Patey, P. (2004). Rating non-technical skills: Developing a behavioral marking system for use in anesthesia. *Cognition Technology Work, 6,* 165–171.

Glynn, P. (2012). Evaluation of senior nursing students' performances with high fidelity simulation. *Online Journal of Nursing Informatics, 16*(3), 1–12. Retrieved from http://ojni.org/issues

Jeffries, P. R. (2012). *Simulation in nursing education: From conceptualization to evaluation* (2nd ed.). New York, NY: National League for Nursing.

Kardong-Edgren, S., Adamson, K. A., & Fitzgerald, C. (2010). A review of currently published evaluation instruments for human patient simulation. *Clinical Simulation in Nursing, 6,* e25–e35. http://dx.doi.org/10.1016/j.ecns.2009.08.004

Kirkpatrick, D. L. (1998). *Evaluating training programs* (2nd ed.). San Francisco, CA: Berrett-Koehler.

Lasater, K. (2007). Clinical judgment development: Using simulation to create an assessment rubric. *Journal of Nursing Education, 46*(11), 496–503.

Lee, F. W., Schaefer, J., Houck, R., Walker, J., & Cason, M. (2014). Cooperative learning in dyads using hybrid task training simulation. Presentation conducted at the International Meeting for Simulation in Healthcare, San Francisco, CA.

McGaghie, W. C., Draycott, T. J., Dunn, F. W., Lopez, C. M., & Stefanidis, D. (2011). Evaluating the impact of simulation on translational patient outcomes. *Simulation in Healthcare, 6,* S42–S47. http://dx.doi.org/10.1097/SIH.0b013e318222fde9

McGaghie, W. C., & Issenberg, S. B. (2009). Simulations in assessment. In S. M. Downing & R. Yudkowsky (Eds.), *Assessment in health professions education* (pp. 245–268). New York, NY: Routledge. doi:http://dx.doi.org

McGaghie, W. C., Issenberg, S. B., Petrusa, E. R., & Scalese, R. J. (2010). A critical review of simulation-based medical education research: 2003–2009. *Medical Education, 44,* 50–63. http://dx.doi.org/10.1111/j.1365-2923.2009.03547.x

Mikasa, A. W., Cicero, T. F., & Adamson, K. A. (2012). Outcome-based evaluation tool to evaluate student performance in high-fidelity simulation. *Clinical Simulation in Nursing,* e1–e7. doi:http://dx.doi.org/10.1016/j.ecns.2012.06.001

Miller, G. E. (1990). The assessment of clinical skills competence performance. *Academic Medicine, 65*(9), 63–67.

Motola, I., Devine, L. A., Chung, H. S., Sullivan, J. E., & Issenberg, S. B. (2013). Simulation in healthcare education: A best evidence practical guide. AMEE Guide no.82. *Medical Teacher, 35,* e1511–e1530. http://dx.doi.org/10.3109/0142159x.2013.818632

Parsons, M. E., Hawkins, K. S., Hercinger, M., Todd, M., Manz, J. A., & Fang, X. (2012). Improvement in scoring consistency for the Creighton Simulation Evaluation Instrument. *Clinical Simulation in Nursing, 8,* e233–e238. doi:10.1016/j.ecns.2012.02.008

Patton, S. K. (2012). A pilot study to evaluate consistency among raters of a clinical simulation. *Nursing Education Perspectives, 34*(3), 194–195.

Polit, D., & Beck, C. (2012). Introduction to nursing research in an evidence-based practice environment. In *Nursing research: Generating and assessing evidence for nursing practice* (9th ed.). Philadelphia, PA: Lippincott Williams & Wilkins.

Rizzolo, M. A. (2014). Developing and using simulation for high-stakes assessment. In P. R. Jeffries (Ed.), *Clinical simulations in nursing education: Advanced concepts, trends, and opportunities* (pp. 113–134). Philadelphia, PA: Wolters Kluwer, Lippincott Williams & Wilkins.

Rosen, M. A., Salas, E., Silvestri, S., Wu, T. S., & Lazzara, E. H. (2008). A measurement tool for simulation-based training in emergency medicine: The simulation module for assessment of resident targeted event responses (SMARTER) approach. *Simulation in Healthcare, 3,* 170–179. http://dx.doi.org/10.1097/sih.0b013e318173038d

Rush, S., Firth, T., Burke, L., & Marks-Maran, D. (2012). Implementation and evaluation of peer assessment of clinical skills for first year student nurses. *Nurse Education in Practice, 12,* 219–226. http://dx.doi.org/10.1016/j.nepr.2012.01.014

Sando, C. R., Coggins, R. M., Meakim, C., Franklin, A. E., Gloe, D., Boese, T., . . . Borum, J. C. (2013). Standards of best practice: Simulation standard VII: Participant assessment and evaluation. *Clinical Simulation in Nursing, 9*(6S), S30–S32. http://dx.doi.org/http://dx.doi.org/10.1016/j.ecns.2013.04.007

Schaefer, J. J., Vanderbilt, A. A., Cason, C. L., Bauman, E. B., Glavin, R. J., Lee, F. W., & Navedo, D. D. (2011). Instructional design and pedagogy science in healthcare simulation. *Simulation in Healthcare, 6,* S30–S41.

Shinnick, M. A., & Woo, M. A. (2013). Does nursing student self-efficacy correlate with knowledge when using patient simulation? *Clinical Simulation in Nursing, 10*(2), e71–e79. http://dx.doi.org/10.1016/j.ecns.2013.07.006

Society for Simulation in Healthcare (SSH). (2014). *Certified healthcare simulation educator handbook.* Retrieved from http://ssih.org/certification/handbook

Tanner, C. A. (2006). Thinking like a nurse: A research-based model of clinical judgment in nursing. *Journal of Nursing Education, 45*(6), 204–211.

Thomas, E. J., Sexton, J. B., & Helmreich, R. L. (2004). Translating teamwork behaviors from aviation to healthcare: Development of behavioral markers for neonatal resuscitation. *Quality Safety Health Care, 13,* 157–164.

Todd, M., Manz, J. A., Hawkins, K. S., Parsons, M. E., & Hercinger, M. (2008). The development of a quantitative evaluation tool for simulations in nursing education. *International Journal of Nursing Education Scholarship, 5,* 1–17. Retrieved from http://www.bepress.com/ijnes/vol5/iss1/art41

Watts, W. E., Rush, K., & Wright, M. (2009). Evaluating first year nursing students' ability to self-assess psychomotor skills using videotape. *Nursing Education Perspectives, 30,* 214–219.

Wilhaus, J., Burleson, G., Palaganas, J., & Jeffries, P. (2014). Authoring simulations for high stakes evaluation. *Clinical Simulation in Nursing, 10*(4), e177–e182. http://dx.doi.org/10.1016/j.ecns.2013.11.006

Operations and Management of Environment, Personnel, and Nonpersonnel Resources

CAROLYN H. SCHEESE

By failing to prepare, you are preparing to fail.
—Benjamin Franklin

This chapter addresses Content Area 4: Managing Overall Simulation Resources and Environments (Society for Simulation in Healthcare [SSH], 2014a).

LEARNING OUTCOMES

- Discuss basic managerial and operational principles associated with delivering simulation activities; management of personnel and nonpersonnel resources
- Identify ways in which the physical environment can be modified to maximize simulation-based learning, including the use of timelines and checklists
- Identify common policies, procedures, and practices of an efficient simulation program
- Discuss effective ways in which one may respond to technical and material issues (e.g., video capture, simulator failures, material supplies) that may occur in the simulation environment

This chapter focuses on the management and operations of a simulation center, including the management of personnel and nonpersonnel (space, supplies, equipment, technology, money, etc.) resources. Whether large or small, completely outfitted with the latest high-fidelity technology or an outdated space stocked mainly with task trainers and low- to mid-fidelity mannequins, there are key operational principles that can apply to almost any setting. This chapter is divided into sections with multiple headings and is intended to serve as a guide and resource, not only to provide sufficient information to aid in passing certification examinations, but as a resource that you can come back to from time to time so you can improve planning, organizing, managing, and executing simulations in your center.

OPERATIONS MANAGEMENT: WHAT IS OPERATIONS?

Operations management is the process of managing and coordinating all resources—personnel and nonpersonnel—and coordinating and managing them in such a way that they are used efficiently and effectively to meet the goals and mission of the institution. Operations provides the support and infrastructure to get things done; it is considered the business side of simulation. Business operations usually includes four key aspects

1. The physical space (location)
2. Equipment and supplies (tools)
3. Personnel (people)
4. Policies, procedures, and processes (Peterson, Jaret, & Schenck, 2013)

Operations is the coordination and management of the many support pieces that are required to put a plan into place, and then execute that plan.

SCHEDULING

Scheduling of the space, personnel, and equipment is one of the biggest challenges and headaches of a simulation center because scheduling events involves a complex set of rules and variables. Scheduling involves matching personnel (faculty, students, volunteers, staff, information technology [IT] support, etc.) and nonpersonal resources (space, technology, mannequins, supplies, etc.) with dates and times. Throughout this section, you will note that scheduled items are referred to as "events." Events can include many things: a simulation scenario, open house or VIP tour, meeting with faculty/instructors, standardized patient (simulated patient [SP]) training, an objective structured clinical examination (OSCE), skills lab training session, open lab time for students, or center closures to install or maintain equipment. Each of these events is unique, yet all require the coordination of personnel and nonpersonnel resources within a date and time.

Methods to Track Scheduling

Many different methods may be used to schedule and track simulation center activities. Paper-and-pencil office scheduling ledgers are available for a minimal cost and may meet the needs of a small center with just a few activities or events per day. Ideally, keep all various pieces related to an event in one location; having items in multiple locations can be frustrating and lead to lost or missing information critical to the event's success.

Advantages of pen–paper scheduling are that it is inexpensive, portable, and easy to use and update. Limitations to this method include

- Limited access—only one person has access to the ledger at a time
- The ledger could become lost, making it difficult to reconstruct upcoming events
- As a center grows, this system can be time-intensive to manage and maintain
- Limited information can be written in the ledger, which may require additional support methods to manage event information, such as the final confirmed date and time, names of students, scenario details, and other resources

Schedules can be maintained through a variety of electronic methods, some of which are free or very low cost such as Google and Outlook Calendars or home-grown methods, whereas other commercially available event managers and scheduling products may cost up to several tens of thousands of dollars. The available features vary according to the product. Some advantages of commercial products may include the following.

- Calendar sharing: greater access and knowledge related to the simulation center-scheduled events because these products can frequently be shared and may have varying levels of access and privileges, according to the audience who is viewing the calendar, such as view-only and full-scheduling rights
- The ability to link communication/e-mails and event information to the scheduled event
- Some systems include the ability to track students, personnel, space, supplies, and equipment to generate detailed invoices reflecting event and center costs
- Some systems house the pre-work and allow instructors access to student and scenario information remotely
- Some systems allow self-registration and automatic event reminders and allow students and faculty to sign in to the center upon arrival (Scheese, 2013)

Scheduling and maintaining the schedule so that the information is disseminated to the level needed for implementation can take a lot of time. So, although the cost of an electronic event manager may be high, it can potentially generate cost savings by saving time and decreasing frustration as well as increase quality and event consistency (Exhibit 20.1).

EXHIBIT 20.1

What to Consider When Scheduling

- Mission
- Priorities
- Resource limits
- Personnel
- Knowledge and skills/skill level
- Availability
- Nonpersonnel
- Physical space
- Equipment/supplies

The Scheduler

The individual who is responsible for the scheduling calendar is potentially one of the most powerful individuals in the center. This individual is your public relations officer. He or she is often the first individual with whom your customers interact. He or she is the face of the business, a gatekeeper who can deter or encourage the use of the center by the very manner in which he or she interacts with those who contact the center. How the scheduler's power is used and managed will to a large extent determine accessibility to the center. If someone is unable to schedule an event, or if the hassle factor is too high or negative in nature, customers will go elsewhere. It stands to reason that unless events are scheduled, you won't run events. Understanding your customers and providing good customer service from the very first encounter is essential to sustained success (Scheese, 2013).

> A business absolutely devoted to service will have only one worry about profits. They will be embarrassingly large.
>
> —Henry Ford

The schedule is a linchpin. The scheduling calendar holds all the information together so that a successful event can occur. A poorly managed schedule creates inefficiencies and frustration for those who use the center as well as those who support the events. An ideal scheduler is detail oriented, good at organizing content and information, proactive, a good communicator, and willingly accepts direction.

Block Scheduling

Block scheduling has been used for many years in operating rooms (ORs) and surgical centers to provide predictability for the "end user" and the facility (Fei, Meskens, & Chu, 2009). Simulation centers have many common elements with these facilities and may benefit from this method of scheduling events. Block scheduling consists of providing/setting aside a block of days or times for an end user. An end user in this situation could refer to a faculty member, course, class, or pass-off/exam where there is predictability in the need for resources. For example, medical students in your center may have OSCEs every 6 weeks. Scheduling these events out even as far as 1 year in advance makes sense, if supporting the education of medical students is consistent with the center's mission. Using block scheduling, SPs, space, staff, and faculty/instructor support may also be scheduled out into the future and made predictable.

The greater the predictability in the schedule, the easier it is to adjust for minor changes and challenges that come along. Block scheduling is based on the principle that if you schedule your highest priority customers first, you can work the lower priority customers into the vacancies that exist.

First, determine what groups have priority and why. This can be determined by an oversight committee and should be consistent with the center's mission, vision, and values. One method is to classify users into three groups, according to definitions of priority: A, B, and C and to schedule As first and Bs second, followed by Cs.

CASE STUDY 20.1

An event that uses SPs will run all day long, 8 hours, for a total of 14 cases. What items should be considered when scheduling this event? Breaks, attire, length and complexity of case, and nature of the case—whether it is invasive or not. SPs' rights—they have the right to be treated with respect and the right to refuse to continue a simulation experience.

Sharing space and other available resources can be challenging. It takes negotiation and open communication. Like filling a jar with various sizes of rocks, pebbles, and sand, if you put the rocks in first, starting with the largest, followed by the pebbles and last of all the sand, then the jar can hold the maximum amount of material. This principle can be applied to scheduling. Fill the schedule with the largest (priority) users first, then fit your other users around them to maximize the capacity of the center.

Disadvantages: This system can be abused and needs a check-and-balance system to be most effective. You may have some users who schedule block time and then don't use it, especially ones who do not cancel with sufficient notice to schedule other users. Users in the C group may feel frustrated at not getting their first choice, or prime slots. Again, assuring that the scheduling process reflects the mission, vision, and values of the center will help in the decision-making process related to this challenge. One way to deal with this is to reassess your users at regular intervals and reprioritize groups as needed. Clearly established policies will help all parties understand expectations.

First Come, First Served Scheduling

First come, first served is another philosophy that can be used when scheduling events. Simply put, customers and events are prioritized and scheduled in accordance to when the request is received. Using a hybrid or combination of both block scheduling and first come, first served is another way to manage the schedule. Regardless of the method chosen, it should be consistent with the mission, vision, and values of the center, clearly communicated to the "communities of interest," and supported by the policies and procedures of the center.

PREPARING FOR DELIVERY OF A SIMULATION EVENT

Preparation and organization are essential to the successful outcome of a simulation experience. Templates may be useful in scheduling events and writing scenarios. Timelines and checklists can be helpful in outlining expectations and organizing events from conception to implementation and final evaluation. Tracking and organizing scenarios can be done electronically, with a physical hard copy, or by a combination of both electronic and hard copies.

Clearly establish timelines and expectations with those who schedule events, so that there is sufficient time for all to prepare for the event (Exhibit 20.2).

EXHIBIT 20.2

Timeline and Checklist for a New Simulation Event

3 to 6 months prior to event

- Determine goals/learners/instructor support (overarching concept of event determined)
- Schedule space and major equipment and supplies needed to support event
- Schedule learners/instructors and support personnel
- Scenario/OSCE writing
- Order needed equipment and supplies

6 to 8 weeks prior to event

- Finalize number and begin to schedule SPs
- Verify request for ordering of any special supplies

4 weeks prior to event

- Finalize event/scenario
- Review plan with those who will be implementing and modify as needed

2 weeks prior to event

- Do a "walk-through": Facilitators/instructors and support staff meet together in the space where the simulation will occur and review the scenario; identify and resolve areas of question or concern or that need to be clarified or modified
- Train SPs 5 to10 days prior

Week of event

- Send reminders to participants and instructors
- Review need for and last-minute changes by facilitators/instructors
- Preevent evaluation and prework sent out and completed by learners

Day prior/day of

- Arrive early
- Set up room
- Team huddle/preprocedure checklist, verify room setup, and modify as needed
- Complete learner postsimulation evaluation and other postwork as assigned

Following the event

- All team members meet to discuss what went well and what can be improved
- Revise scenario and document changes as needed

Events themselves can also have timelines to aid in keeping the event on time and focused on what matters most. Both simple and complex events can benefit from timelines.

Checklists can be used just prior to when the simulation starts to verify that all items are set up and ready to go, much like the OR uses a checklist for a "time-out" prior to surgery or the airlines use a preflight checklist (Exhibit 20.3). This checklist can be a part of the huddle some centers use. The huddle is a short meeting just prior to starting the simulation to ensure that everyone is ready to go, to ensure a common understanding of the sequence of events, and to answer any questions any member of the team may have (Table 20.1).

TABLE 20.1
Simulation Event Timeline

TIMELINE	SEQUENCE OF EVENTS	RESOURCES: FACILITATOR AND ROLES
20 minutes	Orientation to environment Overview and expectations Prework Division of roles	Orient students to simulation room Collect consent from students Review prework, discussion, articles Use PowerPoints with prescenario videos Determine roles Review chart contents/divide into roles
10 minutes	Scenario 1—Patient needs blood Group B participates in scenario	Group A observational engagement
20 minutes	Debrief	All facilitators debrief
15 minutes	Scenario 2—Patient develops acute blood transfusion reaction Group A participates in scenario	Group B observational engagement
20 minutes	Debrief	All facilitators debrief
5 minutes	Wrap-up	Closing remarks, handouts, reminder to do postsurvey and confidentiality
Total time = 1.5 hours		

TRACKING CENTER ACTIVITIES

Simulation is expensive. Those who support simulation financially or by other means will want to know how their contributions made a difference. In business, this is referred to as ROI, return on investment. In other words, what was the benefit of the time, energy, and resources put into this event or center as a whole? In order to provide this information to those who invest in the center, it is important to track usage, productivity, and costs associated with the center. The following are just a few items that can be tracked for each event: number of learners, number of instructors, length of simulation (time/hours), supply costs, equipment and space usage, time required for event setup and breakdown, administrative and support time, and so on. This information can be tracked by individual events and then compiled at the end of the year as a portion of the annual report. Data is invaluable when it comes to asking for continued or additional financial support.

EXHIBIT 20.3

Prescenario Checklist

Simulation Event
- Scenario duration & number
- Sequence of events
- Anticipated end time
- Anticipated breaks/setup Δs
- Simulation room number
- Debriefing room number

Technical
- Video/camera setup
- Video debriefing needs
- Electronic files, location
- Smart board needs

Mannequin
- Type
- Preprogrammed/on-the-fly
- Position/location
- Moulage
- Fluids
- Name & allergy band

Standardized Patient (SP)
- Training/instructions
- Moulage
- Waiting/staging area
- Props/name and allergy band
- 2-Way radio/walkie-talkie
- Time cards/parking validations

Room Setup
- Equipment
- Supplies
- Electronic health record/bedside computer needs
- Props
- Bed type/gurney/crib
- Special needs?

Medications
- Label
- Name
- Dose
- Planned med error?
- Location: OmniCell/refrigerator
- OmniCell programming

Roles & Responsibilities
- Technical roles/responsibilities
- Faculty roles/responsibilities
- Confederate role needed?
- Adequate resources?

Other?

Reprinted with permission from Lassche and Scheese (2013).

Annual Report

Preparing and publishing an annual report is a way to report on and evaluate accomplishments, ROI of the center, to relay information to the many communities of interest and stakeholders, and to measure and track progress on goals. Items that may be listed in an annual report include changes in leadership, instructors, or personnel; income and expense reports; purchases of new equipment; grants received and processed; scholarship activities such as manuscripts submitted and published; type and number of presentations; center event utilization rates; and student/learner contact hours.

> **Simulation Teaching Tip 20.1**
> The number of students times the number of hours present for a learning activity equals learner contact hours.

Business Plan

The business plan is like a road map or navigational chart that provides a plan and summaries of information related to that business. This information may include the purpose and organizational structure of the business, company strategy, the existing market place, a marketing plan, a review of finances, and action plans with a timetable. A business plan can be used not only to help establish a business, but it can also be used to help improve operations, efficiencies, or provide a new direction (Fiore, 2005). It takes time and effort to develop a business plan, and it can be challenging because there are many difficult questions that have to be addressed when putting this plan together. However, it is worth the effort and one of the most important steps you can take for success. A written business plan can help a company stay focused on its purpose (Peterson, Jaret, & Schenck, 2013). Be realistic in establishing a timetable when establishing a new center. Recognize that it takes about 18 months to get a simulation center fully operational (SSH, 2014a). Even once a center has been established, the business plan should be revisited and modified to meet changing needs. The U.S. Small Business Administration (http://www.sba.gov) has many resources for starting and managing small businesses.

Strategic Plan

A strategic plan is a plan for the future that links present and future operations to the organization's mission, vision, and values. Strategic plans are commonly generated for 3 to 5 years into the future, but can be changed more frequently if the business climate is dynamic and in a rapidly changing environment. Annual and semiannual goals are generated to support and achieve the strategic plan. Strategic plans should be reviewed at least annually. Alterations in the marketplace and other factors, such as changes in an administration with a new direction or goals, may necessitate a change in the strategic plan.

Mission, Vision, Values

Businesses (yes, education and simulation can be considered businesses) often create a mission statement to define their purpose and priorities. Many times, but not always, a vision statement and values are also defined. A mission statement is a statement of purpose; it defines the institution's purpose for existence and its focus (Peterson, Jaret, & Schenck, 2013). Vision is the overarching view of purpose—where the company is headed. Key values may also be selected and defined. Examples of values include integrity, quality, collaboration, and so on. Mission, vision, and values help determine what projects to undertake and which ones to decline.

Budget

A budget is a spending plan. Costs must be planned and tracked. Depending on the size of your center, you may have a budget of a few thousand dollars, or in a larger center, your budget may be several million dollars or more. However, the principles of a budget remain the same. Revenue, or money coming in, must not exceed expenses, or money going out. All money coming in and going out must be tracked and accounted for. Costs are usually broken down into personnel and non-personnel cost or salary and nonsalary items. A budget should take into account the depreciation of equipment and plan for the replacement of durable equipment. Other considerations include software licensing and upgrades, equipment repair and maintenance, office supplies, and so on. Computers and technology have a very short life span, about 4 to 6 years. A state-of-the-art center, without a plan and budget to consistently and thoughtfully upgrade, repair, and replace old equipment, will quickly become outdated and enter a state of disrepair.

When creating a budget, plan for both current and future costs and needs. Consider the items that you need to request to keep your center going, not just now, but in the future. Work with your finance administrator or chief financial officer (CFO) to see how your institution can set aside money each year for anticipated purchases and to plan for the replacement of simulators, computers, and other technological devices and equipment. Consider the infrastructure; anticipate needs for growth and updates.

Determine the life span of the equipment in your center; then plan for its replacement. Staggering the replacement of some of these items over a few years can help to level out the cost of this in the overall budget. For example, if you have 21 computers that are aging and need to be replaced within the next 3 years, you can budget for 7 computers per year for 3 years. This can help to even out the overall budget. Likewise, cameras, mannequins/human patient simulators (HPSs), task trainers, and so on, and their life expectancy need to be considered and put into the budget accordingly.

Capital equipment is generally considered durable equipment that has a life expectancy of greater than 1 year and exceeds a certain purchase amount. The amount is usually determined by the institution. For example, it might be defined by an institution as $5,000. So anything that costs more than $5,000 would be considered capital equipment and usually has to go through different channels and processes in order to make that purchase. Some institutions require that all capital purchases go out for bid or may require at least three quotes from competing vendors. In simulation, most HPSs fall into the capital equipment request category of the budget. Don't be shy about asking for what you need to run a good program.

> Asking is the beginning of receiving. Make sure you don't go to the ocean with a teaspoon. At least take a bucket so the kids won't laugh at you.
>
> —Jim Rohn

Recognize that it may take a few budget cycles to get the things you need. Don't give up. Prepare yourself to speak knowledgeably about the proposed purchase and do your research so that you know what features you need and the expected ROI for learners.

One thing to keep in mind when considering approving expenses is learning the restrictions on various funds/revenue accounts. For example, money donated to the center may be restricted to a specific purchase, such as a crib, task trainer, or mannequin. Money from grants may also have strict limitations on how it can be spent. In academic institutions, there are many restrictions on what student fees, state funds, or tuition money can purchase. Tracking and accounting for each type of incoming revenue and the requisite expenses are very important. Misuse of funds may result in embarrassment, loss of trust, and even loss of employment.

Equipment and supplies can also be obtained by networking with those in your community who have access to outdated supplies and equipment. This can save a tremendous amount of money for programs that do not have a budget for these items (Lazzara, Benishek, Dietz, Salas, & Adriansen, 2014). Some equipment can be rented; refurbished rather than new items can be purchased at a fraction of the cost.

Simulation centers can obtain their revenue in a variety of ways, such as student fees, tuition, grants, donors, usage fees, and so on. Some are for profit, whereas others are nonprofit. A cost recovery center or recharge center is a center that is able to recoup costs by charging fees to users such that it is able to compensate the cost of doing business. Other approaches are called "pay to play." In order to use the center, you must first agree to pay. Often the payment is received upfront. No matter the source of the revenue stream, in order for a center to be viable, it must be sustainable. Expenses cannot exceed revenue.

PHYSICAL SPACE

As much as possible, organize the physical space of the center so that items are grouped according to similar supplies and convenient to the site or point of use. For example, locate all moulage supplies in the same area, and group all wound dressings or intravenous (IV) supplies together. Organizing the physical space increases efficiency, reduces frustration in not being able to find needed supplies

FIGURE 20.1 A shelf of labeled supplies.

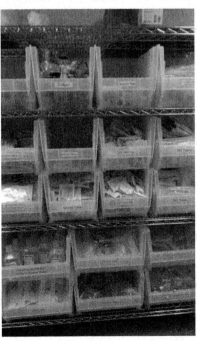

and equipment, and facilitates the ease of tracking the inventory of supplies and equipment. Label everything (Figure 20.1). Supplies for specific scenarios or skills can be organized and placed in containers with their specific inventory sheets/ required supply lists and instructions.

Keep reference materials, such as user manuals, policies and procedure manuals, simulation scenarios, skill equipment checklists, and so on, in a common area that can be accessed by all who may need these reference materials. Create logbooks to track capital equipment inventory, periodic maintenance, and repair histories that can be traced to a particular device/piece of equipment, such as a specific HPS. This history and tracking information is necessary if a piece of equipment ever malfunctions or needs repairs covered by warranty.

Quick setup guides can be created (or may be available from the manufacturer) and filed in a common area or attached to a device as appropriate. A short-list "quick setup"/"troubleshooting guide" can be written up in bullet points and attached to the equipment/device with clear waterproof tape or laminated and attached as appropriate for the end user. Be sure to include the sales representative's name, phone number, and manufacturer contact information.

Modifying the Environment

Assessing and modifying the physical environment is an important part of setting up a simulation. The physical space of a simulated environment can be modified to create realism. Our senses help us form memory. Sight, smell, sound, and temperature can all be a part of an engaging physical setup for simulation. Moulage can be used to create a more realistic experience for the learner. It can be a wig, a fake scar, vomit, urine, or blood, and so on. Moulage is an art that increases realism. Odors can enhance realism, too. For example, combining lemon juice and finely grated parmesan cheese with food coloring can create not only the appearance of vomit; it also has the odor associated with vomit. Sprays can be purchased that simulate feces, iron tablets can be added to fake blood to create odor, and a small amount of ammonia can be added to fake urine to create a realistic odor (Langford, n.d.). The presence of odors can enhance realism and emotionally engage the learner.

A simulation room at the Winter Institute for Simulation and Research (WISER), the Peter Winter Institute for Simulation in Pittsburgh, Pennsylvania, has several sets of ceiling-to-floor curtains with various images from the environment they want to portray, such as a scene of a big city for a group of emergency medical technicians (EMTs) or a scene of an OR, to help immerse their learners in the physical environment.

The Center for Advanced Medical Learning and Simulation (CAMLS, 2014) in Tampa, Florida, has a trauma OR that projects images on the walls, using sights, sounds, and temperature changes in the environment they wish to recreate to increase realism.

HPSs can be dressed in expected attire, and a few pieces of furniture or relevant objects may be brought into the scenario room. For example, the realism of a disaster scenario may be improved with the use of strobe lights and a fog machine.

A balance between learner goals and costs should be considered. Reviewing the goals and learning outcomes of the simulated event can provide clear guidance as to what is required and what is an unnecessary expense. For example, if there is a scenario that includes a patient-controlled anesthesia (PCA) pump and the center does not own a pump (but could rent one with tubing for a month for $350), reviewing the scenario objectives may help to determine whether it is worth the extra cost of renting the pump. If a key component of the scenario objectives includes the setup and use of the PCA pump, it may be worth the additional cost. If the pump plays a very minor role and the setup and use of the PCA pump are minor, then it may not be worth the extra costs. In its place, a mocked-up pump may work to achieve the learning objectives.

The greater the realism in sights, sounds, smells, and temperature, the easier it is for a learner to engage in the realism of the scenario. The use of prescenario video clips or briefs can be effective engagement tools. Of course, the learner has to be willing to engage and suspend disbelief, but the right environment makes it much easier than it would be otherwise.

POLICIES, PROCEDURE, AND PRACTICES

A policy is a brief description of a plan or standard that is used in decision making. A procedure is the step-by-step process or set of instructions outlining how to implement the policy. Procedures are usually used for complex procedures or for procedures that require detail and quality control. Processes are the manner in which things actually occur. Quality improvement assumes that there is a connection between processes and efficiency or quality care. Process audits can be done to evaluate current inefficiencies and to identify efficiencies (Marquis & Huston, 2012).

Every center should have formally written documents, including organizational structure and policies and procedures to help establish an understanding of expectations for facility users, employees, and the communities of interest/stakeholders. Policies can be either formal (written and sanctioned by a formal authoritative body [governing board or perhaps a guidance or steering committee]) or informal, based on historical actions. Written policy is best, as it allows for transparency and consistency. Writing policies can be very time-consuming and often require many drafts before a final policy gains approval, is agreed on, and implemented (Exhibit 20.4).

Basic organizational documents include

- Mission, vision, values
- Organizational chart
- Job descriptions with roles and responsibilities

Core polices should be consistent and support the mission of the facility whether it be research, education/teaching, assessment, or an integration of several of these (SSH, 2014a).

Basic policies, procedures, and processes include scheduling an event, managing tours, retention and access to video (how long video is retained/

EXHIBIT 20.4
Define and Clarify Processes
• What needs to be done? • Who will do it? • How will it be done?

EXHIBIT 20.5
Required Documentation for Accreditation
• Mission and governance • Organization and management • Facilities, technology, simulation modalities, and human resources • Evaluation and improvement • Integrity • Security • Expanding the field • Learning activities • Qualified educators • Curriculum design • Learning environment • Ongoing curriculum feedback and improvement • Educational credit

Adapted from the Society for Simulation in Healthcare (SSH, 2014b).

archived), resolving customer/communities of interest/stakeholder complaints, hours of operation, access to center and admittance criteria, loaning of equipment and supplies, costs/charges, and many others. Human resource policies and procedures may include dress code, payroll and attendance issues (clocking in, scheduling vacation, calling in sick, etc.), role and expectations, and so on (SSH, 2014a). Consider developing policies and procedures related to the accreditation requirements. It will provide a good foundation for your center, even if you choose not to go through the accreditation process (see Exhibit 20.5).

Physical Security—Locked Up

Simulation centers often contain hundreds of thousands of dollars worth of equipment and supplies. In order to protect this investment, security systems with alarms should be put into place and policies adopted that can achieve a balance between protecting the valuable assets and allowing entry into the facility in a manner that is consistent with the mission of the center. Some centers allow access to specific users 24/7, whereas other centers greatly restrict access to standard operating hours. For example, medical residents, desiring to improve their skills with laparoscopic surgery, are among those who may want 24/7 access to the equipment and supplies. Their hours are unpredictable and ready access to the center may be required to meet the needs of the user/learner. Clearly established policies and procedures, along with proper training on the care and use of the equipment are essential to preserving the investment and preventing costly repairs or replacements.

Separation of Simulated and Actual Patient Medications, Supplies, and Equipment

Simulation in situ is a simulation done in the actual clinical setting, for example, within an actual OR, emergency room, or critical care unit at a functioning hospital or clinic. This allows for maximum realism as related to the environment. Simulation in situ is particularly valuable in examining processes.

CASE STUDY 20.2

One center used in situ simulation to identify potential problems with a new policy related to responding to a critical patient incident. Through this simulation they were able to identify equipment and badge-access issues. Another facility used simulation in situ to keep their staff current in responding to codes and other critical patient events. What other applications can simulation in situ have?

When using in situ simulation, there must be a clear separation between actual patient information, equipment, and supplies, and those items used for simulation. Patient safety is of upmost concern. Fake medications and expired or unsterile supplies may be used in simulation, and must be clearly identified "Not for patient use—for simulation use." All simulated medications, supplies, and equipment should be clearly labeled to prevent inadvertent use on an actual patient (see Figure 20.2)

Personnel

"Personnel" or "human capital" are terms that may be used to identify anyone who is employed or volunteers for the simulation center. Personnel is a business's

FIGURE 20.2 Labeling props for simulation.

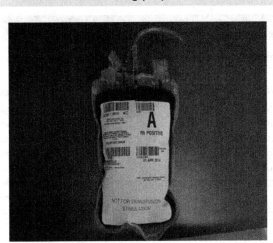

greatest resource because although equipment, supplies, and space (nonpersonnel resources) may depreciate and decline in value over time, personnel can continually improve and increase in value. It is the individual and collective personnel's talents, skills, knowledge, attitudes, and abilities that create the unique nature of each center. Not only are personnel the most valuable asset, they are the most expensive (Lazzara, Benishek, Dietz, Salas, & Adriansen, 2014).

Titles, roles, and responsibilities differ from center to center, but support of essential functions remain: managing, planning and preparing, implementing, cleaning up, and evaluating are all required support activities of a simulation event. Each center determines how best to meet the various needs of its unique center accordingly. Some common titles and roles of simulation center personnel may include simulation technology specialists (STSs)/simulation technologists, information technologists, computer support, faculty/instructors, student workers/teaching assistants, administrative support/secretary, simulation coordinators, managers, program directors, operations directors, administration, SPs /patient actors, and so on.

Stakeholders and Communities of Interest

Every simulation center has an impact on individuals and groups in their community. These individuals and groups are called stakeholders. Stakeholders can be internal or external. Internal stakeholders include people with a direct vested interest in the success of the center, whereas external stakeholders have an indirect interest in the success of the center due to the actual or potential impact of the center (Exhibit 20.6). Stakeholders can have a variety of goals and vested interests in the center (Marquis & Huston, 2012).

Together (the combination of external and internal stakeholders), these groups are sometimes referred to as *communities of interest*. This term, communities of interest, is frequently used in accreditation criteria and by accrediting bodies. These groups are important because they can provide valuable information on how well the center is doing at meeting the expectations of the communities of interest and center goals.

EXHIBIT 20.6

Examples of Stakeholders in an Academic Healthcare Simulation Center

Internal Stakeholders	External Stakeholders
Employees/staff	Local businesses/hiring hospitals
Administration	Accrediting bodies
Financial donors/grantors	Certification agencies
Learners/students	Community leaders
Instructors/faculty	Professional organizations
Board of directors/governing board	Alumni boards
	Malpractice insurance companies

VARIOUS USERS OF A SIMULATION CENTER

Depending on the physical structure, equipment, and personnel, simulation centers have many opportunities to serve various groups and users. A center can specialize, or expand to fit, several audiences depending on its resources. In healthcare simulation, a center may develop a plan to focus on a wide variety of customer groups or users, including interprofessional education (IPE), continuing education, nurse residency programs, certification pass-offs, research, and medical student and resident training and subspecialty training fellowships.

> **Simulation Teaching Tip 20.2**
> Evolving to meet the needs of your community can include purchasing equipment and supplies that are representative of those in the clinical settings in which your learners practice. It will decrease reality shock and the amount of time required to transition to the work setting.

IPE involves a simulated experience with one or more professions. SPs are individuals who are hired to portray a specific disease or condition with consistency so that learners can demonstrate their skills and knowledge in these areas. Training, high-stakes pass-offs, such as a required score to pass a course, or a certification required to obtain or maintain employment, are all other activities present in a simulation center. Centers may also be used to conduct research, not just research on simulations, but research on equipment and how it interfaces with humans, that is, device testing.

> In the end, you're measured not by how much you undertake but by what you finally accomplish.
> —Donald Trump

Managers and Administrators

Managers and administrators have many responsibilities that can keep them at the job for long hours, especially those who are involved in expansion projects, renovations, mergers, or if they are in the process of bringing an entire new center online. It is not easy to work long hours, beyond reason, for extended amounts of time. This can result in fatigue and burnout. Recognize your limitations and ask for the help and support you need. Document your hours and activities, and then review your accomplishments so that you can focus your time and strength on items that have the greatest ROI of time and energy. Align your goals and efforts with those of the upper administration or the board of directors to avoid a mismatch of expectations and resultant conflict. Eliminate those items that are not valued and focus on what matters most. As new projects are added, assess what can be handed off, simplified, eliminated, or negotiated so that workload can be brought back into balance. Administration sets the tone for the business as they control the resources; they determine the priorities and the degree to which quality and safety are emphasized.

Be like Switzerland; don't make enemies with anyone. It is a small world, and you never know when a critical and sensitive negotiation or partnership will depend on the relationships you have established and maintained. Don't view others as competitors. Figure out how you can help support the mission of your center. Look at "value added" by using the simulation center and consider it from the customers' or stakeholders' viewpoint: WIFM—What's in it for me? In other words, how it will benefit them (Center for Medical Simulation, 2011).

PERSONNEL AND NONPERSONNEL ISSUES

Personnel issues are any dealings that have to do with human beings. Nonpersonnel issues are concerned with anything that is not human. For example, equipment, supplies, hardware- or software-related items, and so on. Both personnel and nonpersonnel issues have their unique challenges.

Personnel issues may include

- Hiring
- Orienting
- Training
- Coaching
- Counseling
- Termination

Most centers can tap into human resources to assist them in many of these aspects. It is especially important to involve human resources in the hiring, counseling, and firing of employees so as to ensure that the laws and rights of individuals are not violated anywhere in the process. Each region, state, and country can have varying laws and employee rights. Those in human resources generally have the expertise in this area to ensure compliance with local requirements.

The first 90 days of employment are the most important time in helping the new employee understand job expectations and receive orientation and training for his or her position, knowledge, attitudes, and skills. Opportunities for continuing education and personal development support will help to keep the support staff energized about the role they play in supporting the facilitators and improving operations. Institutional review board (IRB) training for support staff involved in research may be necessary.

Counseling and Termination

Whether counseling an employee or a learner, some common elements should be present. Meet when you are both calm and have sufficient time for the meeting with the employee/learner; clarify and establish expectations, document these expectations, monitor and revisit as needed. If expectations continue to be met, no further action is required. If not, set a meeting during which expectations are again clarified, with documentation of missed expectations/misbehaviors and possible consequences of continued noncompliance, including probable termination/ failure. Be sure to include administration and human resources personnel in these critical meetings. It is important not to hold these meetings alone with the

---

EXHIBIT 20.7

Process of Progressive Discipline for Rule Breakers

The Progressive Discipline Process

1. Informal reprimand or verbal admonishment
2. Formal reprimand or written admonishment
3. Suspension from work
4. Involuntary dismissal or termination

Adapted from Marquis and Huston (2012).

individual who has the concerns. It can turn into a "he said, she said" scenario that is difficult to prove. Involving another individual can help ensure the message is consistent. He or she can also be there as a neutral party, as protection or as a witness (Exhibit 20.7).

When Things Do Not Go As Planned: Understanding and Responding to Technical and Material Issues

There is little as unnerving as when you have spent hours preparing the "perfect" simulation, only to have technical difficulties occur and completely throw you off the scenario. Blood pressure cuffs break, HPSs turn off automatically or lose connection, IV pumps go on the blink, and computers or cameras need to be reset. In addition to technology, learners can respond in unexpected ways (see Exhibit 20.8).

> It's not the people you fire who make your life miserable. It's the people you don't.
> —Dick Grote, *Discipline Without Punishment: The Proven Strategy That Turns Problem Employees into Superior Performers*

EXHIBIT 20.8

Unexpected Events

- Technology does not function correctly
- The learners misunderstand the objectives of the scenario
- The learners have difficulty suspending reality
- The scenario is too easy or complex for the learners' stage of education
- A learner does something that is not in the scenario and changes the progress or the outcome of the scenario
- Debriefing is altered because an unexpected event happened during the scenario

---

Adapted from Dieckmann, Lippert, Glavin, and Rall (2010).

How one chooses to frame or view these situations that can occur from time to time and how one responds to them will have a tremendous impact on the learner and the learning that can take place.

So, what is the best way to respond to these unexpected events? It is important to consider this in two phases, immediate and long term. What is the best immediate response, during the event and when the learners are present? First, consider the core learning objectives you have for the scenario, and as much as possible, use the unexpected event to meet the goals.

Scenario lifesavers can be delivered from inside or outside the scenario. Inside-scenario lifesavers use things from within the scenario used to influence the learners and the direction the scenario is headed so that they can return to the key learning objectives (Dieckmann, Lippert, Glavin, & Rall, 2010).

Dieckmann, Lippert, Glavin, and Rall (2010) suggest that if the unexpected turn of events is a safety issue for the learners or the equipment—such as the possibility of someone being injured with the incorrect use of the defibrillator—you can intervene by making an overhead announcement. This is called a lifesaver from outside the scenario. Another approach is to come up with a plausible background story as to why something may have occurred. This is an example of an inside lifesaver, because it is based on something that occurred inside of the scenario.

If the scenario has gone way off course, or there are critical technology failures, consider stopping the scenario and then restarting it so that the core learner objectives can be met. Lifesavers are also discussed in Chapter 5 of this text.

As a debriefer or simulation instructor, take a deep breath and collect your thoughts before you return to debrief the learners. The learners will often mirror the response of the debriefer. If the debriefer is flustered and complains, the learners will quickly pick up on this and join in, and a teaching moment is lost. On the other hand, if the debriefer is composed and positive, the learners can still walk away with a positive learning experience.

> How we choose to see things and respond to others makes all the difference.
> —Thomas S. Monson

Normalize the feelings of the group—share what it is that groups frequently feel or how they respond in this given situation. Normalizing helps to decrease the feelings of guilt and resistance.

During the debriefing session, as individuals point out the problems that occurred, agree with them quickly. Yes, there was a problem with item A; then quickly bring it back to real life and ask, could that ever happen in the actual clinical setting? Could item A stop working? What actions would be appropriate? What can be learned? Then, redirect the group back to the learning objectives. Agreeing with the learners quickly can diffuse the emotion surrounding the situation. Once the emotion is defused, learning can take place (Center for Medical Simulation, 2011).

What is the best long-term response to technical issues? Troubleshoot the item that caused the problem. Determine the cause, and get the item repaired or find a substitute or work around as quickly as possible so that this does not become a common occurrence. Reschedule other events if an acceptable solution is not possible. Include money for technology repairs in the budget. If the unexpected response comes from the learner, edit the scenario to prevent a recurrence.

> **CASE STUDY 20.3**
>
> The HPS suddenly turns off; the monitor has flat lines. The learner notices this, interprets this as a cardiac arrest, and calls a code. What possible responses can you have? What responses can keep you consistent with the key learning objectives?

Troubleshooting Equipment: General Information

When dealing with technology, troubleshooting has some standard steps.

1. Ensure all cable connections are secure
2. Ensure the device is plugged in/charged
3. Shut down the device and start it back up again
4. Refer to the owner's manual for troubleshooting
5. Call the sales representative/manufacturer
6. Repair or replace the defective item

Create a notebook to log all major pieces of equipment: their purchase, service and repairs, and problems. Document everything. It will become particularly useful if you have to make claims on the warranty of an item. Ensuring that all individuals who use the equipment are adequately trained will decrease the problems and breakage of equipment. Again, be sure to budget sufficient funds to repair and replace the equipment.

SUMMARY

Effective operation of a simulation center is based on principles of leadership, management of personnel and other resources, policies, procedures, and processes. Additional skills include effective troubleshooting when unexpected events occur and good judgment in influencing the scenario from inside or outside sources.

PRACTICE QUESTIONS

1. During a simulation, it is noted that some of the requested supplies and equipment are not in the room and available for learner use. What is the best initial step to take toward addressing this issue?
   A. Stop the simulation and ask the STS why the supplies are not available. Restart the simulation once the proper supplies have been obtained.
   B. Continue the simulation with the STS introducing the supplies and equipment into the scenario, stating that these supplies have just arrived from central supply for this patient.
   C. Continue the simulation observing how the learners adapt to the lack of supplies and equipment.
   D. Stop the simulation and begin the debriefing, explaining to the participants that this is a common occurrence and that they are the unfortunate victims of a poorly managed center.

2. During a simulation, the wi-fi connection to the baby HPS is lost, and the baby becomes unresponsive. The learners believe that the baby has gone into cardiac arrest and begin cardiopulmonary resuscitation (CPR). As a facilitator, what is your best initial course of action?

   A. Stop the simulation and attempt to reestablish the wi-fi connection while you give the learners a break.
   B. Continue the simulation and modify the scenario on the fly as the learning outcomes are related to crew resource management and can be met within this evolving scenario.
   C. Stop the simulation and debrief the scenario based on the objectives the learners have met. Use the debriefing time for the STS to attempt to reestablish connection.
   D. Announce to the students that the wi-fi connection was lost and to please continue the simulation with modified objectives.

3. The individual who schedules events (the scheduler) in your simulation center cancels a high-priority user and, in his place, schedules one of her friends' groups (a midpriority user) in the center. You are the director of the center, and you just received an e-mail complaint from your high-priority user. What is the most appropriate immediate action?

   A. Speak with the scheduler to find out why this action was taken.
   B. Reschedule the event for the high-priority user and cancel the second group.
   C. Do a resource assessment and, if able, negotiate so that both groups can use the center.
   D. Remove or severely restrict scheduling privileges until the scheduler undergoes retraining on scheduling policies and procedures.

4. An important tour is scheduled after normal working hours 2 months from now. Staffing this event has become a challenge because one of the employees in a leadership position has openly refused to modify her schedule to work for or support this event and has encouraged the other employees to refuse to work, as well. Alternate time off and compensation has been offered; their schedules are seldom modified. What resource can best help with this problem?

   A. Human resources personnel
   B. Resource allocation
   C. Benefits specialist
   D. Policies and procedures

5. During a scenario, the STS leaves the center, returning 30 minutes later. You are the instructor/facilitator and are upset because equipment malfunctioned and supplies were missing, creating a very difficult and stressful situation. You had expected the STS to be there to help you if anything went wrong. You are upset and have only 5 minutes to do something about this situation. What is the best course of action?

   A. Report this incident to the director and have her deal with the situation.
   B. Confront the STS, letting the STS know how upset you are at what happened.
   C. Ignore the situation; it just isn't worth the effort to try and resolve.
   D. Schedule a time in the near future to meet with the STS to discuss the incident.

6. Depreciation in relation to a simulation center's budget may be used for all of the following EXCEPT

    A. To represent the loss in value of a piece of equipment
    B. In relation to capital equipment
    C. In calculated loss of value based on the projected lifetime
    D. To represent supply inventory

7. While setting up for a simulation, you note that the HPS is not functioning normally. A few minutes later, it no longer responds to any input. What is the *best* initial course of action?

    A. Shut down and then restart the HPS.
    B. Call your sales rep.
    C. Consult the troubleshooting section of your user's manual.
    D. Check all cords and electrical plugs to ensure the connections are secure.

8. A recently purchased high-fidelity HPS does not function as intended for the third time this week. Each time this occurs, the HPS is turned off and then restarted, after which it begins to work properly. What action should be taken?

    A. Review the troubleshooting section in the HPS manual.
    B. Call the sales rep or manufacturer for customer service.
    C. Report your problems on Facebook.
    D. Accept the fact that this is a normal challenge when working with this HPS.

9. Recommended policies and procedures for a simulation center include all the following EXCEPT

    A. Center hours and scheduling guidelines
    B. Collections of prepackaged scenarios with debrief guide and checklist
    C. Video retention, archiving, and access
    D. Course of action to resolve customer complaints

10. A mission statement is

    A. A statement of global plans and goals
    B. The road map of a simulation center
    C. A statement that briefly describes the purpose for the existence of the center
    D. A comprehensive 3- to 5-year plan

REFERENCES

Center for Advanced Medical Learning and Simulation (CAMLS). (2014). *Surgical and interventional training center.* Retrieved from http://www.camls-us.org/core-components-overview/surgical-and-interventional-training-center-%28sitc%29

Center for Medical Simulation. (2011, November). *Comprehensive simulation instructor workshop.* Workshop held in Boston, MA.

Dieckmann, P., Lippert, A., Glavin, R., & Rall, M. (2010). When things do not go as expected: Scenario life savers. *Simulation in Healthcare, 5*(4), 219–225.

Fei, H., Meskens, N., & Chu, C. (2009). A planning and scheduling problem for an operating theatre using an open scheduling strategy. *Computers & Industrial Engineering, 58*(2010) 221–230. Retrieved February 28, 2009, from www.elsevier.com/locate/caie

Fiore, F. F. (2005). *Write a business plan…. in no time.* Indianapolis, IN: Que.

Langford, J. (n.d.). *Moulage recipes.* Retrieved from http://www.okhealthcareworkforce. com/Conferences/documents/JackieLangford_ArtofMoulage_Recipes.pdf

Lassche, M., & Scheese, C. (2013, June). *Effective team work—More than a game of chance.* Poster presentation at the 12th Annual International Nursing Simulation/Learning (INACSL) Resource Centers Conference: Hit the Jackpot with Evidence Based Simulation, Las Vegas, NV.

Lazzara, E. H., Benishek, L. E., Dietz, A. S., Salas, E., & Adriansen, D. J. (2014). Eight critical factors in creating and implementing a successful simulation program. *Joint Commission Journal on Quality and Patient Safety, 40*(1), 21–29. Retrieved from http:// static.squarespace.com/static/5121177ae4b06840010a00c1/t/531e013ee4b018be29 db8b98/1394475326808/Eight_critical_factors_in_creating_and_implementing_a _successful_simulation_program.pdf

Marquis, B. L., & Huston, C. J. (2012). *Leadership roles and management function in nursing: Theory and application* (7th ed). Philadelphia, PA: Lippincott Williams & Williams.

Peterson, S. D., Jaret, P. E., & Schenck, B. F. (2013). How to define operations in your business plan. In *Business plan kits for dummies.* New York, NY: John Wiley. Retrieved from http:// www.dummies.com/how-to/content/how-to-define-operations-in-your-business -plan.html

Scheese, C. (2013, June). *Strategies for a winning hand in scheduling.* Podium presentation at the 12th Annual International Nursing (INACSL), Las Vegas, NV.

Society for Simulation in Healthcare (SSH). (2014a). *Certified healthcare simulation educator handbook.* Retrieved from http://ssih.org/certification/handbook

Society for Simulation in Healthcare (SSH). (2014b). *Council for accreditation of healthcare simulation programs accreditation standards self-study review.* Retrieved from http://www.ssih .org/Accreditation/Full-Accreditation

Accreditation of Simulation Laboratories

and Simulation Standards

ANTHONY BATTAGLIA, FABIEN PAMPALONI, BETH A. TELESZ,
AND DEBORAH COLTRANE

*Learning by doing, peer-to-peer teaching, and computer
simulation are all part of the same equation.*
—Nicholas Negroponte

This chapter addresses Content Area 4: Manage Overall Simulation
Resources and Environment (Society for Simulation in Healthcare
[SSH], 2014a).

LEARNING OUTCOMES

- Discuss the importance of simulation laboratory accreditation
- Describe the accreditation standards of the Society for Simulation in Healthcare (SSH)
- List the seven standards of best practices in simulation of the International Nursing Association for Clinical Simulation & Learning (INACSL)

As simulation knowledge and theory have evolved, so too has the need to provide standards for simulation education. Today, a popular discussion throughout the simulation community is the pursuit of center accreditation to ensure that standards are met. This chapter provides information on the SSH accreditation process and the standards developed by the INACSL (2014). Both organizations are committed to excellence in simulation education. Both organizations are international and sponsor journals that contain up-to-date simulation teaching, research, and practice. SSH supports interprofessional membership, and INACSL is a nursing-based organization.

ACCREDITATION

The U.S. Department of Education (USDE) defines "accreditation" as "the status of public recognition that an accrediting agency grants to an educational institution or program that meets the agency's standards and requirements" [(R) 602.3, 1999, p. 1].

In the eyes of the public, accreditation is the promise to consumers that the simulation center in the hospital or educational organization has met the highest quality of standards in order for healthcare students to learn. These standards will ultimately be reflected in care provided to patients in associated hospitals.

Accreditation promises to put your simulation center in the spotlight, allowing it to be showcased as a premier center of excellence, which will resonate when opening the door for students, family, and public touring events. As a result, learning continuity, best practices, and standardized processes can be anticipated by Certified Healthcare Simulation Educators™ (CHSEs™), staff, and learners who use the center. In addition, accreditation will lead to

- Improved learning processes for the student
- Probable ease with budgetary preparedness
- Forecasting benefits
- Anticipated fixed assets
- Improvements in business operations

An understanding of the many benefits of simulation center accreditation can serve as a strong motivator to initiate the process. Improved patient safety is the ultimate outcome of center accreditation, and more studies are needed to support this outcome. One of the major benefits of accreditation is to create stronger opportunities for patient safety efforts that are sustainable through the support of standardized simulation modalities.

Developing a simulation laboratory into one that meets the standards of accreditation places the simulation educators in a mentor capacity. Expect to be the new target for other centers that wish to learn from and with you. This exchange of best practices and effective educational strategies fosters networking and mutual growth. Your center will be considered "a center of excellence" for national and international collaborations that may have never existed.

Once accredited, an observable transformation in CHSEs, learners, and community levels of confidence and belief in the quality of services and educational opportunities will be noted. In a society that has reservations about the care provided in today's hospitals, your center will be considered as a highly valid and reliable place where learners "want to learn," CHSEs "want to advance," and one that the community is "proud of."

> **Simulation Teaching Tip 21.1**
> "Accreditation, of course, does not come without determination, dedication and a true investment of time. It is a team effort and involves true commitment," says Dr. John O'Donnell, CRNA, MSN, DrPH, professor and director, University of Pittsburgh School of Nursing Nurse Anesthesia Program, associate director and co-director of Research, WISER (2014, personal communication).

From CHSEs to participants, a growing sense of ownership and enthusiasm will become contagious, and quality improvement efforts will follow. CHSEs will strive to find ways to continuously make improvements that will contribute to best practices and improved patient safety efforts that serve the center's mission, vision, and values.

To ensure success, Dr. O'Donnell (2014, personal communication) also advises the following.

- Designate a project manager who is highly efficient and organized
- Determine the area(s) in which your institution best qualifies for accreditation
- Prepare the appropriate documents to validate the category of accreditation you wish to pursue
- Understand the accreditation standards in each category in order to select the domain for which your center is best suited for accreditation
- Practice strong record keeping and progress mapping to prepare for application submission and onsite visits

Keeping these key principles in mind while reviewing the following standards will open up your pathway to successful accreditation.

THE SOCIETY FOR SIMULATION IN HEALTHCARE

The SSH was established in January 2004 to represent the rapidly growing group of educators, research scientists, and advocates who use a variety of simulation methodologies for education, testing, and research in healthcare. *SSH accredits simulation programs.* As standards and criteria are very specific, most of the following information was directly taken from the SSH guidelines describing the development of a self-study report that must be submitted for the consideration of accreditation.

The self-study report must address the core standards as listed in Exhibit 20.5 in the previous chapter. In addition, one of the following areas must be addressed: assessment, research, or teaching/education. A fourth area may also be addressed, which is "system integration and patient safety" (SSH, 2014b, p. 5). Complete criteria for each area that must be addressed in the self-study can be easily located on the SSH home page (http://www.ssih.org) using the "Accreditation" tab on the top toolbar of the site and using the "Full accreditation" option to locate the materials needed, which include

- An information guide
- A self-study guide
- Application instructions
- Application form

STANDARDS

Standards are established to promote best practice. Simulation programs that meet established standards provide the public with quality programs that are continuously critiqued and evaluated for best practice. The INACSL is an organization

> **EVIDENCE-BASED SIMULATION PRACTICE (EBSP) 21.1**
>
> In the United States, "clinical laboratories" are accredited. Clinical laboratories can be accredited by the College of American Pathologists (CAP) as often as every 24 months, and research laboratories that deal with chemicals can be regulated by the Food and Drug Administration (FDA) as often a three times a month. Many different types of laboratories have a long history of accreditation and regulation to keep them safe for employees and to keep their products and services safe for the consumers (Satyadi, 2011).

devoted to simulation education excellence and has developed best practice standards, which are published and provide an excellent guide for simulation educators.

THE INTERNATIONAL NURSING ACCREDITATION FOR CLINICAL SIMULATION & LEARNING

In 2011, the Board of Directors at the INACSL presented their first standards for best practices. The mission of INACSL is "to promote research and disseminate evidence based practice standards for clinical simulation methodologies and learning environments" (INACSL, 2014, p. 1).

The standards of INACSL accreditation were created, based on a detailed survey geared toward the needs and importance of maintaining an educational homogeneity among clinical practices. The developed standards were published in August 2011 in a special issue of *Clinical Simulation in Nursing* (Volume 7, Issue 4, Supplement, S1–S20). The seven standards of best practice outlined include (INACSL, 2014)

1. Terminology
2. Professional integrity of participant
3. Participant objectives
4. Facilitation methods
5. Simulation facilitator
6. The debriefing process
7. Evaluation of expected outcomes

STANDARDS OVERVIEW

Standard I: Terminology

Adopting a universal terminology is the main focus of this standard (INACSL, 2011a). No matter how many CHSEs are working in your clinical laboratory or the specialty taught in your scenarios, using proper terminology would greatly decrease miscommunication between participants involved in simulation activities. Also, by speaking the same language, CHSEs could constantly improve and ensure consistency in the teaching of simulation theories. *Standardized (simulated) patients, feedback,* or *debriefing* are good examples of terms that are encouraged to be globally and consistently used (INASCL Board of Directors, 2011a).

Standard II: Professional Integrity of Participant

This standard outlines the need for professional behavior and integrity in simulation education to ensure an optimal learning environment. Keeping learners focused during simulation activities can be very challenging at times, and this standard will help them understand the importance of giving each participant an equal learning opportunity. This standard emphasizes the need for the learning environment to be "safe," which means nonthreatening and free form incivility (INACSL Board of Directors, 2011b).

Standard III: Participant Objectives

This standard highlights the importance of using learning objectives to guide the learning experience in the simulation laboratory or environment. Learning should strive to promote clinical reasoning and critical thinking at the appropriate level of the learner. In order to accomplish these standards, learning objectives need to be written at appropriate levels and be measurable (INACSL Board of Directors, 2011c).

Standard IV: Facilitation Methods

Facilitation methods are the learning activities needed to ensure the best learning experience. Assisting students to reach the learning objectives helps them develop confidence in their ability to care safely for patients. A multitude of facilitation methods are available, and endless combinations of simulation strategies exist to promote learning. All activities should consider cultural or holistic beliefs because simulation education is a social experience that affects not only patient care outcomes but learners as well (INACSL Board of Directors, 2011d).

Standard V: Simulation Facilitator

Simulation education must be conducted by an educator who is qualified in simulation education in order to safely accomplish learner goals. An important responsibility held by the facilitator consists of supporting the learners and exposing them to appropriate learning opportunities using simulation. The presence of a skilled facilitator during simulation exercises will also help with unforeseen events and ensure a quality and complete educational learning experience for the learner (INACSL Board of Directors, 2011e).

Standard VI: The Debriefing Process

Debriefing is paramount to the simulation learning process and should be done by a qualified simulation educator. All simulation experiences should include a debriefing session in order for the student to reflect, analyze, and learn from the experience. Debriefing is the pinnacle of simulation learning and necessary to promote self-confidence in clinical decision making (INACSL Board of Directors, 2011f).

Standard VII: Evaluation of Expected Outcomes

Assessment and evaluation of the learning experience in relation to the set learning objectives are necessary to promote best practice. Simulation activities should be used to lead the learner toward the proposed outcomes in a safe and predictable environment (INACSL Board of Directors, 2011g).

SUMMARY

The prestigious recognition of accreditation or meeting standards brings a sense of accomplishment to the staff and simulation educators as participants reap the benefits of learning in a simulation center that has gone the distance and has reached either of these remarkable benchmarks. It is time to take your center to the next level and observe the leadership, learners, competitors, and the public marveling at your accomplishment. It is also time to embrace the new and exciting opportunities that will be presented following your certification. Your center will not only gain respect and admiration from the community, but will also enjoy the recruitment, retention, grant funding, and publication opportunities that will follow. This is an exciting time to be a member of the simulation community and to contribute to its success, development, and advancement.

CASE STUDY 21.1

A newly certified healthcare simulation educator is developing a strategic plan for his interdisciplinary laboratory. The laboratory is a converted skills laboratory in a school of physical therapy. The laboratory has been functioning for a year and has one laboratory technician. How would you advise the simulation educator to go about starting the process for SSH accreditation or meeting INACSL standards? What resources would you recommend to him? How long do you think either process should take?

PRACTICE QUESTIONS

1. A simulation educator is putting together a self-study report for accreditation. His coworker asks him why bother with accreditation. The simulation educator's best answer is

   A. "The provost will see what a good job I am doing."
   B. "The students deserve it."
   C. "This is an excellent simulation laboratory and it should be no problem getting accreditation."
   D. "The goal is quality and safety in patient care."

2. A simulation educator is developing a self-study report for an accreditation process and is describing a simulation about a rapid-response team. This should be integrated in standard

   A. Professional integrity of the participant
   B. Participant objectives
   C. Facilitation methods
   D. The debriefing process

3. Having a systematic plan of evaluation for ongoing excellence includes

   A. Aggregating data as evidence
   B. Collecting data
   C. Making changes based on data
   D. Developing a strategic plan

4. A simulation educator is developing a self-study report for accreditation and includes a section on personnel qualification; this information should be included in

   A. Assessment
   B. Research
   C. Teaching/education
   D. Systems integration

5. The mission statement of a simulation laboratory should be

   A. General so that changes are not noticed
   B. Congruent with the mission of the larger organization
   C. Included in the literature about the laboratory
   D. Detailed so that specifics are understood by the public

6. Protection of learners in the laboratory against Family Educational Rights and Privacy Act (FERPA) violations would be best included in which section of a self-study?

   A. Mission and governance
   B. Facilities, technology, simulation modalities, and human resources
   C. Integrity
   D. Security

7. A standardized (simulated) patient (SP) is doing a critical skills check-off evaluation of a learner. Which educational standard would this practice violate?

   A. Participant objectives
   B. Facilitation methods
   C. The debriefing process
   D. Evaluation of expected outcomes

8. A group of simulation educators are discussing the application for laboratory accreditation, and a member states that her new facility is state of the art, and it should not have to prove that the facility is excellent. The best response is accreditation

   A. "Tells the world how good our facility is"
   B. "Shows that we are experts, so everyone will know"
   C. "Demonstrates expertise in teaching"
   D. "Validates more than just the excellence of the facility"

9. When developing an accreditation self-study report, the simulation educator describes a student grievance incident and the due process that led to a resolution. This should be explained in which standard?

A. Organization and management
B. Evaluation and improvement
C. Integrity
D. Security

10. A key ingredient for a successful accreditation process is to have a

A. Consultant
B. Simulation educator
C. Project manager
D. Accreditation liaison

REFERENCES

International Nursing Association for Clinical Simulation & Learning (INACSL). (2014). *Mission statement.* Retrieved from http://www.inacsl.org/i4a/pages/index.cfm?pageid=3278

International Nursing Association for Clinical Simulation & Learning (INACSL) Board of Directors. (2011a). Standard I: Terminology. *Clinical Simulation in Nursing, 7*(4S), s3–s7. doi:http://dx.doi.org/10.1016/j.ecns.2011.05.005

International Nursing Association for Clinical Simulation & Learning (INACSL) Board of Directors. (2011b). Standard II: Professional integrity of participant *Clinical Simulation in Nursing, 7*(4S), s8–s9. doi:http://dx.doi.org/10.1016/j.ecns.2011.05.006

International Nursing Association for Clinical Simulation & Learning (INACSL) Board of Directors. (2011c). Standard III: Participant objectives *Clinical Simulation in Nursing, 7*(4S), s10–s11. doi:http://dx.doi.org/10.1016/j.ecns.2011.05.007

International Nursing Association for Clinical Simulation & Learning (INACSL) Board of Directors. (2011d). Standard IV: Facilitation methods. *Clinical Simulation in Nursing, 7*(4S), s12–s13. doi:10.1016/j.ecns.2011.05.005

International Nursing Association for Clinical Simulation & Learning (INACSL) Board of Directors. (2011e). Standard V: Simulation facilitator. *Clinical Simulation in Nursing, 7*(4S), s14–s15. doi:http://dx.doi.org/10.1016/j.ecns.2011.05.009

International Nursing Association for Clinical Simulation & Learning (INACSL) Board of Directors. (2011f). Standard VI: The debriefing process. *Clinical Simulation in Nursing, 7*(4S), s16–s17. doi:http://dx.doi.org/10.1016/j.ecns.2011.05.010

International Nursing Association for Clinical Simulation & Learning (INACSL) Board of Directors. (2011g). Standard VII: Evaluation of expected outcomes. *Clinical Simulation in Nursing, 7*(4S), s18–s19. doi:http://dx.doi.org/10.1016/j.ecns.2011.05.011

Satyadi, C. (2011). Overcoming challenges and hurdles of the clinical laboratory accreditation survey—Building a sustained and successful quality system. *Clinical Leadership and Management review, 25*(1), 6–10.

Society for Simulation in Healthcare (SSH). (2014a). *Certified healthcare simulation educator handbook.* Retrieved from http://ssih.org/certification/handbook

Society for Simulation in Healthcare (SSH). (2014b). *Council for accreditation of healthcare simulation programs accreditation standards self-study review.*

U.S. Department of Education. (1999). *Federal aid. Citations: (R)602.3.* Retrieved from http://ifap.ed.gov/regcomps/doc3983_bodyoftext.htm

Fostering Professional Development

in Healthcare Simulation

MARK C. CRIDER AND MARY ELLEN SMITH GLASGOW

Nothing happens until you decide.
Make a decision and watch your life move forward.
—Oprah Winfrey

> This chapter addresses Content Area 5: Engage in Scholarly Activity (Society for Simulation in Healthcare [SSH], 2014).

THE CONTEXT OF PROFESSIONAL DEVELOPMENT

Considering that members of any given profession maintain their professional status at the will of the society they serve, continuous professional expertise development is essential. To maintain professional status, Certified Healthcare Simulation Educators™ (CHSEs™) need to understand their service in the broader context of society.

Sullivan (2005) differentiates professionals from other knowledge workers because of their responsibility in the provision of public goods, such as healthcare. Specified as civic professionals (Sullivan, 2005), the work of these individuals provides added value to the public and is concerned with public values and identity. This then creates the social contract between the profession and the public in which the public grants status and authority to the profession for the service it provides within the society. A profession maintains the trust of society by maintaining civic contributions to society that remain current and beneficial through the profession's efficient and legitimate self-regulation (Sullivan, 2005). Opportunities for dialogue and scrutiny of the profession by society are expected, and thus the profession is compelled to continue to develop and grow in its civic contributions to society. This is accomplished through professional development activities by members of the profession.

As professionals, faculty and clinicians in a simulation environment develop and maintain specified standards of practice in the provision of simulation healthcare education to healthcare providers through their professional organizations and societies. These standards are developed through ongoing critical analysis of best practices in the field of healthcare simulation and are continuously updated through rigorous scrutiny of the discipline. Such updates are then communicated to members of the profession through professional development activities that allow the CHSE to maintain current in the discipline and meet its obligation to society as civic professionals.

STAYING CURRENT AND USING EVIDENCE IN HEALTHCARE SIMULATION

With an understanding of the importance of engagement in professional development by CHSEs, it is possible to explore how this can be accomplished by members of the profession. Staying current in practice is a matter of desire and curiosity. As professionals, the CHSEs maintains a desire to provide the most effective educational experiences to healthcare providers, who have a variety of learning styles. This desire is motivated by a curiosity that propels the CHSE to search for the most current evidence in the practice of its specialty. Keep in mind that evidence supporting development of current professional practice takes a variety of forms, including the development of techniques, interpersonal and intrapersonal skills, and leadership and management skills. Most significant to the professional development of CHSEs is the importance of maintaining communication and support among CHSEs. Independent, isolated professional development strategies must be further discussed among CHSEs well after the development event. With ongoing collegial support, professional development events will have a direct impact on the practice of CHSEs (Lee, 2011).

Evidence of this is noted by Guillemin, McDougall, and Gillam (2009) who recognized the importance of desire and curiosity in stimulating professional development, particularly in the health professions due to the ever-changing healthcare environment. They note that continuing professional development (CPD) provides the development of other necessary skills for success as a professional in the healthcare environment, such as communication. Also, as health professionals gain expertise within their discipline, there is a need for CPD in areas such as leadership and management. These authors focus specifically on the use of CPD in helping health professionals develop ethically (Guillemin, McDougall, & Gillam, 2009).

And yet focusing on professional development of the professional may be limited as discovered by Heller, Daehler, Wong, Mayumi, and Miratrix (2012). These researchers examined the relationships among professional development, teacher knowledge, practice, and learner achievement in a randomized study of 270 elementary school teachers and 7,000 students in 6 states. What the authors found was that professional development experiences may provide better educational outcomes when there is integration of learning content, student learning, and teaching. With this understanding, the CHSE is likely to benefit best from professional development activities that go beyond focusing solely on developing the professional, but rather by including exploration of knowledge acquisition and learner experiences.

An example of the use of evidence specific to the practice of the CHSE is provided by Brink, Back-Pettersson, and Sernert (2012). These authors provided an example of a simulated situation and the use of group supervision as a method in learning in the simulation environment. This was a qualitative study that explored participant perceptions of the simulated group supervision experience. Brink, Back-Pettersson, and Sernert found that participants demonstrated a sense of security in their engagement of the process, a positive response with collegial dialogue, a direct impact on values and attitudes, and a desire to further develop professional skills. Understanding this evidence, the CHSE can use the interventions used by Brink, Back-Pettersson, and Sernert to enhance his or her own practice in the development and provision of simulation scenarios.

Providing another example of the use of evidence to support the professional development of CHSEs, Roche, Pidd, and Freeman (2009) explored the need and use of workforce training in developing skills in health professionals. Although their work focused on drug and alcohol care, the concepts they presented are transferable to the professional development needs of the CHSE, specifically the need for development to include acquisition of knowledge, attitudes, and skills. As CHSE, it is important to use educational skills that are flexible enough to assess, develop, and adjust to any number of individual factors that influence a learner's ability to grow from a simulation experience.

Roche, Pidd, and Freeman (2009) also recognized that education and training occur within an overarching organizational system, rich with culture, policies, and procedures, which can serve to enhance or hinder the success of a healthcare simulation program. Thus, it is important for CHSEs to develop an understanding of organizational structures, systems, and culture, as well as the influence of policies and strategies that influence working conditions. This knowledge will help the CHSE in identifying opportunities within organizations to enhance his or her success.

PROMOTING AND LEADING EVIDENCE-BASED HEALTHCARE SIMULATION IN AN ORGANIZATION

As mentioned earlier, professional development includes a variety of topics. Understanding that healthcare simulation practices are most likely to occur within organizational systems, it is prudent for the CHSE to take advantage of professional development opportunities that enhance understanding of the context within which he or she practices. It has been noted that organizations can be considered to be social entities involving the interplay of individuals in reaching specified goals (Scott, 1998). In order for CHSEs to succeed within the structures of organizations, it is important for them to develop skills to navigate the elements of healthcare organizations.

Mulvey (2013) provided a perspective on the unique interplay among professional practitioners, their professional entities, and the employer as a triad in CPD. The CHSE needs to understand the tensions of all of these in order to effectively obtain and maintain resources, meet professional and organizational accrediting needs, and recruit and engage health professionals. An example of this is provided by Mulvey (2013); the employer focus is on finance, including the cost of training employees, their time away from work, and the coverage needed when the employee is in simulation training. The employer's other concern is the financial investment and the risk of training an employee who then leaves the organization (Mulvey, 2013). The CHSE needs to understand this fiscal perspective and be prepared to present a cost–benefit analysis within the organization system, shifting the employer's perspective to "What if she stays and is not trained?" (Mulvey, 2013).

An example of the importance for the professional development of CHSEs in organizational leadership is provided by Kubitskey and colleagues (2012). Their study identified that the attrition among teacher participants fell under three general categories

1. A teaching assignment change
2. Organizational challenges
3. Personal challenges

Understanding these challenges upfront provides the CHSE an opportunity to take a leadership role in addressing these during the development of proposals for organizational implementation. Further, this is an example of the use of evidence in the development of the CHSE. This study could be easily replicated to provide evidence of the positive outcomes of simulation education, thus supporting the cost-analysis benefits necessary for program sustainability within an organization.

Simmons and colleagues (2011) provided an example of the impact of an interprofessional educational program. The authors examined the use of five modules in teaching different topics using a variety of learning methods and teaching strategies. The authors noted the important role of immersion and experiential learning, interprofessional development in supporting practice, and anticipating change in educational and clinical practices. With an understanding of the evidence provided by Simmons and colleagues (2011), the CHSE can articulate to organizational leaders the significant role they can play in providing cost-effective educational programming, making a broader impact on patient care.

CULTIVATING AND COMMUNICATING ONE'S PROFESSIONAL DEVELOPMENT EXPERTISE

Continuous self-improvement and learning are essential to improve health. In order to acquire the requisite competencies, professional development competencies need to be integrated in all levels of the health profession's curricula along with the appropriate experiences and mentoring, as professional development is critical to advancing health. Healthcare providers need to learn to advocate for patients and engage in *crucial conversations* on behalf of patients in many instances. Crucial conversations are focused on tough issues, the conversations that people normally shy away from. In the professional realm, these conversations concern such issues as safety, productivity, diversity, and quality (Patterson, Grenny, McMillan, & Switzer, 2011). Healthcare simulation is an ideal forum to practice crucial conversations.

Professional development refers to a "positive change process" that healthcare providers experience in role performance, job roles, and better relationships with colleagues (Ismail & Arokiasamy, 2007). Safety, quality, and excellence underscore the need for healthcare providers to keep their skills and competencies current through ongoing professional development and career advancement (Adeniran, Smith Glasgow, Bhattacharya, & Xu, 2013). The influence of mentorship and self-efficacy on professional development deserves careful consideration.

Mentors provide their protégés access to social networks that include sources of knowledge and professional contacts not available through normal channels. Self-efficacy influences how healthcare providers set career goals, which influences not only the initiation of behavior, but also the persistence of behavior in the presence of adversity. Moreover, self-efficacious individuals accept their roles as protégés with greater receptivity and willingness to engage in professional development activities, enhancing their capabilities and competencies (Adeniran et al., 2013).

Self-efficacy as a concept evolved from Albert Bandura's social cognitive theory (SCT) of behavior (Bandura, 1977). SCT contends that individuals learn from the observation of others in a shared social environment. Learning occurs if the role model is relevant, credible, and knowledgeable. In the context of mentoring, protégés benefit from mentors who have the expert knowledge, social reference, credibility, and authority that lead to empowerment (Bandura, 1977). Self-efficacy is considered one of the most powerful motivational predictors of success in one's career (Abele & Spurk, 2009).

In the context of healthcare simulation, the organizational leader in simulation needs to use best practices and maintain currency in the field as well as serve as a role model. This can be accomplished in a variety of ways.

- Conferences
- Professional organizations
- Continuing education
- Literature on simulation
- Mentors
- Portfolio development

A list of resources, although not exhaustive, would include

- International Nursing Association for Clinical Simulation & Learning (https://inacsl.org)
- Society for Simulation in Healthcare (SSH; http://ssih.org)
- International Meeting on Simulation in Healthcare (http://www.ssih.org/Events/IMSH-2015)
- *Simulation in Healthcare* (http://journals.lww.com/simulationinhealthcare/pages/default.aspx)
- *Clinical Simulation in Nursing* (http://www.journals.elsevier.com/clinical-simulation-in-nursing)
- *Journal of Simulation* (http://www.palgrave-journals.com/jos/journal/v3/n3/full/jos200910a.html)

In addition, there are simulation conferences associated with academic health centers and universities and experts in simulation who can provide consultation. Specific attention to one's professional development in simulation can lead to increased knowledge, skill, and confidence in leading simulation scenarios in an organization. As mastery is obtained, the simulation expert has a responsibility to share the expertise via conferences, journal articles, and in a mentoring or consultant role.

THE MENTORING ROLE

Mentors support protégés to gain new competencies in a broad spectrum of skills, providing them challenges and opportunities to grow (Lombardo & Eichinger, 2009). Mentors promote learning and competencies that contribute to the healthcare provider's vitality and career success. Koberg, Boss, and Goodman (1998) found that those who received mentoring reported higher levels of self-esteem and confidence than nonmentored healthcare professionals. Further, mentoring facilitates critical thinking and forms a connection to practice, which supports professional development. Ultimately, this can influence healthcare. This is especially true in the faculty–student role with respect to simulation. Further, Walton, Chute, and Ball (2011) note that faculty, who in their respective roles function as role models and mentors, also need to use evidence-based teaching in their simulation activities to effectively convey the art and science of simulation. Walton, Chute, and Ball (2011) argue that faculty do not have adequate evidence-based resources on how students learn through simulation. They suggest the use of a midrange conceptual model, Negotiating the Role of the Professional Nurse, as this particular model of the professional socialization assists faculty in facilitating students' development during simulation learning activities addressing such concepts as

- Feeling like an imposter
- Trial and error
- Taking the role seriously
- Transference
- Professionalization

Faculty strategies for each concept phase include "validating students' feelings, debriefing with gentleness, role modeling expectations, asking questions about self-improvement, and assisting students with visualizing goals" (p. 301).

Benner, Sutphen, Leonard, and Day (2010) support a three-pronged approach needed in the professional role. These three attributes (Figure 22.1) are vital in the development of critical reasoning and professional development.

Additionally, fostering the professional development of healthcare providers requires experiential and situated learning, best conducted in a simulated environment, as these individuals must be prepared for the actual clinical situations or crucial conversations marked by uncertainty in the real world (Crider & McNiesh, 2011).

DEVELOPMENT OF THE PORTFOLIO

Packaging one's self to effectively communicate and capture one's work is very important to advance one's career. The professional portfolio/dossier is a vehicle to display one's work when applying for appointments, certifications, promotions,

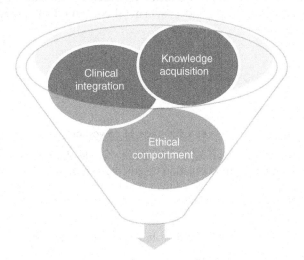

Figure 22.1 Benner, Sutphen, Leonard, and Day's three-pronged approach required in the professional role.

Professional role development

and tenure. A portfolio or dossier should include sample publications, grant submissions, awards, syllabi, evaluations, simulation scenarios, photos, and recommendation letters. A portfolio or dossier is also a practical way to reflect on and document one's work with respect to teaching, research, and service. The value of self-reflection of one's work cannot be underscored. The process lends itself to deep self-analysis—it provides a lens for the individual and reviewer to analyze one's accomplishments in the area of simulation (Seldin & Miller, 2009). In recent years, electronic portfolios have come into use in institutions as a means for students to display their work and demonstrate competency related to writing, clinical objectives, and so on. The portfolio should involve the efforts of the individual and the advice of the mentor in order to showcase the candidate's work in the best possible light in addition to providing the reviewer with insight into the candidate's strengths, accomplishments, and work. Many institutions have requirements for the portfolio in terms of format and content. Typically, a philosophy, objectives, examples of work, reflections, and so on are required at some level (Wittmann-Price, 2012).

SUMMARY

The process of professional development is best conducted in the formative years of one's education so that healthcare providers can have maximum impact on the healthcare profession. It is also known that professional development is largely

Simulation Teaching Tip 22.2
Professional development: Ensure that teachers "think out loud" and make their cognitive "struggles" with difficult issues visible to students so that students can see how one "thinks like a nurse" (Valiga, 2012, p. 423). Role model, role model, role model!

contextual—different settings will require different expectations and different practices. Therefore, a variety of professional developmental experiences is recommended in one's educational journey. Simulation provides a *dress rehearsal* for *real* leadership concerns, crucial conversations, ethical dilemmas, and advocacy issues.

CASE STUDY 22.1

Your Role

Colleague who takes advantage of coworkers

Dr. Sykes is frequently absent due to family obligations and is constantly asking you to cover the simulation healthcare experience that she is providing to occupational therapy learners. You have worked with her for 3 years, but this is getting old. She always has an emergency or an excuse. You feel as though you are being taken advantage of.

Note: This case can be adapted to any work setting.

Case Study Objective

Engage in a crucial conversation with your colleague regarding her behavior.

Checklist

- Objectively stated personal experience with concrete examples in a clear, concise manner
- Addressed personal feelings
- Used "I" statements
- Remained calm
- Listened actively
- Summarized crucial conversation that the colleague would no longer rearrange the schedule

---

CASE STUDY 22.2

Your Role

Mentor and faculty colleague for a junior CSHE

You are participating in a laboratory session with your colleague, Dr. Pinter, who teaches another section. You note that Dr. Pinter becomes very defensive and sarcastic with learners when they ask what you believe to be appropriate questions. At one point, Dr. Pinter is borderline hostile. You are embarrassed.

Case Study Objective

Engage in a crucial conversation with your colleague regarding her defensive and sarcastic behavior.

CASE STUDY 22.2 (continued)

Checklist

- Objectively summarized observations in a private setting
- Explicitly addressed unprofessional behavior
- Used "I" statements
- Remained calm
- Listened actively
- Role modeled appropriate way to respond to questions
- Offered faculty development resources
- Summarized crucial conversation that the colleague must maintain a professional demeanor and open/trusting learning environment for students and the consequences if not maintained

---

PRACTICE QUESTIONS

1. Professional development activities for simulation educators include all of the following EXCEPT

   A. Attendance at healthcare simulation conferences
   B. Membership in professional healthcare simulation organizations
   C. Obtaining a higher degree
   D. Reading journal articles on healthcare simulation

2. The professional portfolio/dossier is used for the following

   A. Appointments
   B. Certifications
   C. Promotions and tenure
   D. All of the above

3. Benner, Sutphen, Leonard, and Day support a three-pronged approach to health profession education, which includes all of the following EXCEPT

   A. Knowledge acquisition
   B. Career ladders
   C. Clinical integration
   D. Ethical comportment

4. A portfolio or dossier is also a practical way to reflect on and document one's work with respect to

   A. Teaching
   B. Research
   C. Clinical service
   D. All of the above

5. The development of critical reasoning and professional development is best addressed via

   A. Healthcare simulation
   B. Didactic classroom sessions
   C. Role-playing
   D. Professional portfolio development

6. The process of professional development is best conducted in

   A. The formative years of healthcare education
   B. Doctoral study
   C. Clinical environment
   D. Continuing education

7. Simulation is the most appropriate pedagogy for addressing

   A. Crucial conversations
   B. Résumé building
   C. Career ladders
   D. Content deficits

8. Which of the following is considered one of the most powerful motivational predictors of success in one's career?

   A. Education
   B. Self-efficacy
   C. Advocacy
   D. Occupation

9. The simulation expert has a responsibility to share expertise via a

   A. Mentoring or consultant role
   B. Clinical ladder
   C. Advocacy role
   D. Ethics training

10. The engagement in professional development by simulation educators is best evaluated by

   A. Use of evidence-based simulation strategies
   B. Subscription to a professional journal
   C. Attendance at health-related conferences
   D. Attendance in a graduate program

REFERENCES

Abele, A. E., & Spurk, D. (2009). The longitudinal impact of self-efficacy and career goals on objective and subjective career success. *Journal of Vocational Behavior, 74*(1), 53–62.

Adeniran, R., Smith Glasgow, M. E., Bhattacharya, A., & Xu, Y. (2013). Career advancement and professional development in nursing. *Nursing Outlook, 61,* 437–446. Retrieved from http://dx.doi.org/10.016j.outlook.2013.05.009

Bandura, A. (1977). Self-efficacy: Toward a unifying theory of behavioral change. *Psychological Review, 84*, 191–215.

Benner, P. (2012). Educating nurses: A call for radical transformation—How far have we come? (Guest Editorial). *Journal of Nursing Education, 51*(4), 183–184.

Brink, P., Back-Pettersson, S., & Sernert, N. (2012). Group supervision as a means of developing professional competence within pre-hospital care. *International Emergency Nursing, 20*(2), 76–82. doi:http://dx.doi.org/10.1016/j.ienj.2011.04.001

Crider, M., & McNiesh, S. (2011). Integrating a professional apprenticeship model with psychiatric clinical simulation. *Journal of Psychosocial Nursing & Mental Health Services, 49*(5), 42–49. doi:10.3928/02793695-20110329-01

Guillemin, M., McDougall, R., & Gillam, L. (2009). Developing "ethical mindfulness" in continuing professional development in healthcare: Use of a personal narrative approach. *Cambridge Quarterly of Healthcare Ethics, 18*, 197–208. doi:10.1017/S0963180 10909032X

Heller, J. I., Daehler, K. R., Wong, N., Mayumi, S., & Miratrix, L. W. (2012). Differential effects of three professional development models on teacher knowledge and student achievement in elementary science. *Journal of Research in Science Teaching, 49*(3), 333–362. doi: http://dx.doi.org/10.1002/tea.2100

Ismail, M., & Arokiasamy, L. (2007). Exploring mentoring as a tool for career advancement of academics in private higher education institutions in Malaysia. *Journal of International Social Research, 1*(1), 135–148.

Koberg, C. S., Boss, R. W., & Goodman, E. (1998). Factors and outcomes associated with mentoring among health-care professionals. *Journal of Vocational Behavior, 53*(1), 58–72.

Kubitskey, B. W., Vath, R. J., Johnson, H. J., Fishman, B. J., Konstantopoulos, S., & Park, G. J. (2012). Examining study attrition: Implications for experimental research on professional development. *Teaching and Teacher Education, 28*(3), 418–427. doi:http://dx.doi .org/10.1016/j.tate.2011.11.008

Lee, N. (2011). An evaluation of CPD learning and impact upon positive practice change. *Nurse Education Today, 31*(4), 390–395. doi:http://dx.doi.org/10.1016/j.nedt.2010.07 .012

Lombardo, M. M., & Eichinger, R. W. (2009). *FYI for your improvement: A guide for development and coaching* (5th ed). Minneapolis, MN: Lominger International: A Korn/Ferry Company.

Mulvey, R. (2013). How to be a good professional: Existentialist continuing professional development (CPD). *British Journal of Guidance & Counseling, 41*(3), 267–276. doi:10.108 0/03069885.2013.773961

Patterson, K., Grenny, J., McMillan, R., & Switzer, A. (2011). *Crucial conversations: Tools for talking when the stakes are high*. New York, NY: McGraw-Hill.

Roche, A. M., Pidd, K., & Freeman, T. (2009). Achieving professional practice change: From training to workforce development. *Drug and Alcohol Review, 28*(5), 550–557.

Scott, W. R. (1998). *Organizations: Rational, natural, and open systems*. Englewood Cliffs, NJ: Prentice Hall.

Seldin, P., & Miller, J. E. (2009). *The academic portfolio: A practical guide to teaching, research, and service*. San Francisco, CA: Jossey-Bass.

Simmons, B., Oandasan, I., Soklaradis, S., Esdaile, M., Barker, K., Kwan, D., & Wagner, S. (2011). Evaluating the effectiveness of an interprofessional education faculty development course: The transfer of interprofessional learning to the academic and clinical practice setting. *Journal of Interprofessional Care, 25*(2), 156–157. doi:http://dx.doi.org /10.3109/13561820.2010.515044

Society for Simulation in Healthcare (SSH). (2014). *Certified healthcare simulation educator handbook*. Retrieved from http://ssih.org/certification/handbook

Sullivan, W. M. (2005). *Work and integrity: The crisis and promise of professionalism in America* (2nd ed.). San Francisco, CA: Jossey-Bass.

Valiga, T. (2012). Nursing education trends: Future implications and predictions. *Nursing Clinics of North America, 47*(4), 423–434.

Walton, J., Chute, E., & Ball, L. (2011). Negotiating the role of the professional nurse: The pedagogy of simulation: A grounded theory study. *Journal of Professional Nursing, 27*(5), 299–310.

Wittmann-Price, R. A. (2012). *Fast facts for developing a nursing academic portfolio.* New York, NY: Springer Publishing Company.

The Role of Research in Simulation

JUDY I. MURPHY

If we knew what it was we were doing,
it would not be called research, would it?
—Albert Einstein

This chapter addresses Content Area 5: Engage in Scholarly Activity (Society for Simulation in Healthcare [SSH], 2014).

LEARNING OUTCOMES

- Discuss the importance of research in simulation for healthcare educators
- Identify the current state of simulation research
- Identify gaps in simulation research
- Discuss research knowledge via case study and practice questions

Although healthcare simulation has been around for more than 40 years, its movement to the forefront in academe and practice is fairly recent. Simulation literature and research are increasing at an astounding rate. Yet, there are many things that we don't know. This chapter discusses the importance of research in simulation, provides a summary of the current state of the research on simulation, identifies gaps in the literature, and provides Teaching Tips and application exercises.

One of the hottest topics being debated and studied is "How much clinical time can be substituted with simulation?" Several state boards of nursing have limited the number of hours of simulation that can be substituted for clinical time. In 2010, the National Council of State Boards of Nursing (NCSBN) surveyed 1,729 nursing programs in the United States (Hayden, 2010; Kardong-Edgren, Wilhaus, Bennett, & Hayden, 2012). Sixty-two percent of the programs from all 50 states and the District of Columbia responded. Overall, 87% reported using either high or medium fidelity in their programs. Fifty-five percent used simulation in five or more courses. The response to the question of whether simulation can or should replace clinical time was affirmative by 77% of respondents. Faculty indicated that 25% of clinical time could be replaced with simulation. However, some state boards of nursing require that a specific amount of time be spent in direct care. In Ohio, simulation hours cannot be counted as clinical hours, whereas in Florida, no more than 25% of clinical time can be replaced with clinical simulation.

Using Weinger's conceptual framework (2010), the pharmacology of simulation to inform simulation research, we still do not know the best dose of simulation needed to get the best response from the learners. The need to answer these questions will be a driving force in simulation research as research findings support the use of simulation, its effectiveness, and its relationship to patient safety. For this review, the current state of the research on simulation is divided into the three components of simulation: pre-briefing/orientation, simulation, and debriefing.

PRE-BRIEFING

According to Standards of Best Practice: Simulation Standard I: Terminology of the International Nursing Association for Clinical Simulation & Learning (INACSL), pre-briefing is "an orientation session held prior to the start of a simulation-based learning experience in which instructions of preparatory information is given to participants. The purpose of the pre-briefing or briefing is to set the stage for a scenario and assist participants in achieving scenario objectives. Suggested activities . . . include an orientation to the equipment, environment, roles, time allotment, objectives and patient situation" (Meakim et al., 2013, p. S7).

Pre-briefing is important to set the tone and focus learners on the main objective, which is learning. Healthcare professionals tend to focus on performance outcomes rather than learning. Learners are disappointed if they do not meet their performance expectations. Standard II: Professional Integrity of Participants (Gloe et al., 2013, p. S13) outlines guidelines and criteria that are essential to support mutual respect, professional integrity, and confidentiality. What happens in simulation and debriefing stays in simulation and debriefing. If learners fear that their performance will be discussed outside of simulation, they will be more anxious and will focus on the outcome of simulation rather than learning (Dieckmann, Molin Friis, Lippert, & Ostergaard, 2009).

Anxiety is a common emotion expressed by learners participating in simulation. Cato (2013) found that high learner anxiety related to simulation was associated with fear of making a mistake, being filmed, being observed by faculty and peers, and discriminating between what is real and what is simulation. Preparation was identified as being critically important to confidence in simulation. Learners in this study requested that they be alerted as to what skills will be used in a simulation in advance so they could practice if needed.

> **Simulation Teaching Tip 23.1**
> Healthcare simulation educators are usually not aware of recent or past life experiences of learners that may influence how they respond in simulation. Has a loved one been in the intensive care unit recently, or has there been a death in the family? Learners need to be briefed early on that simulation may trigger some strong emotions for them. Because research shows that observers learn as much as participants (Jeffries, 2012), learners should be given the option to observe rather than participate in a simulation that may be an emotional trigger.

Facilitators to learning from simulation identified by learners include

- Orientation
- Preparation
- Safe environment
- Feedback during debriefing

There is very little research on the effect of pre-briefing/orientation on student learning. Cato's recent unpublished doctoral research provides initial evidence as to the importance of adequate preparation prior to a simulation.

SIMULATION

Simulation is a method of pedagogy using one or more typologies to promote, improve, or validate a participant's progression from novice to expert (Benner, 1984; Decker, 2007). According to the National League for Nursing (NLN) and Jeffries's theoretical framework, simulation has five components

1. Teacher
2. Learner
3. Educational practices
4. Design characteristics
5. Simulation interventions and outcomes (Ravert & McAfooes, 2013)

For the purpose of this review, this section focuses on outcomes of simulation. A systematic review of simulation research conducted by Cant and Cooper (2010) provides an extensive evaluation of the evidence behind simulation as an educational tool in nursing. The review includes 12 quantitative studies that compared the effectiveness of medium- to high-fidelity simulations compared to other methods of education, such as lecture, group interaction, case studies, debriefings, or tests.

Only one study was a randomized controlled trial; most were pre- and post-test experiments with a comparison group. Seven studies included a validated assessment measure. The authors found that "all 12 studies reported statistical improvements in knowledge, skill, critical thinking ability and/or confidence after simulation education" (Cant & Cooper, 2010, p. 6). Kirkpatrick's evaluation model (2006) is used to present examples of research on evaluation. In Kirkpatrick's model, the four levels of evaluation consist of

1. Reaction
2. Learning
3. Behavior
4. Results

Learner satisfaction and self-confidence (Level 1), both reactions to simulation, are the measures that have been the most heavily researched. Learners' reaction to simulation has been overwhelmingly positive (Jeffries, 2012). According to

Chickering and Gamson (1987), learner performance is higher when learners are satisfied with learning experiences. In simulation, students learn to think critically and solve problems in a safe environment. They can make mistakes, from which they will learn without putting patients at risk. The opportunity to be "the nurse" instead of the learner helps to promote self-confidence. In a comparative study, Alfes (2011) found that learners who participated in a simulation were more self-confident than the control group.

Kirkpatrick's learning (Level 2) has been measured in cognitive (Lasater, 2007; Radhakrishnan, Roche, & Cunningham, 2007), affective (Bambini, Washburn, & Perkins, 2009; Schoening, Sittner, & Todd, 2006), and psychomotor domains (Murray, et al., 2007; Rosen, Salas, Silvestri, Wu, & Lazarra, 2008). In all of these simulation studies, significant learning occurred when best practices of simulation were used. Lasater (2007) developed a rubric to measure clinical judgment by scoring learners on a scale that rated

- Noticing
- Interpreting
- Responding
- Reflecting

Learners were rated as beginning, developing, accomplished, or exemplary on this tool.

Radhakrishnan and colleagues (2007) developed the Clinical Simulation Evaluation Tool (CSET), a clinical performance tool, to measure

- Basic and problem-based assessment
- Prioritization
- Delegation
- Communication
- Interventions and safety

When measuring learning in the cognitive domain, it is important to design the simulation so that learners will be able to demonstrate learning by applying knowledge to make decisions in the scenario.

Evaluation in the affective domain is more subjective. Affective learning and Kirkpatrick's reaction (Level 1) overlap. Many authors have developed both quantitative and qualitative instruments to measure learners' perceptions of simulation. Bambini and colleagues (2009) measured confidence before and after a simulation. Likewise, Schoening and colleagues (2006) also measured learners' perceptions of a maternal–child simulation. Although the literature shows (Bandura, 2000; Zimmerman, 2000) that self-efficacy has been a predictor of learners' motivation and learning, simulation research is lacking in making the connection.

Studies in the psychomotor domain measure a range of skills from basic to complex. There is an overlap between the cognitive and psychomotor domain because one must have the knowledge in order to complete the skill (Adamson, Jeffries, & Rogers, 2012). Instruments to measure performance of medical learners and medical residents were developed by Rosen and colleagues (2008) and Murray and colleagues (2007). Both instruments were specifically designed for performance measurement in simulation. Although these psychomotor tools are specific to medical skills, the American Heart Association Basic Life Support (BLS) and Advanced Cardiac Life Support (ACLS) performance tools may be used for research across professions.

Kirkpatrick's last two levels, behavior (3) and results (4) have not been studied as extensively as satisfaction and learning. Behavior measures change in job performance resulting from the learning process, whereas results measure the tangible outcome of the learning process in relation to cost, quality, and efficiency. Collectively, this work is considered translational science (McGaghie, Issenberg, Petrusa, & Scalese, 2010). In the critical review of simulation-based medical education research of McGaghie and colleagues, the researchers found that studies that show transfer to practice outcomes are difficult to design and execute. Some promising work in this regard has been found with medical residents who trained to mastery with central line insertions in a simulation lab. These residents had significantly less procedural complications in an intensive care unit than those who did not train to mastery in simulation (Barsuk, McGaghie, Cohen, O'Leary, & Wayne, 2009).

Examining the design and pedagogy of simulation as an educational intervention, Shaefer and colleagues (2011) reviewed the literature from 1990 to 2010. Their review included publications from nursing education, hospital and prehospital domain, virtual reality, task training, and hybrid use of standardized (simulated) patients. They examined the validity and reliability of the simulator and of the performance evaluation tool, the study design, and the translational impact. From their review, they concluded that there is a lack of sufficient well-designed studies to draw consensus. However, they identified well-designed studies that translated to clinical practice and improved patient safety.

In summary, the gaps in simulation research on learning outcomes include the need to explore and quantify sources of measurement error, develop defensible scoring rubrics and methodologies, establish and quantify the relationship between performance in simulation scenarios and in patient care situations, and investigate the impact of implementing high-stakes testing using simulation (Boulet et al., 2011).

DEBRIEFING

According to the INACSL Standard I: Terminology, "Debriefing is an activity that follows a simulation experience and is led by a facilitator" (Meakim et al., 2013, p. s5). Participants' reflective thinking is encouraged, and feedback is provided regarding the participants' performance while various aspects of the simulation are discussed. Simulation is the vehicle that takes participants to learning, which is what occurs in debriefing. There is a variety of methods of debriefing, such as

- Plus-delta debriefing
- Advocacy inquiry
- Debriefing for Meaningful Learning© (DML©)

According to INACSL Standards of Best Practice: Simulation, "The facilitator needs to be competent in the debriefing process; conduct debriefing in a trusting environment; observe the simulation; base debriefing on a structured framework;

and align debriefing with the objectives and outcomes of the simulation-based learning experience" (Decker et al., 2013, pp. s27–s29).

Although debriefing is a critical component of simulation, the literature indicates there is a need for studies focused on debriefing principles (Neill, & Wotton, 2011; Raemer et al., 2011). In a systematic review of the literature in nursing on debriefing, Neill and Wotton found that the format of debriefing varied across institutions; there was no agreement on one developmental framework or on the recommended amount of time spent in debriefing in relation to time spent in simulation. In a review of the medical literature, McGaghie and colleagues (2010) found that instructor training is an important component of effective simulation debriefing (see Chapter 16). In their review, they found that the instructor and learner did not need to be from the same profession. Gaps in understanding include whether simulation instructors should be certified for various devices, and what the appropriate learning models are for simulation instructors.

Salas, Cooke, and Rosen (2008) found evidence to support that debriefs must be diagnostic and provide a supportive learning environment. The facilitator should

- Be educated on the art and science of leading debriefs
- Focus on just a few critical performance measures during debriefing
- Provide process feedback early and outcome feedback later
- Shorten the delay between task performance and feedback

From the extensive simulation literature in both nursing and medicine, several gaps in our knowledge on debriefing exist. What is the best dose and model of debriefing? Do some methods provide more efficient learning, thus requiring fewer resources and yielding longer lasting results?

RESEARCH

Two research paradigms are described in Table 23.1. These paradigms assume different philosophies in relation to our understanding of reality. Although this chapter is not meant to provide comprehensive information on research frameworks, a review of the basics will help readers see the benefit in both paradigms and how a synthesis of research involving both paradigms enhances our understanding.

EVIDENCE-BASED SIMULATION PRACTICE (EBSP) 23.1

Lasater (2007) investigated nursing students using simulation in a qualitative research study. First-term nursing students using high-fidelity simulation as part of the regular curriculum perceived that it assisted them in the development of clinical judgment.

TABLE 23.1
Research Frameworks

RESEARCH PARADIGM	OVERVIEW	BENEFITS	CHALLENGES
Quantitative	Assumes that reality is objective, measurable, value-free, and unbiased using deductive reasoning	Uses reliable and valid instruments and clearly describes the population to make results generalizable	Requires valid and reliable measuring tools The environment and learner differences may not allow for experimental design
Qualitative	Assumes that reality is subjective, varying as seen by study participants, value-laden, and biased, using inductive reasoning	Emerging design provides flexibility to study according to themes identified in the process Is a good design for pilot study to identify key concepts and variables that may influence outcomes	Data analysis is labor intensive Findings may not be generalizable or reproducible in a different environment with a different population

---

EVIDENCE-BASED SIMULATION PRACTICE (EBSP) 23.2

Sullivan-Mann, Perron, and Fellner (2009) studied associate degree nursing students' ($N = 53$) critical thinking scores before and after simulation experiences. The tool used was the Health Sciences Reasoning Test (Facione & Facione, 2006). Learners exposed to simulation experienced an increase in critical thinking scores compared to a control group.

EVIDENCE-BASED SIMULATION PRACTICE (EBSP) 23.3

Shapiro and colleagues (2004) used a mixed-method approach to study simulation with interprofessional students who would respond in an emergency. One group was exposed to simulation education and another was not. The simulation-trained group scored slightly higher in observed behavior and rated the simulation learning experiences as valuable.

Simulation research can be looked at from the overall design perspective or from the type of methods used. So although the reasoning may be inductive or deductive, a mixed-method design in which both qualitative and quantitative methods are used adds to the richness of the data. Until we have valid, reliable tools that can be used across professions, using a mixed-method approach will enhance our understanding of the effect of simulation on learning.

SIMULATION RESEARCH RESOURCES

Keeping Current

One of the most important ways to keep up to date on the research in simulation is by joining one or more of the simulation societies. The two organizations that are most active in simulation research, accreditation, and developing standards of best practice are the INACSL and the SSH. Both organizations publish a monthly journal devoted to simulation. The journal articles are peer reviewed and indexed in medical and nursing databases. Other associations that may be helpful include the Association of Standardized Patient Educators (ASPE) and SimLEARN. The organizational mission or goals are listed in Table 23.2. All four organizations provide a community of practice in which a group of individuals share a common interest, craft, or profession (Lave & Wenger, 1991).

In 2004, the SSH was established to represent the rapidly growing group of educators and researchers who use a variety of simulation techniques for education, testing, and research in healthcare. The SSH is the organization that provides the certification examination and accredits simulation programs. Programs that comply with core standards and fulfillment of standards applied to one or more of the areas of assessment, research, teaching/education, and/or systems integration are eligible for application. The SSH goal is to lead in facilitating excellence in (multispecialty) healthcare education, practice, and research through simulation modalities.

On July 17, 2009, the acting undersecretary for health authorized the establishment of a national simulation training and education program for the Veterans Health Administration (VHA). Dubbed the "Simulation Learning, Education and Research Network," or SimLEARN, the program is improving the quality of healthcare services for America's veterans through the application of simulation-based learning strategies in clinical workforce development. The program operations and management are aligned with the VHA Employee Education System (EES) in close collaboration with VHA's Office of Patient Care Services (PCS) and Office of Nursing Services (ONS). Although the use of simulation for healthcare training and education is not new to VHA, it has become critical for VHA to develop an integrated approach to better realize the maximum benefits of simulation for VHA staff and the veterans they serve.

These simulation practice communities decrease the learning curve for those new to simulation and help to avoid reinventing the wheel. INACSL, SSH, SimLEARN, and ASPE use the collective expertise of their leaders and membership to advance the science of simulation.

> **Simulation Teaching Tip 23.2**
> Although I have been using simulation as a teaching/learning pedagogy for more than a decade, I find that I learn something new each time I engage with INACSL, SimLEARN, or SSH. Thus, even for the expert in simulation, these resources provide a place to learn and cocreate simulation knowledge, skills, and best practices (https://inacsl.org/learn/journal).

In summary, although simulation is increasingly being used in education and practice, the strength of the evidence is not yet strong. Gaps in the research exist in

TABLE 23.2
Simulation Organizations for Healthcare Educators

ORGANIZATION	MISSION/GOALS	PUBLICATION
INACSL	INACSL promotes research and disseminates evidence-based practice standards for clinical simulation methodologies and learning environments. The organization is a community of practice, a place where novice and expert practitioners can network, share ideas, and learn from and with each other about the knowledge, skills, and attitudes necessary for best practices in the use of simulation.	*Clinical Simulations in Nursing*
SSH	The SSH mission is to improve performance and reduce errors in patient care using all types of simulation, including task trainers, human patient simulators, virtual reality, and standardized (simulated) patients (SPs). The SSH is a multidisciplinary, multispecialty, international society with ties to many medical specialties, nursing, allied health paramedical personnel, and industry (http://ssih.org/about-ssh).	*Simulation in Healthcare*
ASPE	ASPE is the international organization of simulation educators dedicated to • Promoting best practices in the application of SP methodology for education, assessment, and research • Fostering the dissemination of research and scholarship in the field of SP methodology. • Advancing the professional knowledge and skills of its members • Transforming professional performance through the power of human interaction (http://www.aspeeducators.org/node/117)	Many web resources; ASPE recently announced its collaboration with MedEdPORTAL to house SP cases.
SimLEARN	The Simulation Learning, Education and Research Network (SimLEARN) is the VHA's program for simulation in healthcare training. Serving as the largest integrated healthcare system in the world, VHA's SimLEARN provides an ever-growing body of curricula and best practices that improve healthcare for our nation's veterans (http://ssih.org/about-ssh).	SimLEARN newsletter

ASPE, Association of Standardized Patient Educators; INACSL, International Nursing Association for Clinical Simulation & Learning; VHA, Veterans Health Administration.

the orientation, simulation, and debriefing areas. Evidence as to learner satisfaction, self-confidence, and perception of simulation is fairly strong. Questions that still need to be answered include

- How much simulation can replace clinical time?
- How much time should be spent in simulation?
- How much time spent in debriefing?
- How do we measure learning from simulation?
- How do we know if what students learn in simulation is transferred to actual practice?

In order to be up to date on the research, simulation educators and simulation personnel need to stay connected with simulation societies, attend simulation conferences, and read the simulation literature. As this pedagogy continues to diffuse through practice and academia, continued research and lifelong learning will be essential to ensure excellence in simulation.

CASE STUDY 23.1

Mary is an experienced nurse educator, but is new to simulation. One of her students confides that recently she lost a child and is concerned that she might not be able to effectively provide emergency care. Mary tells the learner that the simulation is essential to the course and that she must participate. Does this format follow recommendations of simulation research? How would you counsel Mary to improve her simulation educator skills?

CASE STUDY DISCUSSION

Mary's response does not follow recommendations. As observers who are actively engaged get just as much out of simulation as participants, Mary should give the learner a choice to observe rather than participate in this emotionally charged simulation. Mary should address the possibility of emotional triggers in the orientation/prebrief. Learners should be given the choice to observe rather than participate in the simulation if they think that participation may be too painful.

PRACTICE QUESTIONS

1. A new physician has heard about your simulation laboratory and is interested in scheduling a simulation. The physician would like to do a mock code. Based on simulation research and best practice, what should you have the physician do first prior to running the simulation?

   A. Develop a scenario
   B. Develop objectives
   C. Observe a mock code simulation
   D. Notify participants as to date and time

2. An instructor who is new to simulation is pressed for time. In order to provide sufficient time for debriefing, the instructor skips the orientation. Why is orientation important? Orientation gives the learners

   A. A chance to identify roles
   B. Time to plan their course of action
   C. Assistance in meeting objectives
   D. An opportunity to observe the environment

3. Unless the simulation is for high-stakes testing, the main objective in simulation is

   A. Patient outcome
   B. Learner outcome
   C. Task mastery
   D. Learning

4. A learner approaches you and confides that she has just had a death in her family. Her infant died after being in neonatal intensive care. She is not sure that she can handle participating in a simulation. The *best* course of action is to

   A. Send her for counseling.
   B. Have her play a secondary role in the simulation.
   C. Give her the opportunity to watch the simulation.
   D. Tell her to come back another day.

5. Which of Kirkpatrick's levels of evaluation has been *most* heavily researched in simulation?

   A. Level 1, reaction
   B. Level 2, learning
   C. Level 3, behavior
   D. Level 4, results

6. The simulation researcher wants to study the live experience of the learner in a complex, interprofessional simulation. Which method should the researcher choose?

   A. Quantitative method
   B. Survey method
   C. Mixed method
   D. Qualitative method

7. Which of these is *not* a credible source for up-to-date, simulation research information?

   A. INACSL
   B. SSH
   C. ASPE
   D. Simulator vendors

8. Which debriefing method has *not* been found to be the *most* effective?

   A. Advocacy–inquiry
   B. Critical judgment
   C. Plus–delta
   D. DML

9. What does the research on debriefing indicate?

   A. Effective debriefers should provide process feedback early.
   B. Effective debriefers should initially focus on whether outcomes were met.
   C. The debriefing should include a comprehensive review of all critical outcomes.
   D. An instructor who is a content expert will be an effective debriefer.

10. Which norm will promote a quality simulation experience?

    A. A consistent template to develop scenarios
    B. Ensuring that all participants have the same knowledge base
    C. Use of a confidentiality contract
    D. An enforced time limit

REFERENCES

Adamson, K. A., Jeffries, P. R., & Rogers, K. J. (2012). Evaluation: A critical step in simulation practice and research. In P. Jeffries (Ed.), *Simulation in nursing education: From conceptualization to evaluation* (2nd ed.). New York, NY: National League for Nursing Press.

Alfes, C. M. (2011). Evaluating the use of simulation with beginning nursing students. *Journal of Nursing Education, 50*(2), 89.

Bambini, D., Washburn, J., & Perkins, R. (2009). Outcomes of clinical simulation for novice nursing students: Communication, confidence, clinical judgment. *Nursing Education Perspectives, 30*(2), 79–82.

Bandura, A. (2000). Exercise of human agency through collective efficacy. *Current Directions in Psychological Science, 9*(3), 75–78.

Barsuk, J. H., McGaghie, W. C., Cohen, E. R., O'Leary, K. J., & Wayne, D. B. (2009). Simulation-based mastery learning reduces complications during central venous catheter insertion in a medical intensive care unit. *Critical Care Medicine, 37*(10), 2697–2701.

Benner, P. (1984). *From novice to expert: Power and excellence in nursing practice.* Palo Alto, CA: Addison-Wesley.

Boulet, J. R., Jeffries, P. R., Hatala, R. A., Korndorffer, J. R., Jr., Feinstein, D. M., & Roche, J. P. (2011). Research regarding methods of assessing learning outcomes. *Simulation in Healthcare, 6*(7), S48–S51.

Cant, R., & Cooper, S. (2010). Simulation-based learning in nursing education: Systematic review. *Journal of Advanced Nursing, 66*(1), 3–15.

Cato, M. (2013). *Nursing student anxiety in simulation and its effect on learning.* Paper presented at the National League for Nursing Education Summit, Washington, DC.

Chickering, A. W., & Gamson, Z. F. (1987). Seven principles of good practice in undergraduate education. *AAHE Bulletin, 39*(7), 5–10.

Decker, S., Fey, M., Sideras, S., Caballero, S., Rockstraw, L. R., Boese, T., . . . Borum, J. C. (2013). Standards of best practice: Simulation standard VI: The debriefing process. *Clinical Simulation in Nursing, 9*(6), S26–S29.

Decker, S. I. L. (2007). *Simulation as an educational strategy in the development of critical and reflective thinking: A qualitative exploration.* Denton, TX: Texas Woman's University.

Dieckmann, P., Molin Friis, S., Lippert, A., & Ostergaard, D. (2009). The art and science of debriefing in simulation: Ideal and practice. *Medical Teacher, 31*(7), e287–e294.

Dreifuerst, K. T. (2009). The essentials of debriefing in simulation learning: A concept analysis. *Nursing Education Perspectives, 30*(2), 109–114.

Facione, N. C., & Facione P. A. (2006). *Health Sciences Reasoning Test (HSRT): A test for critical thinking skills for health care professionals. Test manual.* Millbrae, CA: California Academic Press.

Gloe, D., Sando, C. R., Franklin, A. E., Boese, T., Decker, S., Lioce, L., . . . Borum, J. C. (2013). Standards of best practice: Simulation standard II: Professional integrity of participant(s). *Clinical Simulation in Nursing, 9*(6), S12–S14.

Hayden, J. (2010). Use of simulation in nursing education: National survey results. *Journal of Nursing Regulation, 1*(3), 52–57.

Jeffries, P. R. (2012). *Simulation in nursing education from conceptualization to evaluation* (2nd ed.). New York, NY: NLN Press.

Kardong-Edgren, S., Adamson, K. A., & Fitzgerald, C. (2010). A review of currently published evaluation instruments for human patient simulation. *Clinical Simulation in Nursing, 6*(1), e25–e35.

Kirkpatrick, D. L., & Kirkpatrick, J. D. (2006). *Evaluating training programs* (3rd ed.). San Francisco, CA: Berrett-Koehler.

Lasater, K. (2007). High-fidelity simulation and the development of clinical judgment: Students' experiences. *Journal of Nursing Education, 46*(6), 269–276.

Lave, J., & Wenger, E. (1991). *Situated learning: Legitimate peripheral participation.* Cambridge, UK: Cambridge University Press.

McGaghie, W. C., Issenberg, S. B., Petrusa, E. R., & Scalese, R. J. (2010). A critical review of simulation-based medical education research: 2003–2009. *Medical Education, 44*(1), 50–63.

Meakim, C., Boese, T., Decker, S., Franklin, A. E., Gloe, D., Lioce, L., Sando, C. R., & Borum, J. C. (2013). Standards of best practice standard I: Terminology. *Clinical Simulation in Nursing, 9*(6), 3–11. doi:10.1016/j.ecns.2013.04.001

Murray D. J., Boulet, J. R., Avidan M., Kras J. F., Heinrich B., & Woodhouse J., (2007). Performance of residents and anesthesiologists in simulation-based skill assessment. *Anesthesiology, 107*(5), 705–713.

Neill, M. A., & Wotton, K. (2011). High-fidelity simulation debriefing in nursing education: A literature review. *Clinical Simulation in Nursing, 7*(5), e161–e168.

Radhakrishnan, K., Roche, J. P., & Cunningham, H. (2007). Measuring clinical practice parameters with human patient simulation: A pilot study. *International Journal of Nursing Education Scholarship, 4*, Article 8.

Raemer, D., Anderson, M., Cheng, A., Fanning, R., Nadkarni, V., & Salvadelli, G. (2011). Research regarding debriefing as part of the learning process. *Simulation in Healthcare 6*(Suppl S), 52–57. doi:10.1097/SIH.0b013e31822724d0

Ravert, P., & McAfooes, J. (2013). NLN/Jeffries simulation framework: State of the science summary. *Clinical Simulation in Nursing, 10*(7), 335–336.

Rosen, M. A., Salas, E., Silvestri, S., Wu, T. S., & Lazarra, E. H. (2008). A measurement tool for simulation-based training in emergency medicine: The simulation module for assessment of resident targeted event responses (SMARTER) approach. *Simulation in Healthcare, 3*(3), 170–179.

Salas, E., Cooke, N. J., & Rosen, M. A. (2008). On teams, teamwork, and team performance: Discoveries and developments. *Human Factors: The Journal of the Human Factors and Ergonomics Society, 50*(3), 540–547.

Schaefer, J. J., III, Vanderbilt, A. A., Cason, C. L., Bauman, E. B., Glavin, R. J., Lee, F. W., & Navedo, D. D. (2011). Literature review: Instructional design and pedagogy science in healthcare simulation. *Simulation in Healthcare, 6*(7), s30–s41.

Schoening, A. M., Sittner, B. J., & Todd, M. J. (2006). Simulated clinical experience: Nursing students' perceptions and the educators' role. *Nurse Educator, 31*(6), 253–258.

Shapiro, M. J., Morey, J. C., Small, S. D., Langford, V., Kaylor, C. J., Jagminas, L., . . . Jay, G. D. (2004). Simulation based teamwork training for emergency department staff: Does it improve clinical team performance when added to an existing didactic teamwork curriculum? *Quality and Safety in Health Care, 13*(6), 417–421.

Society for Simulation in Healthcare (SSH). (2014). *Certified healthcare simulation educator handbook.* Retrieved from http://ssih.org/certification/handbook

Sullivan-Mann, J., Perron, C. A., & Fellner, A. N. (2009). The effects of simulation on nursing students' critical thinking scores: A quantitative study. *Newborn and Infant Nursing Reviews, 9*(2), 111–116.

Weinger, M. B. (2010). The pharmacology of simulation: A conceptual framework to inform progress in simulation research. *Simulation in Healthcare, 5*(1), 8–15.

Zimmerman, B. J. (2000). Self-efficacy: An essential motive to learn. *Contemporary Educational Psychology, 25*(1), 82–91.

Practice Test

RUTH A. WITTMANN-PRICE, LINDA WILSON, AND SAMUEL W. PRICE

Twenty years from now you will be more disappointed by
the things that you didn't do than by the ones you did do.
So throw off the bowlines. Sail away from the safe harbor.
Catch the trade winds in your sails. Explore. Dream. Discover.
—Mark Twain

This practice test "simulates" the certification test. There are 115 questions. Try to answer them in 120 minutes. Read the rationales when you have completed the test and score yourself when you are done. Good luck!

1. One of the *most* important learning processes of simulation is

   A. High fidelity
   B. Debriefing
   C. Teamwork
   D. Suspending disbelief

2. Foundational to providing appropriate feedback is the concept that feedback

   A. Is provided by the instructor to the learner
   B. Contains things done well and improvements needed
   C. Is a cycle of information and reaction
   D. Does not always respond with performance improvement

3. A learning difference that is not attributed to adult learners includes

   A. Flexibility in conceptualization
   B. Ingrained personality traits
   C. Previous experiences with learning
   D. Relationship patterns

4. When discussing contextual factors that influence feedback, the simulation educator must think about

   A. The content to be discussed
   B. The place of the feedback session
   C. The aim of the feedback
   D. The feedback recipient

5. An attribute of traditional education includes

    A. Teamwork
    B. Experiential learning
    C. Constructivism
    D. Unidirectional communication

6. The novice simulation educator needs additional mentoring because he is providing weak feedback to the learners as demonstrated by the statement

    A. "I was able to observe the entire procedure."
    B. "Let's review the learning objective before we begin."
    C. "I will reobserve you performing the procedure."
    D. "I heard from the simulation technician that it went well."

7. Of the seven elements of debriefing defined by Lederman (1984), what or who produces the impact of the experience?

    A. The debriefer
    B. The participants
    C. The recollection
    D. The simulation scenario

8. The best method to objectively evaluate learner performance when doing a specialty examination would be

    A. Reflective writing
    B. Peer evaluation
    C. Concept map
    D. Performance checklist

9. When debriefing, the scenario may be interpreted differently from what happened if

    A. Excessive time has passed.
    B. The learners are at varied stages.
    C. The debriefer lacks experience.
    D. The objectives were not met.

10. When evaluating learners' simulation performance, the evaluation tool should demonstrate interrater reliability, which is

    A. Different learners score similarly on the evaluation tool.
    B. The evaluation tool works the same, group after group.
    C. Different evaluators rate the same performance similarly.
    D. The items on the tool are deemed appropriate by experts.

11. The art of debriefing occurs when the debriefer moves the discussion from the personal accounts of the scenario to

    A. The "hot-seat" participant's account
    B. A descriptive account of the event
    C. An objective global perspective
    D. A subjective descriptive account

12. A standardized (simulated) patient (SP) is used to demonstrate abnormal breath sounds. The SP has chronic obstructive pulmonary disease (COPD). This type of simulation is referred to as

    A. A symptomatic SP
    B. An asymptomatic SP
    C. Nonhealthcare provider instructor
    D. Confederate

13. A debriefing session should be tailored to the characteristics of the participants and

    A. The characteristics of the debriefer
    B. The details of the experience
    C. The learning objectives
    D. The feelings of the group

14. The three critical components found that influence learning in the simulation laboratory are

    A. Fidelity of the simulation, demeanor of the faculty, and debriefing
    B. Adequate preparation, skill of the faculty, and debriefing
    C. Fidelity of the simulation, demeanor of the faculty, and reflection
    D. Adequate preparation, demeanor of the faculty, and debriefing

15. The best teaching role for debriefers to assume is

    A. Authoritarian
    B. Instructor
    C. Facilitator
    D. Observer

16. The simulation situation that depicts a formative evaluation of learning is

    A. Specific body system examinations for a course grade
    B. The objective structured clinical examinations (OSCEs) for medical students
    C. A midterm evaluation of a procedure
    D. A scenario in which the simulation educator uses a final patient safety checklist

17. The debriefer who takes a "back seat" during a debriefing session and only guides the group when absolutely necessary is said to be taking a(n)

    A. High level of facilitation
    B. Intermediate level of facilitation
    C. Low level of facilitation
    D. Lassie-faire commitment

18. The best simulation method for a summative evaluation of a sterile dressing change is to

    A. Observe the learners in a group format assisting each other.
    B. Videotape the procedure using a high-fidelity mannequin.
    C. Have an SP scenario.
    D. Observe them on a task trainer using an objective checklist.

19. The novice debriefer is telling the team all about his impressions of the simulation event. The best response by the experienced debriefer would be

    A. "Thank you for the impressions, please continue."
    B. "The students need to tell their impressions."
    C. "Thank you, let's hear from the students."
    D. "Can you sum up the experience for us?"

20. Scenario "lifesavers" are used primarily to

    A. Decrease the stress during a simulation scenario.
    B. Preserve the learning objectives of the scenario.
    C. Keep the SP on track.
    D. Change the content of the scenario as needed.

21. The debriefer of a simulation scenario develops a tool for the students that includes a column titled "What went well" and a second column titled "What can we change?" This type of facilitation is described as

    A. Framing
    B. Target focused
    C. Advocacy–inquiry
    D. Plus–delta

22. The novice simulation educator needs better understanding of using a scenario "lifesaver" when the expert simulation educator asks him why he changed the scenario and he states

    A. "The learners did something wrong, but it was not life threatening."
    B. "The learners did not understand the scenario."
    C. "The learners were having difficulty suspending disbelief."
    D. "The scenario was too complex for the learners' level."

23. The debriefer says to a learner, "I observed you checking the patient's identification band once before you administered the medication. That makes me uncomfortable because it is a double-check process. Can you tell me what you were thinking at the time?" This form of reflection is known as

    A. Framing
    B. Target focused
    C. Advocacy–inquiry
    D. Plus–delta

24. An example of a simulation scenario "lifesaver" from "within" would be

    A. Stopping the scenario to get learners back on track
    B. Changing the patient's vital signs in order to demonstrate decomposition
    C. Telling the learners over the microphone that the IV is wide open
    D. Coming into the simulation room and providing an instruction in intubation

25. When there is more than one debriefer, a technique that is effective to prevent opposing sides is

    A. Good cop–bad cop
    B. Target focused
    C. Advocacy–inquiry
    D. Plus–delta

26. An example of a scenario "lifesaver" from "outside" would be

    A. Changing the electrocardiogram (EKG) pattern on the monitor
    B. Telling the learners, through the mannequin, that he has a pain level of 8
    C. Having the SP demonstrate signs of an acute abdomen
    D. Stopping the scenario to clarify the difference between respiratory wheezes and rhonchi

27. An expert who brings specialized instruction postscenario to an experienced group of learners may be

    A. An advanced student
    B. A simulation technician
    C. A simulation educator
    D. A content debriefer

28. One of the main learning strategies used in debriefing is

    A. Information gathering
    B. Reflective learning
    C. Discussion
    D. Socratic questioning

29. The novice simulation educator needs further orientation when he stops a scenario for "in-scenario" debriefing, when he states

    A. "Let's start that procedure over because the field is contaminated."
    B. "Stop the procedure; the mannequin is malfunctioning."
    C. "Let's stop and talk about how you are feeling about the event."
    D. "Stop the procedure to realign the catheter in order for it to work."

30. During debriefing, the type of reflective learning that is used is

    A. Reflection in action
    B. Reflection on action
    C. Reflective consciousness
    D. Reflective reasoning

31. When debriefing a large group of participants, it may be more effective if the debriefer(s)

    A. Ask them to write their reflections.
    B. Break them into small groups and debrief one group after another.
    C. Have them all sit in a classroom and pass around a microphone.
    D. Break them into small groups with different debriefers.

32. A constructivist theory of learning includes

    A. Establishing baseline knowledge for the learner
    B. Group analysis that assists the learning process
    C. Learning that is individually constructed
    D. New knowledge that is categorized simplistically

33. The following setup depicts the "fishbowl" method of debriefing (Steinwachs, 1992)

    A. Arrange the learners in an inner and outer circle.
    B. Arrange the learners in a large circle.
    C. Arrange the learners in three or more concentric circles.
    D. Arrange the learners in two semicircles facing each other.

34. One of the main purposes of interprofessional simulation experiences is to foster

    A. Communication
    B. Procedural competence
    C. Role definition
    D. Scope of practice

35. During simulation debriefing, it is important to avoid creating "energy gaps." Therefore, simulation educators should try to (Steinwachs, 1992)

    A. Keep the group engaged.
    B. Show enthusiasm.
    C. Seat learners next to each other.
    D. Have learners make eye contact when speaking.

36. Using simulation to identify "tacit team voice" with interprofessional teams that have been together for a time is helpful to accommodate

    A. Differences in culture
    B. Differences in roles
    C. Conflict
    D. Newcomers to the team

37. One of the major ways that debriefing contributes to simulation education is that it

    A. Provides the debriefer's instructions to the group
    B. Helps learners to increase procedural proficiency
    C. Brings closure to the experience
    D. Develops individual self-efficacy

38. Kneebone (2005) describes simulation as a method of learning with which of these four key aspects for healthcare providers?

    A. Assisted learning, psychomotor skills learning, situated learning, and affective learning
    B. Assisted learning, psychomotor skills learning, cognitive learning, and professional role development
    C. Professional role development, skills learning, cognitive learning, and affective learning
    D. Psychomotor skills learning, affective learning, team learning, and situated learning

39. The novice in simulation education needs further instructions about debriefing when she states that debriefing

    A. "Tells the entire scenario all over again."
    B. "Focuses on perceptions."
    C. "Provides closure for the learners."
    D. "Adds useful insights."

40. Successful deliberate practice (DP) involves four components, which include

    A. Knowledge facilitation, skill assessment, feedback, and reflection
    B. Repetitive performance, skill assessment, feedback, and increased skill performance
    C. Knowledge facilitation, skill performance, reflection, and increased skill performance
    D. Repetitive performance, reflection, feedback, and increased skill performance

41. After a simulation scenario, the learners rate their own performance and use the rating as a talking point in the debriefing session. This is referred to as

    A. Pre-debriefing
    B. Self-debriefing
    C. Peer debriefing
    D. Reflection

42. When developing an evaluation instrument, *content validity* includes

    A. Items that are equitable in difficulty
    B. Items that measure the elements of the construct being tested
    C. Items that yield the same results over and over
    D. Items that discriminate learners who do not know the content

43. A tool used to distribute roles and responsibilities among simulation learners during a scenario that can be used to promote active learning for all the participants, is a

    A. Rubric
    B. Content module
    C. Team description
    D. Collaborative script

44. Evaluating instrument *reliability* offers simulation educators the knowledge that the instrument can

    A. Test the construct it is meant to test.
    B. Test the content it is meant to test.
    C. Yield the same results in different groups.
    D. Yield the same results in the same group at a later date.

45. A simulation educator understands that to produce the best physical fidelity, the scenario about a motor vehicle accident trauma victim's arrival to the emergency department should be conducted

    A. In a simulation laboratory set up as a trauma bay
    B. In a simulation laboratory set up like an examination room
    C. In an emergency department
    D. On the road where the accident occurred

46. Curriculum recommendations for using simulation learning experiences for healthcare professionals include

    A. Use of simulation in clinical courses
    B. Simulation of interprofessional events to promote communication
    C. Use of simulation throughout the curriculum
    D. Simulation for key procedures needed by each profession

47. The simulation educator is trying to increase the psychological fidelity for a scenario that deals with end-of-life issues. The best mechanism to do this would be to

    A. Hire an actor who is educated as an SP.
    B. Use a high-fidelity mannequin that can simulate tears.
    C. Videotape the scenario to use in debriefing to evaluate emotions.
    D. Have other learners act as family members around the bedside.

48. Virtual reality (VR) simulators are *most* effectively used for

    A. Common procedures
    B. Complex procedures
    C. Interpersonal skills
    D. Decision making

49. The simulation educator is worried about the feel of the granulated skin on a mannequin that is simulating a burn patient. The simulation educator is concerned about the

    A. Physical fidelity
    B. Environmental fidelity
    C. Equipment fidelity
    D. Psychological fidelity

50. The simulation educator is developing a scenario for healthcare learners to focus on health history taking. The best simulation method to develop would be

    A. A high-fidelity mannequin
    B. A task trainer
    C. VR
    D. An SP

51. The simulation educator is setting up the simulation room to depict the room of a confused patient. The simulation educator is ensuring

    A. Physical fidelity
    B. Environmental fidelity
    C. Equipment fidelity
    D. Psychological fidelity

52. The best method of simulation to use to combine communication and procedural skills is

    A. High-fidelity and low-fidelity mannequins
    B. Task trainer and VR
    C. Task trainer and SP
    D. VR and high-fidelity mannequin

53. The simulation educator understands that the novice simulation educator needs additional mentoring when she states

    A. "I think that student learning outcomes will be better if the mannequins look more real."
    B. "I think that this fidelity is adequate for the objectives of this simulation."
    C. "I believe that the method of simulation must be coherent with the learning objectives."
    D. "The student learning outcomes may be able to be met with different simulation methods."

54. Scaffolding scenarios and feedback to learners provide the learners with

    A. Different perspectives
    B. Progressive knowledge building
    C. More reflective time
    D. Self-pacing

55. The learners describe the respirations of the SP in breaths per minute. This is describing the simulation "realism" in which mode?

    A. Fidelity
    B. Physical
    C. Semantical
    D. Phenomenal

56. Serious gaming can be described as

    A. Designed learning experiences
    B. Free-flow decisional experiences
    C. Fun learning with self-developed objectives
    D. Interactive fun activities

57. A scenario is set up so the learners find a patient who is unresponsive, and they need to react to the situation and start cardiopulmonary resuscitation. This scenario prompts a cognitive structure process for learners to understand that they need to acknowledge the situation. This would be a

    A. Secondary affective-promoting frame
    B. Modulation of a skill
    C. Social primary frame
    D. Natural primary frame

58. Creating an avatar to interact in a learning game is establishing a(n)

    A. Learning objective
    B. Identity
    C. Pseudonymity
    D. Dual role

59. Learners in the simulation lab are briefed on a scenario. The simulation educator asks them to sign a contract that states they will treat this scenario as a real situation. The simulation educator is asking them to

    A. Acknowledge an informed consent
    B. Regulate their behavior and not laugh
    C. Suspend disbelief
    D. Interact professionally

60. In serious gaming, endogenous games include games that

    A. Have context and game play linked
    B. Have context outside the actual game play
    C. Provide context before the game
    D. Contain "in situ" instructions during the game

61. A simulation scenario calls for a patient with an allergic reaction to an antibiotic. The SP asks the healthcare learner to look at the rash on his chest, which is not actually present. The healthcare provider examines the chest of the SP. By doing so, the healthcare learner is supporting which of the following simulation concepts?

    A. Moulage
    B. DP
    C. Realism
    D. As if

62. The SP is trained to demonstrate hyporeflexia for learners when they are checking deep tendon reflexes. The SP is considered

    A. An asymptomatic SP
    B. A symptomatic SP
    C. A confederate
    D. A hybrid situation

63. A simulation educator asks the learners to sign a statement that they will treat the scenario as if it is a real patient situation. The document they sign is referred to as a

    A. Fiction contract
    B. Informed consent
    C. Suspending disbelief contract
    D. Promise document

64. A healthcare learner needs to perform a summative physical assessment evaluation. The best simulation mode for this evaluation would be

    A. A high-fidelity mannequin
    B. A task trainer
    C. An asymptomatic SP
    D. A VR avatar

65. One of the key learning elements of simulation is that it can provide learners with

    A. Historical patient scenarios
    B. Common patient problems
    C. Uncommon patient problems
    D. Futuristic healthcare ideas

66. Types of test validity can be drawn from all of the following analyses EXCEPT

    A. Testing the constructs
    B. Test content
    C. Relationship of test scores to other instruments
    D. The relationship of test items to each other

67. Nurse anesthesia learners need to practice how to do a spinal tap on a patient for a blood patch. The best type of simulation to teach this would be

A. A high-fidelity mannequin
B. A torso task trainer
C. An SP
D. VR

68. A form of simulation in which a person spontaneously demonstrates a personality trait or a characteristic of a patient–provider interaction is called

A. An asymptomatic SP
B. Role-playing
C. Hybrid simulation
D. A symptomatic SP

69. The novice simulation educator needs further instruction about simulation when she states simulation is an asset because

A. "There is no risk to actual patients."
B. "Uncommon patient problems can be presented."
C. "Simulation can be stopped for teaching purposes."
D. "Each simulation scenario cannot be standardized."

70. During an SP interaction, the simulation educator calls a "time-out" in order to have the

A. SP describe what is happening
B. Learners reflect on what they are feeling
C. Provide instruction by himself or herself
D. Confederates redo their parts

71. Nursing learners are learning how to insert a sterile urinary catheter. The best method of simulation to teach this procedure would be

A. Male and female torso task trainers
B. SPs
C. High-fidelity mannequins
D. VR

72. During a simulation "time-out," the SP

A. Is removed from the room
B. Discusses the diagnosis
C. Remains in role and speaks
D. Goes into suspended animation

73. Combining a task trainer in a simulation environment with an SP, simulation educators can

A. Deliver low-fidelity learning
B. Simulate VR in a simulation room
C. Change a low-fidelity simulator into a high-fidelity experience
D. Provide a DP situation

74. The design of the simulation scenario should be determined by

   A. The simulation educator
   B. The level of the learners
   C. The fidelity of the mannequins
   D. The learning objectives

75. The last phase of the Simulation Learning Pyramid (Doerr & Murray, 2008) is

   A. Debriefing
   B. Simulation plan
   C. Transference
   D. The simulation

76. During a scenario, using a high-fidelity mannequin as a recovering alcoholic, a faculty member takes the role of the patient's belligerent spouse. The role being played by the faculty member is that of a

   A. Standardized patient
   B. Simulated patient
   C. Confederate
   D. Extra

77. To develop a simulation plan, the simulation educator understands that the first step is to

   A. Decide on a case to develop
   B. Script the SPs
   C. Develop the objectives
   D. Establish time limits

78. An important aspect of briefing learners is to

   A. Have them decide what they need to learn
   B. Develop the scenario
   C. Discuss debriefing expectations
   D. Orient them to the equipment

79. "Confederates" used in simulation scenarios are actually

   A. Other people in the scenario besides the learners and SPs
   B. SPs
   C. Mannequins with moulage
   D. The learners who have secondary roles in the simulation experience

80. A learner is able to perform a procedure with real patients after DP in the simulation laboratory. This demonstrates which step of Kilpatrick's (1998) four-level training evaluation model?

   A. Reaction
   B. Learning
   C. Behavior
   D. Results

81. One excellent method used to enhance transference of knowledge is to

    A. Develop realistic moulage.
    B. Use SPs with symptoms.
    C. Have the simulation experience "in situ."
    D. Have the simulation experience in a well-equipped laboratory.

82. Directive feedback provides the learner with

    A. Questions to reflect on
    B. Items that require correction
    C. Suggestions so learners can facilitate their own correction
    D. A grade for the experience

83. Simulation educators understand that a tenet of adult learning theory is that adults

    A. Do not need to know why they should learn something; they just need to know how to do it
    B. They are interdependent learners
    C. Like things that are immediately applicable
    D. Like subject-centered rather than life-centered learning

84. Facilitative feedback provides the learner with

    A. Questions to reflect on
    B. Items that require correction
    C. Suggestions so learners can facilitate their own correction
    D. A grade for the experience

85. According to Kolb's experiential learning theory (1984), learning is

    A. Sequential
    B. Newly found knowledge
    C. Involves transaction between people
    D. A holistic process

86. A *fundamental attribution* error of a learner during a feedback session is

    A. Blaming external factors
    B. Not understanding the objectives
    C. Admitting to being unprepared
    D. Discussing the scenario with peers

87. According to Kolb's experiential learning theory (1984), four different abilities are needed by the learner. The ability to become involved in a simulation scenario fully without bias is which ability?

    A. Concrete experience (CE)
    B. Reflective observation (RO)
    C. Abstract conceptualization (AC)
    D. Active experimentation (AE)

88. Using *interactional justice* during a feedback session means

    A. Describing what went right and then wrong
    B. Balancing the feedback with the psychological needs of the learner
    C. Providing negative feedback only when necessary
    D. Providing positive feedback only

89. A simulation learner gives concentrated glucose during a scenario that simulates a diabetic patient in severe hypoglycemia. The learner is demonstrating which learning ability identified by Kolb (1984)?

    A. CEs
    B. RO
    C. AC
    D. AE

90. Feedback provided to learners is more beneficial if it is

    A. Specific
    B. General
    C. Conceptual
    D. Overarching

91. The goal of DP is

    A. Performance improvement
    B. Getting practice before clinical experience
    C. Developing intricate skills
    D. Pure repetition

92. The biggest disadvantage of using SPs is

    A. Preparation
    B. Differences in acting for different learners
    C. Cost
    D. Recruitment

93. A primary goal of a simulation educator is to

    A. Develop a realistic simulation scenario
    B. Establish teacher–student boundaries
    C. Create a safe environment
    D. Decrease mistakes during simulation experiences

94. Trained SPs are able to provide

    A. Assessment feedback
    B. Course grade
    C. Learning objectives
    D. Summative evaluations

95. Kneebone (2005) believes that simulation educators should do all of the following EXCEPT

    A. Encourage DP
    B. Provide peer tutoring
    C. Correlate simulation with real-life experiences
    D. Maintain a learner-centered environment

96. SPs have their roles and script provided by

    A. Simulation educators
    B. Patient instructors
    C. Lead actors
    D. Theater coaches

97. The first level of Kirkpatrick's (1959) four-level learning theory is

    A. Learning
    B. Results
    C. Reaction
    D. Behavior

98. A simulation scenario is about delivering bad news to family members of a motor vehicle accident victim. The best simulation methodology would be

    A. A high-fidelity mannequin
    B. A low-fidelity mannequin
    C. VR
    D. An SP

99. The last level of Kirkpatrick's (1959) four-level learning theory is

    A. Learning
    B. Results
    C. Reaction
    D. Behavior

100. Characteristics of an SP that need to be considered for realism include

    A. Height and weight
    B. Age and ethnicity
    C. Hair and skin color
    D. Education and articulation

101. The best simulation method to promote changes in learner behavior in the affective domain is

    A. High-fidelity mannequins
    B. Task trainers
    C. SPs
    D. VR

102. The best simulation method to promote changes in learner behavior in the psychomotor domain is

    A. High-fidelity mannequins
    B. Task trainers
    C. SPs
    D. VR

103. A learning method used during debriefing that leads learners to the higher order of critical thinking is

    A. Faculty instruction
    B. Peer discussion
    C. Direct questioning
    D. Reflection

104. The *best* role for a debriefer to assume is

    A. Instructor
    B. Coach
    C. Advisor
    D. Facilitator

105. The choice of fidelity when planning a simulation-based learning (SBL) experience should depend on the

    A. Skill of the simulation educator
    B. Learning outcomes
    C. Equipment available
    D. Cost

106. The *best* simulation method to use to teach professional behavior and decision making for an ethical issue is

    A. Low-fidelity mannequins
    B. Task trainers
    C. SPs
    D. VR

107. Clinical management of the simulation laboratory by the simulation educator includes all of the following aspects EXCEPT

    A. Scheduling
    B. Management of equipment
    C. Content expertise
    D. Budgeting

108. Factors that influence the SBL experience include all of the following EXCEPT

    A. Active learning
    B. Cost of equipment
    C. Faculty–student interaction
    D. Realism

109. Psychological fidelity can best be ensured by using

    A. SPs
    B. The learning outcomes to guide the simulation experience
    C. Experienced simulation educators
    D. A learner-centered approach

110. The *best* simulation method to teach tracheotomies to otolaryngology residents is to use

    A. Patients who need the procedure
    B. Task trainers
    C. Intermediate-fidelity mannequins
    D. VR

111. The *best* simulation method to use for a delicate open-heart surgical procedure is

    A. Patients who need the procedure
    B. Task trainers
    C. Intermediate-fidelity mannequins
    D. VR

112. Positive outcomes of interprofessional simulation education include all of the following EXPECT

    A. It decreases anxiety in emergencies
    B. It increases autonomy
    C. It promotes communication
    D. It promotes retention of skills

113. When using volunteers as SPs, the simulation educator must

    A. Offer some compensation
    B. Maintain confidentiality
    C. Get institutional review board (IRB) approval
    D. Have insurance to cover any health issues diagnosed

114. An interprofessional healthcare team is responding to an SP emergency. The team does not recognize the need for a critical airway on the patient and it fails to call the anesthetist. The simulation educator would best intervene by

    A. Stopping the scenario
    B. Giving instructions through the microphone
    C. Giving the team a hint from the doorway
    D. Providing a written note to a team member to check the airway

115. The simulation educator develops environmental fidelity when he

    A. Adds moulage to the mannequin
    B. Uses a hybrid SP and a task trainer
    C. Uses a high-fidelity mannequin as the speaking patient
    D. Sets up the room to resemble an emergency department bay

BIBLIOGRAPHY

Alinier, G. (2011). Developing high-fidelity health care simulation scenarios: A guide for educators and professionals. *Simulation and Gaming, 42*(1), 9–26.

Archer, J. C. (2010). State of the science in health professional education: Effective feedback. *Medical Education, 44,* 101–108.

Barrows, H. S. (1993). An overview of the uses of standardized (simulated) patients for teaching and evaluating clinical skills. *Academic Medicine, 68*(6), 443–451.

Boulet, J. R., Jeffries, P. R., Hatala, R. A., Korndorffer, J. R., Feinstein, D. M., & Roche, J. P. (2011). Research regarding methods of assessing learning outcomes. *Simulation in Healthcare, 6,* S48–S51.

Cant, R. P., & Cooper, S. J. (2009). Simulation-based learning in nursing education: Systematic review. *Journal of Advanced Nursing, 66*(1), 3–15.

Cantell, M. A. (2008). The importance of debriefing in clinical simulation, *Clinical Simulation in Nursing, 4,* e19–e23.

Cleveland, J. A., Abe, K., & Rethans, J. (2009). The use of simulated patients in medical education: Amee Guide No 42. *Medical Teacher, 31*, 477–486.

Dieckmann, P., Gaba, D., & Marcus, R. (2007). Deepening the theoretical foundations of patient simulation as social practice, *Simulation in Healthcare, 2*(3), 183–193.

Diekmann, P., Lippert, A., Glavin, R., & Rall, M. (2010). When things do not go as expected: Scenario life savers. *Simulation in Healthcare, 5*, 219–225.

Doerr, H., & Murray, W. B. (2008). How to build a successful simulation strategy: The simulation learning pyramid. In R. R. Kyle & W. B. Murray (Eds.), *Clinical simulation: Operations, engineering and management* (pp. 771–785). London, UK: Elsevier/Academic Press.

Dorton, L. H., Lintzenich, C. R., & Evans, A. K., (2014). Simulation model for tracheotomy education for primary health-care providers. *Annals of Otology, Rhinology, & Laryngology, 123*(1), 11–18.

Dreifuerst, K. T. (2009). The essentials of debriefing in simulated learning: A concept analysis. *Nursing Education Perspectives, 30*(2), 109–114.

Elfrink, V. L., Nininger, J., Rohig, L., & Lee, J. (2009). The case for planning in human patient simulation. *Nursing Education Perspectives, 30*(2), 83–86.

Fanning, R. M., & Gaba, D. M. (2007). The role of debriefing in simulation-based learning. *Simulation in Healthcare, 2*(2), 115–125.

Forsythe, L. (2009). Action research, simulation, team communication, and bringing the tacit into voice society for simulation in healthcare. *Simulation in Healthcare, 4*(3), 143–148.

Handley, R., & Dodge, N. (2013). Can simulated practice learning improve clinical competence? *British Journal of Nursing, 22*(9), 529–535.

Hughes, R. (2013). Multi-disciplinary simulation training for anaesthetic practitioners. *Journal of Perioperative Practice, 23*(6/7), 167–170

Inch, J. (2013). Perioperative simulation learning and post-registration development. *British Journal of Nursing, 22*(20), 1166–1172.

Issenberg, S. B., McGaghie, W. C., Petrusa, E. R., Gordon, D. L., & Scalese, R. J. (2005). Features and uses of high-fidelity medical simulations that lead to effective learning: A BEME systematic review. *Medical Teacher, 27*(1), 10–28.

Kardong-Edgen, S., Adamson, K. A., & Fitzgerald, C. (2010). A review of currently published evaluation instruments for human patient simulators. *Clinical Simulation in Nursing, 6*, e25–e35.

Kirkpatrick, D. L. (1998). *Evaluating training programs: The four levels* (2nd ed.). San Francisco, CA: Berrett-Koehler.

Kneebone, R. (2005). Evaluating clinical simulations for learning procedural skills: A theory-based approach. *Academic Medicine, 80*(6), 549–553.

Knowles, M., Holton, E. F., & Swanson, R. A. (2005). *The adult learner: The definitive classic in adult education and human resource development* (6th ed.). Boston, MA: Elsevier,

Kolb, D. A. (1984). *Experiential learning: Experience as the source of learning and development.* Englewood Cliffs, NJ: Prentice Hall.

Lederman, L. (1984). Debriefing: A critical reexamination of the post experience analytic process with implications for its effective use. *Simulation Games, 15*, 415–431.

May, W., Park, J. H., & Lee, J. P. (2009). A ten-year review of the literature on the use of standardized (simulated) patients in teaching and learning: 1996–2005. *Medical Teacher, 31*, 487–492.

McGaghie, W. C., Issenberg, S. B., Petrusa, E. R., & Scales, R. J. (2010). A critical review of simulation-based medical education research: 2003–2009. *Medical Education, 44*, 50–63.

Nelles, L. J., Smith, C. M., Lax, L. R., & Russell, L. (2011). Translating face-to-face experiential learning to video for a web-based communication program. *Canadian Journal for the Scholarship of Teaching and Learning, 2*(1), 1–13.

Squire, K. (2006). From content to context: Videogames as designed experience. *Educational Researcher, 35*(19), 19–29.

Steinwachs, B. (1992). How to facilitate a debrief. *Simulation Gaming, 23*, 186–195.

Stillman, P. L., Ruggill, J. S., Rutala, P. J., & Sabers, D. L. (1980). Patient instructors as teachers and evaluators. *Journal of Medical Education, 55*, 186–193.

Swanson, D. B., & Stillman, P. L. (1990). Use of standardized (simulated) patients for teaching and assessing clinical skills. *Evaluation and the Health Professions, 13,* 79–103.

Van de Ridder, J. M. M., Stokking, K. M., McGaghie, W. C., & ten Cate, O. T. J. (2008). What is feedback in clinical education? *Medical Education, 42,* 189–197.

Wang, E. E. (2011). Simulation and adult learning. *US National Library of Medicine, Disease of the Month, 57*(11), 664–678.

Wordsworth, A. (2013). Realising the potential of simulation: Integrating simulation into nursing programmes at Whitireia, New Zealand. *Whitireia Nursing and Health Journal, 20,* 11–18.

Answers and Rationales to

End-of-Chapter Practice Questions

CHAPTER 2 PRACTICE QUESTIONS

1. A new simulation educator is hired in the simulation laboratory. The simulation educator who has been working at the laboratory for 5 years should be aware that when orientating the novice educator, the best method would be to

   A. Describe the purpose of simulation globally and then locally—NO, novices are not ready to take in the "big picture."
   B. Have the novice educators observe first—NO, although this has some value, it may not assist them in functioning.
   C. Teach the novice educator to evaluate learners—NO, this is a skill that needs to be developed after experience.
   D. Discuss step-by-step procedures for the activity—YES, novice educators are procedure oriented.

2. A healthcare educator is interviewing for a job as a simulation coordinator at a small, private institution. The educator asks about the simulation laboratory budget, and the administrative interviewer tells the educator that the budget has been set and that all the supplies needed have been purchased. The educator understands this type of leadership is

   A. Transactional—YES, decisions were made at the top and handed down.
   B. Situational—NO, this usually happens in a crisis situation.
   C. Laissez-faire—NO, the administrator took charge of the budget.
   D. Transformational—NO, the administrator did not indicate there was input from others.

3. An administrator discusses the development of a simulation laboratory with a healthcare educator and states that the needs of the community must also be considered. What aspect of leadership is this demonstrating?

   A. Negotiation—NO, this is more of a needs assessment.
   B. Resources management—NO, this happens within the institution.
   C. Strategic planning—YES, this is planning the long-term usage of the simulation laboratory.
   D. Governance—NO, this is associated with the mission, and it would have already been decided that a simulation laboratory fits the institution's mission.

4. An expert simulation educator is hired and states that at his previous place of employment, they used highly effective high-fidelity simulation and that this institution would benefit from purchasing a better equipped mannequin. You know that the current budget will not allow the purchase; therefore, your best answer is:

   A. "We can put it on our wish list."—NO, this does not address the issue of narrow-mindedness.
   B. **"There are many methods to do effective simulation."—YES, this demonstrates openness to alternative methods.**
   C. "Can you think of a way to raise funds?"—NO, this is often not the activity of a simulation educator.
   D. "We don't have the money for that."—NO, this is a close-ended statement.

5. Which of the following activities by a simulation educator would not be considered as professional development?

   A. **Taking the role of the standardized (simulated) patient (SP) in a culturally sensitive situation—YES, this is participation not development.**
   B. Presenting a poster about simulation at a general education conference—NO, this is professional development.
   C. Developing a simulation education portfolio to demonstrate to other educators the depth and breadth of simulation learning—NO, this is professional development.
   D. Surveying learners about their anxiety pre- and postsimulation experience—NO, this is professional development.

6. During a scenario debriefing, a learner is questioning the simulation educator about his simulation evaluation grade. The educator describes the learner's behavior and tells him, calmly and professionally, that the behavior is inappropriate. The simulation educator asks the learner to dialogue with her about appropriate ways to address the issue. This situation best describes

   A. Mentoring—NO, the simulation educator and learner are not in a mentor–mentee relationship.
   B. Leadership—NO, this has to do with leading the simulation team.
   C. Educating—NO, this is not facilitation for the acquisition of new information.
   D. **Role modeling—YES, this is facilitating the development of appropriate and inappropriate behavior by displaying proper management skills.**

7. An educator is asked to play a belligerent family member during a scenario and states the he is uncomfortable playing that role in front of learners because it may cause them to disrespect him. As a seasoned simulation educator your best response would be

   A. "I understand your concern but it is important that you participate."—NO, this is close-ended and authoritarian.
   B. "You should not worry about such things; we are pretending."—NO, this downgrades the concern.

C. "The simulation laboratory is safe space, so do not worry."—NO, this downgrades the concern.

D. "All learners have been instructed on the nature of the simulation environment."—YES, this recognizes the concern, but puts into perspective that it is an educational experience.

8. A learner tells the novice simulation educator who is demonstrating on a task trainer that he is doing the procedure wrong. The best response to the learner would be

A. "This is the way we do it in practice."—NO, this is inappropriate.

B. "I think I have more experience than you."—NO, this is inappropriate and uncivil.

C. "Please do not interrupt during the procedure; we can discuss it afterward."—NO, this is inappropriate because it does not address the concern.

D. "Please show me the procedural steps in your textbook."—YES, seek information and always be a learner too.

9. The education department's leader tells the simulation team that he can envision the simulation program growing and eventually making money for the institution by doing simulated team-building exercises for local organizations. The simulation team members regard the leader as

A. Transactional—NO, this is not visionary.

B. Transformational—YES, this is visionary.

C. Hierarchical—NO, this is involving others.

D. Inspirational—NO, although it is inspirational, this is not a leadership label.

10. The simulation educator has been in her role for several years but needs a better understanding when she states that simulation resources involve

A. "Administrative support"—NO, these do involve administration support.

B. "Current financial concerns of the institution"—NO, they do involve current fiscal status.

C. "Legal and ethical concerns"—YES, these are issues, not resources.

D. "Laboratory personnel"—NO, personnel are resources.

CHAPTER 3 PRACTICE QUESTIONS

1. At a faculty meeting, a healthcare educator states that simulation cannot take the place of "real" clinical practice. The best response would be that simulation

A. "Is not meant to take the place of clinical practice"—NO, this is true, but not the best answer to explain the role of simulation to another healthcare educator.

B. "Is more productive than clinical practice"—NO, this is not true.

C. "Has advantages and disadvantages like all learning activities"—NO, this is true but, again, may not be the best way to depict it as a learning activity.

D. "Is an adjunct to clinical practice"—YES, it is an adjunct or support for clinical practice; neither is exclusive of the other.

2. A goal that high-fidelity simulation education does not usually support is

   A. Providing standardization for evaluation of learners—NO, this is one of the evaluation goals.
   B. **Self-learning strategies—YES, high-fidelity simulation usually does not involve just one person.**
   C. Improved quality patient care—NO, this is a goal.
   D. Effective patient safety initiatives—NO, this is a goal.

3. Candidates eligible to sit for the Certified Healthcare Simulation Educator™ (CHSE™) exam may

   A. Be a healthcare administrator who has a simulation lab in the organizational structure—NO, this is management; not actual working with simulation.
   B. Have a master's degree in a healthcare education discipline—NO, baccalaureate or equivalent healthcare educators are eligible to take the examination.
   C. Understand the importance of simulation—NO, understanding does not always include taking part in the simulation experiences.
   D. **Develop simulation scenarios for healthcare learners—YES, this is one of the expected roles for a candidate.**

4. An important goal of simulation is

   A. **Learner assessment—YES, validating that learning has taken place.**
   B. Managing simulation resources—NO, this is not the content that weighed the highest on the examination.
   C. Understanding simulation principles—NO, this is not the content that weighed the highest on the examination; it is second highest.
   D. Developing professional values—NO, this is not the content that weighed the highest on the examination.

5. An effective method of studying for many examination candidates would be

   A. Independent studying—NO, study groups are more effective.
   B. **Using mnemonics—YES, this is helpful.**
   C. Memorizing details—NO, understanding concepts is more helpful.
   D. Elevating anxiety to a point for action—NO, only mild anxiety assists.

6. A candidate taking a computerized test is anxious because the questions appear to be progressing in difficulty, and the candidate can narrow the answers down to two distracters for each question. The candidate is probably experiencing questions written at which level of Bloom's taxonomy?

   A. **Application—YES, this type of question requests the test taker to make a clinical decision.**
   B. Comprehension—NO, this is knowing why something is true.
   C. Knowledge—NO, this is recalling data.
   D. Understanding—NO, this is basically remembering facts.

7. A reason to become certified as a simulation healthcare educator is to

   A. Better understand teaching with simulation—NO, this is for a learner before the certification test.
   B. Develop scenarios that can be widely used by others—NO, this is for a learner before the certification test.

C. Publish about simulation techniques—NO, certification does not ensure publication.

D. Validate expertise in an area—YES, it demonstrates expertise.

8. The ultimate goal for having an interdisciplinary certification for healthcare simulation educators rather than discipline-specific certification is to

A. Promote interdisciplinary conferences—NO, this may happen, but is not a focus.

B. Clarify roles in patient care—NO, this may happen, but is not a focus.

C. Promote quality patient care—YES, this is the ultimate goal.

D. Develop collaboration—NO, the goal of collaboration is quality patient care.

9. Clinical learning differs from simulated clinical experiences for healthcare in the concept of

A. Patient safety—NO, both are concerned with patient safety.

B. Procedural accuracy—NO, both are concerned with accuracy.

C. Interprofessional communication—NO, both are concerned with safe communication.

D. Deliberate practice—YES, only simulation can provide this.

10. During a simulation experience, the learner is asked to review the patient's complete laboratory data, x-rays, and health history, and come up with a diagnosis. This type of scenario develops clinical decision making and uses a skillset on which level of Bloom's taxonomy?

A. Evaluation—YES, multiple data must be assessed to make a decision.

B. Application—NO, because an assessment and integration of data must be done before an intervention is applied.

C. Comprehension—NO, it is more than just interpreting data.

D. Knowledge—NO, it is more than just memorizing facts.

CHAPTER 4 PRACTICE QUESTIONS

1. An experienced simulation educator wants to include simulation in a community-based course that does not currently use simulation as a teaching strategy. The course leader states that it is not feasible to include simulation because it is too difficult to schedule another course activity in the simulation lab. What is the best response?

A. "There may be too many activities in your course already."—NO, this may be a separate issue but does not impact the ability to include simulation.

B. "The simulation lab personnel will need to cancel another course to accommodate this activity."—NO, simulation can work within the confines of available resources.

C. "There are many kinds of simulated activities that would not require time in the simulation lab."—YES, there are many activities that do not require physical lab space.

D. "Simulation might not be the right fit for your course."—NO, simulation can be molded to fit almost any course objectives.

2. A course leader is looking for a way to supplement a clinical experience. There is concern that the current experience is observational and not interactive for the learners. The course leader has had some experience with simulation in the past, but has never designed a scenario. What is the best way to mentor this educator?

   A. Refer the educator to some training resources and offer to help design a scenario that has clear objectives and addresses low-volume, high-risk clinical situations.—YES, this fits the model of a strong mentor.
   B. Design the new scenario based on a conversation with the manager of the clinical site.—NO, objectives should be developed by the educator.
   C. Decline to assist because independent learning through trial and error is the best way to gain experience.—NO, not when there is an experienced simulation educator to act as a mentor.
   D. Show the educator how to use the high-fidelity simulator.—NO, this may be one step in the process but does not encompass mentorship.

3. An administrator wants to increase the amount of clinical time in an educational program. This will require additional simulation educators. Which of the following statements by the administrator demonstrates an understanding of simulation educator development?

   A. "I can ask the clinical educators to help out because they already have the experience."—NO, clinical education is a different learning strategy from simulation.
   B. "I will need to replace my current educators and hire experienced simulation educators."—NO, current educators can be trained to be simulation educators.
   C. "I will identify educators who are interested in the role and have them work with the more experienced simulation educators."—YES, this demonstrates acknowledgment of available mentorship.
   D. "Anyone interested in becoming a simulation educator will need time off from work to go back to school."—NO, further education may be useful but it will not require enrollment in a formal education program.

4. A new simulation educator has been working with experienced educators and is now running simulation scenarios independently. According to Benner's stages, how would you describe the level of this educator?

   A. Novice—NO, technical training may be appropriate at this level.
   B. Competent—NO, observation and practice are expected at this level.
   C. Advanced beginner—NO, beginning to understand the methodology at this level.
   D. Proficient—YES, the simulation educator should be able to function independently at this level.

5. A new simulation educator is facilitating a scenario involving a diabetic patient in a medical–surgical area. The learner administers a potentially lethal dose of medication after committing a medication calculation error. The best response by the educator is to

   A. Intervene when the learner is calculating the incorrect dose.—NO, this is part of the experiential learning.
   B. Stop the learner from administering the medication.—NO, this is part of the experiential learning.

C. **Intervene as the critical care response team and administer the reversal agent.—YES, allowing the learner to make mistakes is important, but being able to engage the "escape plan" is also important.**

D. Program the simulator to go into cardiac arrest.—NO, unplanned death in simulation can impact the learning environment.

6. A simulation educator is running a scenario about diabetic ketoacidosis, and the students interpret the glucose sliding scale wrong and give too much insulin. The students realize the mistake and adjust the glucose intravenous (IV) drip. The simulation educator uses this as a teaching scenario during the debriefing and understands that this type of situation, when it arises in simulation, is referred to as

A. An "as-is situation"—NO, this creates a realistic patient situation (Dieckmann, Gaba, & Rall, 2007).

B. A "critical incident"—NO, this is not the terminology used in this case because it was rectified.

C. **A "what if"—YES, this is a "what if situation" that arises and needs to be discussed during the debriefing.**

D. An "escape plan"—NO, this is needed if the patient is deteriorating to the point of no return.

7. A simulation educator is running the same scenario about diabetic ketoacidosis, and the students interpret the glucose sliding scale wrong and give too much insulin. The students do not realize the mistake. The simulation educator uses this as a teaching scenario during the simulation by sending in an experienced SP to question the dose. This type of situation, when it arises in simulation, is referred to as

A. An "as-is situation"—NO, this is not part of developing the reality of the scenario.

B. A "critical incident"—NO, although the medication error could be conceived as a critical incident, by rectifying the incident the simulation educator produces an escape plan.

C. A "what if"—NO, this is a more serious variation.

D. **An "escape plan"—YES, this is a plan to prevent the patient from dying.**

8. The simulation educator is providing first-year medical students and freshman nursing students with a scenario about a geriatric patient who has pneumonia. The patient's condition is declining, and the students discuss types of appropriate oxygenation. The appropriate progression of the scenario for this level of healthcare students would be to

A. Discuss the scenario after it is done and let it progress.—NO, this would not provide the learners with an escape plan.

B. Let the scenario progress uninterrupted.—NO, again, it would not provide an escape plan.

C. **Intervene and prompt them to the appropriate treatment.—YES, this would get the scenario back on track.**

D. Allow the patient to deteriorate and observe the students' behavior.—NO, this may be traumatic for beginning learners.

9. A novice simulation educator has developed a scenario about a critically ill patient, and the students have not received the didactic content for overwhelming sepsis. As the mentor, you should

A. Ask the novice simulation educator to redo the entire scenario.—NO, a revision may suffice.

B. Teach all the variables that the students will need to know.—NO, this may not be possible.

C. Simplify the scenario for the novice simulation educator.—NO, the novice is the developer.

D. Direct the novice simulation educator to re-examine the learning objectives.—YES, have the novice simulation educator review what objectives need to be accomplished.

10. A novice simulation educator develops a scenario for interprofessional learners. The scenario is well developed and at the appropriate level. As the mentor, you review the scenario for the novice simulation educator. In which part of the scenario would you provide guidance to the novice simulation educator?

A. The "what if" that is worked into the scenario—NO, this is a good strategy to anticipate variables in a scenario.

B. The 10 objectives that the scenario should facilitate—YES, this is too many objectives to accomplish.

C. The environmental description of the resources needed for the scenario—NO, this is needed.

D. The role of the learners participating in the scenario—NO, this is needed.

CHAPTER 5 PRACTICE QUESTIONS

1. During a role-play simulation about poverty, a healthcare learner excuses himself and leaves the simulation laboratory. On the evaluation form he states that the scenario was humiliating, and people don't really understand what poverty is like. As the simulation educator, how would you first address this with the learner?

A. Discuss with him that his reality contract was signed and that he needs to abide by it.—NO, this is not demonstrating cultural sensitivity.

B. Ask him why he felt the scenario was insensitive.—YES, this may assist the learner and the simulation educator to understand better how role-playing may affect some learners and to prepare better for the next poverty simulation.

C. Discuss his lack of achieving the learning outcomes.—NO, this is not demonstrating cultural sensitivity.

D. Develop a plan to achieve the outcomes in a different format.—NO, this may be completed after the issues are discussed.

2. A simulation educator is approached by an ESL learner who asks whether she can have the full written evaluative scenario in her hands because it is difficult for her to understand the patient's voice over the microphone. The simulation educator would best reply by

A. Providing the entire script to the learner—NO, this disrupts the integrity of the evaluation process.

B. Explaining to the learner that it is copyrighted and would be giving her an unfair advantage—NO, this is not demonstrating cultural sensitivity and may be challenged in an academic setting.

    C. Reviewing the scenario with her beforehand—NO, this disrupts the integrity of the evaluation process.

    D. Asking another learner in the scenario to repeat the patient responses— YES, this would provide a reasonable accommodation, yet not disrupt the integrity of the scenario for evaluative purposes.

3. During a scenario, a group of four interdisciplinary learners arrives at the wrong conclusion for the patients' manifestations. As the patient is reporting postsurgical pain of 10 on a scale of 1 to 10, the group discusses the possibility of an infection when, in fact, a hematoma is developing in the surgical site. The simulation educator overseeing the scenario decreases the body temperature and increases the pulse above 120 bpm. This technique is referred to as

    A. Adjusting the primary frame—NO, this occurs before the scenario so that learners can make sense out of the situation.

    B. Adjusting the secondary frame—NO, this is not a valid term.

    C. Adjusting from within—YES, providing changes and clues during the scenario.

    D. Adjusting from outside—NO, this is stopping the scenario to explain.

4. During a scenario, a learner stands in the background but does participate in the role assigned. When assessing the video replay of the scenario, the simulation educator discusses the actions of this learner as those that could possibly exemplify which learning style?

    A. Verbal (linguistic)—NO, this learner type likes to talk things through.

    B. Tactile—NO, this learner type would jump in and manipulate the equipment.

    C. Global—NO, this learner type is spontaneous.

    D. Reflective—YES, this learner type wants to quietly process information.

5. During an interdisciplinary scenario, a learner who is in the role of the nurse tells the learner in the role of a physician that the procedure being considered is not the best choice for the patient's condition. In reviewing the scenario, the simulation educators discuss the possible learning style of the learner in the role of the nurse as

    A. Sequential—NO, this learner type is procedurally driven.

    B. Tactile—NO, this learner type likes to adjust equipment.

    C. Global—YES, this learner type is spontaneous and will jump in.

    D. Reflective—NO, this learner type likes to process information quietly.

6. During a hybrid simulation scenario, the learner tells a family member that she needs to give the healthcare professional team "a minute to think" when the family member keeps asking what is wrong with her son. The simulation educator decides that the best debriefing method for this learner would be to

    A. Have him review the video and write a reflection—NO, the learner may not see this as unprofessional if it is a lifelong communication style.

    B. Individually counsel him on professionalism—YES, the learner needs to understand this is not acceptable in a professional role.

    C. Have a group review of all aspects of the scenario—NO, this is an individual issue.

    D. Send him to student services for counseling—NO, this may need to be done, but not after one incident.

7. An interdisciplinary healthcare team of learners is experiencing its first scenario together, and one learner giggles frequently during the simulation scenario. The simulation educator understands that this may be a symptom of which of the following phases of learner development?

A. Transference—NO, this is when the learner is assuming a professional role.

B. Trial and error—NO, this is when the learner is invested in a professional role.

C. Professionalism—NO, this is the outcome of understanding and internalizing a professional role.

D. **Feeling like an imposter—YES, this is lack of confidence in the professional role, and giggling is a symptom of being unsure how to act.**

8. During a high-fidelity simulation scenario, a beginning learner is reluctant to place the monitor leads on the mannequin, turn on the cardiopulmonary monitor, and adjust the computer screen so the recording is visible. The simulation educator understands that this learner is most likely from which of the following generational groups?

A. Millennials—NO, this generation is familiar with technology.

B. Generation X—NO, this generation is familiar with technology.

C. Generation Y—NO, this generation is familiar with technology.

D. **Baby boomers—YES, this is a generation of older people who are the least familiar with technology.**

9. During a high-fidelity simulation, the interdisciplinary learners are drawing the wrong conclusion as the case is unfolding, and the simulation educator stops the case and provides some educational information. The educational technique is referred to as

A. Modulation framing—NO, this is considering individual learner differences.

B. **Lifesaving from outside—YES, this is stopping the scenario before it goes too far off course.**

C. Preventing cognitive dissonance—NO, this is when learning and cultural values are at odds with each other.

D. Demonstrating authority in the educator role—NO, this is just a teaching style.

10. A learner requests to use an amplified stethoscope during the scenario. The simulation educator allows her to use it because

A. Many learners are able to hear better with one.—NO, this may be true but is not the rationale for allowing them.

B. It is an American with Disabilities Act mandate.—NO, there are no mandates for individual devices.

C. It demonstrates cultural sensitivity.—NO, this is not a cultural issue; it is a diversity issue.

D. **It is a reasonable accommodation.—YES, this is a reasonable accommodation.**

CHAPTER 6 PRACTICE QUESTIONS

1. A novice nurse educator reports to the department chair that there are three learners in the back of the room who are chattering during class, and the nurse educator finds it very distracting. The nurse educator tells the department chair that the next step is to "call them out" and send them to the department chair's office to be "written up" for unprofessionalism. The best response by the department chair is

   A. "Calling them out in front of their peers should take care of the problem."—NO, this is not role modeling professional behavior and it is dehumanizing.
   B. "I will tell them that if they are unprofessional again, they will be excused from the program."—NO, the director is not the first person in the chain of command.
   C. **"Before the next class, move their seats to separate areas."—YES, this addresses the problem before it occurs again.**
   D. "After the next class, speak with them and explain how their behavior is affecting you."—NO, although this addresses the problem it does not do it before the next class.

2. The nurse educator is developing a test and formulating a test item at an application level on Bloom's taxonomy. Which type of test question would best evaluate the learner's cognitive level of understanding?

   A. A true/false question that has two different interventions—NO, true/false questions provide a 50/50 chance for guessing.
   B. **A hot spot that asks the learner to place an X on an anatomical part— YES, this is knowledge based.**
   C. A multiple-choice question that asks for the best nursing assessment of a patient with costovertebral tenderness—NO, this evaluates the learner's comprehension of what assessment would be appropriate for a manifestation.
   D. A select-all-that-applies question that asks for the appropriate nursing interventions for a postoperative abdominal hysterectomy—NO, choosing the interventions is applying the knowledge to nursing care.

3. A nurse educator has submitted a syllabus with the following learning outcomes. Which learning outcome is written at the highest level of Bloom's taxonomy?

   A. Demonstrate caring to geriatric patients—NO, this is at the level of applying the learning outcomes.
   B. Discuss common healthcare concerns of geriatric patients—NO, this is at the level of understanding the learning outcomes.
   C. **Evaluate geriatric patients' understanding of home safety—YES, this is at the level of evaluating the learning outcomes.**
   D. Formulate a plan of care for a geriatric patient—NO, this is at the level of creating the learning outcomes.

4. During a curriculum meeting, a nurse educator states, "I think we should coordinate the clinical skills checklists for all the classes to make sure they are appropriately leveled and each is measurable." The philosophical foundations for this analysis would be

   A. Narrative pedagogy—NO, this is a philosophy that derives meaning from words.
   B. Behaviorism—YES, this calls for measurable and observable outcomes.
   C. Constructivism—NO, this exemplifies the learners creating their own goals.
   D. Feminism—NO, this is concerned with equality in education.

5. During a faculty interview, the nurse educator candidate states a preferred learning activity to facilitate learner understanding is storytelling. What nursing educational philosophy or theory is indicated by this learning activity?

   A. Narrative pedagogy—YES, narrative pedagogy includes dialogue and storytelling.
   B. Behaviorism—NO, this looks for outcomes that can be measured.
   C. Constructivism—NO, this uses hands-on activities.
   D. Feminism—NO, this bases its content on decreasing oppressive forces.

6. A nurse educator would like learners to each become responsible for a section of a case study and to articulate how their work contributes to the patient care picture. An active learning activity that would best accomplish this outcome would be

   A. An unfolding case study approach—NO, this can be done in a group but is usually an individual activity.
   B. Socratic questioning—NO, this usually occurs between learner and educator.
   C. A learning circle—NO, this is more of a sharing activity.
   D. A jigsaw activity—YES, this facilitates learners taking a part in the activity and contributing to the whole.

7. A nurse educator states at a faculty meeting that switching from traditional care planning to concept mapping will not teach the learners the nursing process. Which statement by the department director would address this concern?

   A. Ask the other faculty members what they think.—NO, this is just opening the floor to opinion without evidence.
   B. Request the nurse educator making the comment to provide evidence.— YES, evidence will assist the group to make an informed decision.
   C. Ask the group to vote on one of the learning tools, care plans, or concept maps.—NO, this is just opening the floor to opinion without evidence.
   D. Tell the faculty that the evidence shows that concept mapping increases critical thinking.—NO, critical thinking was not the nurse educator's concern, it was learner knowledge of the nursing process.

8. When interviewing for a job, a nurse educator is asked about her education philosophy, and she says that she is primarily concerned with equality in the classroom. This nurse educator most likely subscribes to the philosophy of

   A. Phenomenology—NO, this has to do with the learners' previous life experiences.
   B. Emancipatory education—YES, this is concerned with social equality.

    C. Narrative pedagogy—NO, this is concerned with meaning derived from words.

    D. Constructivism—NO this is concerned with learner knowledge being built on past learning.

9. At a faculty retreat, a nurse educator is telling the group about her philosophy and says, "I believe in rewarding learners for good behavior and doing well on tests." What philosophy is the educator a proponent of?

    A. Realism—NO, this is based on quantitative analysis.

    B. Essentialism—NO, this is based on the traditional education belief that knowledge is passed form teacher to learner.

    C. Perennialism—NO, this based on drilling down to the basics: reading, writing, and math.

    D. Behaviorism—YES, this is about stimulus response.

10. Which statement by a learner should alert a nurse educator to consider using another learning activity to increase learner comprehension?

    A. "I have never been given such low grades before."—YES, this statement describes a discrepancy in the comprehension process.

    B. "I read the book before class."—NO, this is expected learner behavior.

    C. "I do extra questions every night."—NO, this is expected learner behavior.

    D. "I understand the material in class, but cannot pick the right test answer."—NO, this describes a testing difficulty.

CHAPTER 7 PRACTICE QUESTIONS

1. Which of the following is well established regarding integrating simulation into the curriculum?

    A. Integrate with other learning events—YES, simulation is one part of a curriculum needed to prepare healthcare professionals for today's practice.

    B. Simulation can be substituted with lectures—NO, it is an active learning strategy.

    C. Clinical experience can substitute for immersive simulation—NO, simulation is different from clinical experience.

    D. Educational objectives are not required for case scenarios—NO, learning outcomes are needed for evaluation of learning.

2. Which of the following best describes a complete needs assessment?

    A. Identify the problem or educational gap—NO, this is just one aspect.

    B. Identify the current approach (who is doing what, when, how, resource limitations)—NO, this is only one aspect.

    C. Identify the ideal approach—NO, this is only one aspect.

    D. Ideal – current approach = general assessment—YES, this is a complete assessment.

3. Which of the following learning domains is not evaluated through simulation?

    A. Affective—NO, this can be evaluated.

    B. Constructive—YES, this is not a learning domain.

    C. Psychomotor—NO, this can be evaluated.

    D. Cognitive—NO, this can be evaluated.

4. Realism for technical skill assessment would be best assessed by which of the following?

   A. Full-body mannequin—NO, this may be a method, but not the best method.
   B. Standardized patient—NO, this may be a method, but not the best method.
   C. Task trainer—YES, this would be the best method to demonstrate.
   D. Computer-based interactive activity—NO, this may be a method, but not the best method because the actual skill is not being done in real time.

5. Which of the following organizational barriers can prevent simulation implementation in the curriculum?

   A. Lack of administrative support—NO, this is a barrier, but does not include all barriers.
   B. No dedicated space for simulation—NO, this is a barrier, but does not include all barriers.
   C. No time in the curriculum—NO, this is a barrier, but does not include all barriers.
   D. All of the above—YES, all are barriers.

6. In which step of the educational model of Kern and colleagues (2009) should the faculty member "identify the learners, level of training, previous experience, current performance, learning styles and preferences"?

   A. Step 1—NO, this is problem identification.
   B. Step 2—YES, the learners are assessed.
   C. Step 3—NO, goals are established.
   D. Step 4—NO, educational strategies are chosen.

7. "Deliberate practice" as discussed by Ericsson is best described as which of the following in simulation?

   A. Practice once per week with an instructor—NO, this may not ensure competency.
   B. Practice in class only—NO, this may not ensure competency.
   C. Practice until competency is achieved—YES, this is the goal of deliberate practice.
   D. Practice scheduled for student—NO, this may not ensure competency.

8. Which type of validity best describes the process of establishing that an action accurately represents the concept being evaluated in simulation?

   A. Construct validity—YES, this answers the question, "Is this testing what it is supposed to be testing?"
   B. Content validity—NO, this has to do with topics.
   C. Objective validity—NO, this has to do with statistics on an item.
   D. Implementation validity—NO, this is about using a concept in practice.

9. Which of the following is a primary benefit of assessing technical skills using simulation modalities?

   A. Shorter time—NO, it may take just as long.
   B. Patient safety—YES, this is a safe environment for learning.
   C. Cost efficient—NO, simulation equipment is costly.
   D. Faculty training time—NO, simulation requires faculty training.

10. Simulation can be effectively integrated into the curriculum in which of the following areas?

   A. Basic sciences—NO, this is just one aspect.
   B. Basic clinical assessment—NO, this is just one aspect.
   C. Crisis management training—NO, this is just one aspect.
   D. All of the above—YES, all can be effectively integrated into the curriculum.

CHAPTER 8 PRACTICE QUESTIONS

1. A learner is of a religious belief that does not allow video recording, and all other learners have agreed to recording for debriefing purposes. The simulation educator should

   A. Explain to the learner that it will be destroyed after debriefing—NO, this does not address the concern of being video recorded.
   B. Make an exception and not video record the learner, but ask the learner to write a summary reflection—NO, this does not meet the student learning outcome (SLO) in a fair manner.
   C. Explain to the learner that the learner cannot meet course objectives and will not pass the scenario—YES, if video recording is a critical part of the debriefing, then the learner cannot meet the SLO.
   D. Explain to the learner it is for educational purposes only—NO, this does not address the concern of being video recorded.

2. The simulation educator overhears learners talking outside the simulation room about the scenario, using information specific to the diagnosis, treatment, and outcomes. The first action the simulation educator should take is

   A. Arrange a meeting with the participants in a private place and discuss the situation—NO, this does not stop the behavior when it needs to be stopped.
   B. Inform the participants they have failed the scenario due to unprofessional behavior—NO, this is not the first action to be taken.
   C. Give the participants a written warning for unprofessional behavior—NO, this is not the first action to be taken.
   D. Ask the participants to immediately stop the conversation and address the unprofessionalism—YES, this is first; the simulation educator must stop the violation immediately.

3. Following a formative simulation session, the team identifies a mechanical issue that did not allow the session to be video recorded. The simulation educator planned to use the video recording as part of the debriefing. What action should the simulation educator take now?

   A. Cancel the debriefing because there is no recording—NO, because this is not a summative evaluation, the recording may not be critical to the process of learning.
   B. Conduct the debriefing without the video—YES, the formative evaluation can be done as a learning process without the video.
   C. Present the key points of the simulation to the participants—NO, this does not meet the purpose of debriefing.
   D. Reschedule the session when the mechanical issue has been fixed—NO, this will mean losing a valuable learning opportunity.

4. A participant arrives to the simulation lab late after the session has begun without having completed the preclass assignment. The simulation lab policy states that all readings must be completed before class. The best action for the simulation educator is to

A. Allow the learner to participate and require the learner to complete an additional simulation assignment—NO, this is not addressing unprofessional behavior.

B. Allow the learner to participate and extend the session to make up the time—NO, this is not addressing unprofessional behavior and can place the patient at risk.

C. **Not allow the learner to participate and agree to discuss alternatives after the session—YES, this is addressing the learner's having placed the patient at risk as well as unprofessional behavior.**

D. Not allow the learner to participate until the preclass assignment is completed—NO, this is not addressing unprofessional behavior and can place the patient at risk.

5. A journalist requests to observe, record, and interview participants in the simulation lab. Your institution does not have a policy regarding outside observers. The best response by the simulation educator to this request is

A. **"No, but I will be willing to give you a tour and answer any questions."—YES, this does not place the learners at risk.**

B. "Yes, this is a summative evaluation, and I will need to get permission from the participants to be recorded."—NO, there is no established policy; the learners should not be placed at risk.

C. "Yes, but you will need to come back next week after our policy is finalized."—NO, there is no policy, and one should be drafted with thoughtful input by all stakeholders.

D. "Yes, absolutely; here is a list of simulations that would be best for your report."—NO, there is no established policy; the learners should not be placed at risk.

6. The simulation lab's policy states that videos will be destroyed after 5 days unless necessary for a research project approved by the institutional review board (IRB). To protect the learners, videos are stored on a secure password-protected server. A faculty member contacts the simulation team and asks to save a class simulation video for a future class scheduled in 14 days. The faculty member has spoken with all of the participants and has received verbal consent to use the video. Which of the following is the best response to the request?

A. Because the video was an excellent example to use in the classroom, an exception to the policy will be made.—NO, this is a violation of the learning contract.

B. The participants have all given verbal consent; therefore, the video will be saved for the faculty member.—NO, this is a violation of the learning contract.

C. The video can only be used for the next 10 days, and then it will be deleted.—NO, this is a violation of the learning contract.

D. **The video was created to use in the classroom only and it will be deleted per policy.—YES, the policy was created to protect learners.**

7. A simulation evaluation that is used to assess learners competency for a degree, award, or against a criteria is called

   A. Formative evaluation—NO, this is usually used to promote self-assessment and provide learner feedback.
   B. Cumulative evaluation—NO, this is not a term that is used.
   C. Peer evaluation—NO, this is not usually used to grant the end judgment.
   D. Summative evaluation—YES, this assesses the end result.

8. A simulation evaluation that is used to promote self-assessment, guide learners, clarify misconception, and provide feedback is called

   A. Formative evaluation—YES, this is provided with the intent to promote future success.
   B. Cumulative evaluation—NO, this is a final evaluation.
   C. Peer evaluation—NO, this is when learners assess each other.
   D. Summative evaluation—NO, this is a final evaluation.

9. A benefit for healthcare simulation educators when using formative evaluation in simulation-based learning (SBL) is to

   A. Improve the learner's performance—YES, this is done to promote improvement and success.
   B. Determine whether the competency was achieved—NO, this is a summative evaluation.
   C. Assign a final grade—NO, this is a summative evaluation.
   D. Require the learner to figure out the scenario independently—NO, this is a method used when there is subjective data to be considered in an evaluation.

10. While conducting team simulation activities, communication, collaboration, and trust of the teams may be enhanced during the session when

   A. The same team leader is used every time—NO, this is not practical.
   B. Learners are criticized for their mistakes—No, this will intimidate learners.
   C. A safe learning environment is created—YES, this will assist learners to feel comfortable about participating.
   D. Learners are encouraged to practice in silos—NO, this will not promote communication, collaboration, and trust among the interprofessional teams.

CHAPTER 9 PRACTICE QUESTIONS

1. Which of the following best describes SBAR (situation, background, assessment, and recommendation) communication?

   A. A concise method of documenting the current status of a patient's condition—NO, SBAR is used to communicate verbally.
   B. A communication technique that evokes the two-challenge rule when one party is in disagreement with the intended action—NO, SBAR should not evoke a challenge, it should be a cooperative communication.
   C. A dialogue between physicians and nurses—NO, SBAR is used among all healthcare professionals.
   D. A brief two-way exchange of information that includes a recommendation for action—YES, this is done to report and receive information.

2. When a learner puts a tourniquet on a simulator and the simulated blood vessel becomes engorged with fluid, what type of fidelity is this associated with?

A. Functional fidelity—NO, this is how operational the system is.
B. Task fidelity—YES, this is learning a task.
C. Physical fidelity—NO, this is the environmental setup.
D. Psychological fidelity—NO, this is the perception of the learner.

3. A technique that replicates real-life experiences with scenarios that immerse the learner in an environment that attempts to closely duplicate the clinical environment best describes

A. SBL—YES, this tries to simulate the real clinical event.
B. Perfect practice—NO, all practice has room for remediation if needed.
C. Deliberate practice—NO, this is intentional practice of a skill.
D. Adult learning theory—NO, this is a learning theory with many concepts.

4. Simulation principles include principles of adult learning theory proposed by Malcolm Knowles (1950), also known as

A. Pedagogy—NO, this refers to the method of traditional teaching.
B. Deliberate practice—NO, this is intentional practice of a skill.
C. Andragogy—YES, this was coined as the method of teaching adults.
D. Team training—NO, this has to do with group processes.

5. During a simulation scenario a learner informs the group that she is applying a nonrebreather oxygen mask to the patient at 10 L/minute and reports that the pulse oximetry improved from 92% to 96%. This is an example of

A. Perfect practice—NO, this allows for repeat attempts at simulation.
B. Closed-loop communication—NO, this is a communication style.
C. Adult learning theory—NO, this is a theory for teaching adult learners.
D. Situational awareness—YES, the learners are taking care of a specific patient situation.

6. When a member of the healthcare team communicates information to another team member and is unsatisfied with the response, the next step is to

A. Document the incident in the medical record—NO, this is not an issue that should be in a patient's chart.
B. Invoke the two-challenge rule—YES, tell the member again.
C. Follow the chain of command—NO, try to tell the member again.
D. Complete the action on his own—NO, the team must work together.

7. Having a high-fidelity mannequin make vomiting sounds during a simulator simulation is an example of what kind of fidelity?

A. Physical fidelity—YES, this is enacting what might happen to a real patient.
B. Functional fidelity—NO, this speaks about the operation of the system.
C. Task fidelity—NO, this is used for specific procedures.
D. Psychological fidelity—NO, this is the perception of realness by the learner.

8. Simulation learners are using deliberate practice on a task training to learn intubation, and one learner keeps repeating the same mistakes. The appropriate instructions to the learner by the simulation educator would be

A. "Keep trying to do the skill until you are successful."—NO, this would be deliberate practice.

B. "Review the physiology of the trachea before you try again."—NO, this would be remediation.

C. **"What part of the procedure do you find is difficult for you and why?"—YES, this promotes reflection, which is a concept in deliberate practice.**

D. "Please stop, and you should watch your colleagues before trying again."—NO, this does not always report reflection.

9. An adult learner in a simulation experience is most apt to

A. Understand the pathophysiology behind a skill.—NO, this is not always applicable.

B. Demonstrate exact skill execution.—NO, this is not a concept of adult learning.

C. Be hesitant to perform a skill.—NO, this is not a concept of adult learning.

D. **Understand the need for being successful at a skill.—YES, adult learners need skills that are directly applicable.**

10. During a team simulation exercise, one learner provides another healthcare learner with information about the patient. The other learner does not acknowledge the information. The first learner tells the team member who is role-playing the nursing supervisor that critical information is missing. The learner playing the nursing supervisor should

A. Reprimand the learner who did not acknowledge the information.—NO, this is not following the two-challenge rule.

B. Repeat the information to all the learners.—NO, this is not following the two-challenge rule.

C. Stop the scenario and restart with clearer ground rules.—NO, this is not following the two-challenge rule.

D. **Tell the learner to repeat the information a second time.—YES, this is the next step.**

CHAPTER 10 PRACTICE QUESTIONS

1. A new simulation coordinator has recently read an article on the use of moulage in simulation and intends to incorporate it into upcoming scenario events. The coordinator realizes that the most important consideration to implementing moulage as a methodology is

A. The additional expense and justification that must now be incorporated into the cost of the simulation—NO, although these are considerations, they will not be the largest initial impact.

B. Breaking the news to the SPs that they will now be wearing makeup and responsible for cleanup—NO, although it is a change, in the process of simulation for this center this is a small change in job responsibilities.

C. Performing an inventory of the types of mannequins to ensure compatibility of moulage and plastics—NO, although this is helpful, it is not the most important consideration.

D. Adjusting the timing of the simulation sessions to include the preparation time needed for moulage—YES, this is the most impactful concern especially early in the implementation of moulage into a program. The increased time needed will necessitate a reassessment of the time required to conduct simulation sessions and will impact many of the aspects of planning.

2. The best makeup to use on a mannequin is

A. A product that has a low concentration of parabens as a base—NO, this is generally not an issue.

B. A product that has been tested on a hidden area of mannequin skin— YES, this is the safe and effective way to determine the best makeup to use on mannequins.

C. A product that mixes well with an even base of petroleum jelly—NO, this does not confirm that the makeup in question will work well on the mannequin.

D. A product that uses a small amount of red dye number 4—NO, although the less red dye used generally means the less amount of staining, this information alone will not determine the best makeup to use.

3. A simulation educator and moulage proponent is hired and states that at her previous place of employment they sculpted and molded their own wounds. You know that the current staff does not have the skillset to accomplish this, the department does not have the materials on hand, and acquiring them will incur an additional expense; therefore, your best answer is

A. We can review the possibility after considering the costs of materials and training. YES, keeping an open mind and exploring new moulage concepts lends support while recognizing the limitations.

B. Our budget and current staffing doesn't allow for onsite manufacturing or construction.—NO, this is limited in response and supports the incorrect idea that moulage requires unreasonable resources.

C. It is a questionable prospect because we do not have sculptors on staff.— NO, this does not allow for the enrichment of the staff at the center and the exploration of new techniques.

D. The store-bought wounds and sticky notes work just fine.—NO, this is not the best answer as it supports a simplistic approach to moulage and not an investment in realism. Although this may be a good beginning, thought should be given to growth.

4. A faculty member has just returned from a moulage conference and is very excited about a new recipe that she has learned for creating pus and infection. She wants to add an infected wound to an upcoming end-of-life simulation to see how the students will react. She feels that it will have a big impact, especially if she can add the right odors. The best response to her would be

A. That is a great idea, but only if it is very realistic and we add treatment materials.—NO, although it is good to consider the degree of realism and provide for treatment interventions, for the case described, the moulage is not logical or indicated.

B. **The suggested moulage does not support nor is it indicated by the objectives of the case.—YES, the moulage must support the learning outcomes for the given simulation.**

C. Putting makeup on actors carries too much risk of allergic reaction and staining. –NO, these issues are possible, although very controllable.

D. It is not a good idea as it will add expense to the scenario and cause excessive cleanup.—NO, initial investment in moulage can be small, and the benefit outweighs the cost.

5. A simulation educator who has been in his role for several years indicates that he does not have a good understanding of the educational concepts supporting the use of moulage in simulation by the following comment

A. "Simulation is a fabrication and not real; so the environment is not important as long as the students are successful."—NO, the degree of fidelity can positively impact the success of the students in the scenario.

B. "The students do not know the difference; regardless of how the simulation is laid out, we just need to keep the process moving."—NO, although there are not very many studies that speak specifically about moulage use, there is evidence that the degree of realism is not lost on the students.

C. "Adding a realistic vague distracting wound to the simulation keeps the students on their toes."—NO, moulage simply for the sake of moulage does not support the objectives of the case and can have a negative impact if it is not logical to the case.

D. **"As simulation is a representation of a realistic event, the more realistic the simulation, the more impact there is on the learning process."—YES, as simulation is supported by experiential learning theory, the degree of realism or fidelity that is built into the scenario helps support the student's processing of the event.**

6. A novice simulation educator needs more mentoring when she tells you

A. **"Simulation is just as effective without using moulage."—YES, this may not be true.**

B. "Moulage adds to the learners' perception of the situation."—NO, this is true.

C. "Moulage is part of simulation preparation."—NO, this is true.

D. "SPs are effective with moulage."—NO, this is true.

7. It is important to have an SP understand the importance of protecting the moulage that was done on him because

A. It is costly.—NO, this is a concern but not the major one.

B. It is a work of art that should not be destroyed.—NO, it is more than art, it is part of an intended program.

C. Many students can learn from one moulaged SP.—NO, although this may occur, it is not the most important reason.

D. **It is time-consuming.—YES, it is costly in human time.**

8. When unsure of the type of material a high-fidelity mannequin is made of, which needs to be made up for a scenario, the best method is to

A. Apply the makeup lightly.—NO, this may stain.

B. **Test a small section.—YES, this is the safest method.**

C. Use a plastic cover.—NO, this would be difficult at best.

D. Provide pictures of a person around the mannequin.—NO, this does not produce the realism that may be needed.

9. A simulation educator requests a budget to buy moulage supplies, but only half of the finances are received. The best action would be to

A. Try again in the following year's budget to secure the money.—NO, this does not help for the current year.

B. Use no moulage.—NO, this may decrease realism.

C. Buy supplies and wait for reimbursement.—NO, this may cost the simulation educator out-of-pocket money.

D. **Use inexpensive makeup for the fiscal year.—YES, this would be the best alternative.**

10. Understanding moulage is important, and applying appropriate moulage to the simulation scenario should be guided by

A. The equipment being used—NO, this is not an indicator.

B. The financial status of the laboratory—NO, this should not be an indicator.

C. **The learning objectives—YES, the goal of the learning session is most important.**

D. The artist's capability—NO, this should not be an indicator.

CHAPTER 11 PRACTICE QUESTIONS

1. A simulation educator is planning to start using SP simulation in the simulation lab. Where should the educator look to find SPs?

A. Advertise for SPs through the school website —NO, this is just one method, but may be effective.

B. Contact another simulation center in the area for advice —NO, this is just one method, but may be effective.

C. Check with the drama department at the university —NO, this is just one method, but may be effective.

D. **All of the above—YES, all of the above are ways to recruit SPs.**

2. When an SP is used with a human-patient simulator (HPS) scenario, this type of simulation is often referred to as

A. SP simulation—NO, this only refers to SP simulation.

B. HPS—NO, this only refers to HPS simulation.

C. **Hybrid simulation—YES, combining HPS and SP simulation is often referred to as hybrid simulation.**

D. Double simulation—NO, this is not a term used to describe simulation.

3. When developing an SP simulation scenario, the maximum time limit for the length of the scenario is

A. Fifteen minutes—NO, there is no limit.

B. Thirty minutes—NO, there is no limit.

C. Forty-five minutes—NO, there is no limit.

D. **There is no maximum time limit—YES, the SP simulation experience can be as long or short as you want it to be; there is no limit.**

4. What is the best method for SP training?

   A. Review of the case scenario—NO, this is just part of the eduction needed.
   B. Demonstrate the assessment techniques—NO, this is just part of the eduction needed.
   C. Role-playing—NO, this is just part of the eduction needed.
   D. All of the above—YES, all of the above are excellent methods included in SP training.

5. During a simulation scenario, the student, completing the assessment, proceeds to examine the patient's eye with the otoscope. The patient should

   A. Not do anything.—NO, the patient could be injured.
   B. Tell the student the wrong scope is being used.—NO, that would be out of character for the patient.
   C. Scream—NO, this would not be appropriate.
   D. State, "I do not want you to examine my eyes."—YES, to protect eye safety, the individual as a patient can refuse any procedure.

6. During an SP scenario, the SP notices the student looking at a piece of paper in her pocket. After the session is over, the SP should

   A. Do nothing.—NO, the student could be cheating.
   B. Make a note on the student checklist.—NO, this may not been seen in a timely fashion.
   C. Ask the student about the note.—NO, that would be out of character.
   D. Notify the simulation educator.—YES, this is important because the student could possibly be cheating.

7. After an SP simulation experience, a student comes out of the room crying. The simulation educator should

   A. Do nothing.—NO, the emotional status of the student must be addressed.
   B. Wait until after the feedback session and approach the student.—NO, the feedback session will not be beneficial if the student is upset.
   C. Take the student aside and speak to the individual in a private area.— YES, it is important to find out why the student is upset in private.
   D. Ask the student to leave the simulation lab.—NO, the student's emotional state must be addressed.

8. The SP role in the evaluation of students is

   A. To grade the student—NO, that is the role of the faculty.
   B. To complete the checklist to document what the student did and did not do—YES, the completion of the checklist provides the faculty with the data they need to grade the experience.
   C. The SP has no involvement in student evaluation—NO, completion of the checklist provides the information for the faculty to determine the student grade.
   D. To compare the student performances against each other—NO, students are not compared against each other to determine success.

9. The acronym SP stands for standardized patient. What other word is sometimes substituted for the word "standardized"?

   A. Super—NO, this is not a descriptor.
   B. Stupendous—NO, this is not a descriptor.

C. Simulated—YES, SP simulation is sometimes referred to as simulated patient.

D. Steadfast—NO, this is not a descriptor.

10. The simulation educator wants the SP to have a blood pressure of 190/100 for the scenario. How can the educator make this happen?

A. Have the SP drink a lot of caffeine before the scenario.—NO, this can make the SP sick and it will not guarantee a specific blood pressure.

B. It is not possible—NO, there are definitely ways this can be done.

C. Have the SP hand a Post-it note with the words "BP 190/100" to the student after the student takes the blood pressure—YES, this is one way to tell the student the specific blood pressure wanted for the scenario.

D. Have the SPs do a strenuous exercise class prior to the scenario—NO, this can make the SP sick and it will not guarantee a specific blood pressure.

CHAPTER 12 PRACTICE QUESTIONS

1. The goal of using hybrid simulation is to

A. Assess student learning—YES, all simulation teaches and can be used for evaluation.

B. Develop different modalities of teaching—NO, this is not the goal.

C. Construct reality for practice—NO, this is not the goal.

D. Assist in programmed evaluation—NO, this is not the goal.

2. A discipline that used simulation effectively and was a forerunner of healthcare simulation efforts included

A. Medicine—NO, this was not the first.

B. Architecture—NO, this was not the first.

C. Automobile companies—NO, this was not the first.

D. Aviation—YES, this was the first.

3. An appropriate role for a standardized participant would be

A. A prisoner who is a brought to the emergency room with appendicitis—NO, this is an SP.

B. A mother who is in labor—NO, this is an SP.

C. A child having an asthma attack—NO, this is an SP.

D. A sitter watching a patient with Alzheimer's—YES, a participant is usually someone other than the patient.

4. A simulator that represents part of the human anatomy would best fit the description of

A. Virtual—NO, this is computer based.

B. Simulator—NO, this is usually full body.

C. Human—NO, this is usually full body.

D. Task trainer—YES, this is usually part of a body.

5. Students are being taught to deal effectively with end-of-life issues in an intensive care unit (ICU). In order to best facilitate their learning, the simulation educator must develop

   A. Constructed reality—NO, this is not the most important aspect for this particular scenario.
   B. Physical fidelity—NO, this is not the most important aspect for this particular scenario.
   C. Environmental fidelity—NO, this is not the most important aspect for this particular scenario.
   D. Psychological fidelity—YES, this is important in end-of-life scenarios because of the human emotions involved.

6. The highest fidelity constructed is portrayed in which of the following situations by using

   A. A part-task trainer (PTT) to learn Foley catheter insertion in a simulated hospital room—NO, this is a skills setup for learning a procedure.
   B. Virtual reality (VR) to perform a delicate laparoscopic procedure—NO, this is computer based.
   C. SP to portray a patient in drug withdrawal in a simulated clinical examination room—NO, the environment is simulated.
   D. An obstetrical emergency with a mannequin in an actual labor suite in a hospital—YES, because it is in the actual environment.

7. The first consideration to incorporating simulation into a curriculum is

   A. Developing the teaching strategies—NO, this is developed after the learning outcomes.
   B. Deciding on the simulation equipment—NO, this is done after the learning outcomes.
   C. Developing the learning outcomes—YES, the experience must meet learning outcomes.
   D. Financing the simulation laboratory—NO, this is done after the learning outcomes are written and the methodology is decided on.

8. Research is being conducted using two groups; one group of learners is using a mannequin with an SP to learn suturing, and the other group is using a PTT. The person entering the data into the spreadsheet should be a(n)

   A. Mannequin-patient simulation specialist—NO, this person writes scenarios.
   B. Mannequin-patient technician—NO, this person fixes equipment and maintains the laboratory.
   C. SP educator—NO, this person teaches SPs the role they are to play.
   D. Psychometrician—YES, this person works with data.

9. Healthcare team training is best accomplished by using

   A. VR—NO, this is usually one person although it can be used with groups.
   B. Mannequins—YES, mannequins can be used in team scenarios.
   C. PTTs—NO, this is used usually to practice a skill with one person.
   D. Role-play—NO, this is usually one person although it can be used with groups.

10. During a scenario, the mannequin malfunctions. The best person to address the technical problems would be a(n)

 A. Mannequin-patient simulation specialist—NO, this person writes scenarios.
 B. **Mannequin-patient technician—YES, the technician understands the working of the equipment.**
 C. SP educator—NO, this person teaches SPs the role they are to play.
 D. Psychometrician—NO, this person enters and analyzes data.

CHAPTER 13 PRACTICE QUESTIONS

1. The novice simulation educator needs more mentoring when he states

 A. **"The students learn better when they use the mannequin."—YES, this is not true.**
 B. "The learning outcomes should guide the equipment we use."—NO, this is true.
 C. "Keeping the part-task training in a climate-controlled room is important,"—NO, this is true.
 D. "Being available at all times to assist and watch students using the part-task trainer (PTT) is important."—NO, this is true.

2. PTTs can be used in a hybrid format with other modalities. To teach communication skills, the best method would be to use a PTT with

 A. VR—NO, this is computer based.
 B. **An SP—YES, this adds a real person to converse with.**
 C. A mannequin—NO, this is not as effective as a real person.
 D. Another PTT—NO, this is not as effective as a real person.

3. PTTs can be all of the following except

 A. Manufacturer made—NO, they can be manufactured.
 B. Developed by the simulation educator—NO, they can be invented.
 C. Made from household items—NO, they can be made from common objects.
 D. **Part of a high-fidelity mannequin—YES, this is usually not done because dismantling a high-fidelity mannequin may damage it.**

4. When using learning stations in the simulation laboratory

 A. PTTs should not be used.—NO, they are usually used.
 B. Stations should each have a debriefing.—NO, this is for simulation scenarios.
 C. The simulation educator only oversees the flow of learners.—NO, the simulation educator facilitates the learning.
 D. **PTTs can be peer supervised.—YES, students may run this station alone.**

5. Adding texture to the PTT adds

 A. Developmental fidelity—NO, adding texture is physical fidelity.
 B. Psychological fidelity—NO, adding texture is physical fidelity.
 C. Emotional fidelity—NO, adding texture is physical fidelity.
 D. **Physical fidelity—YES, this increases the physical realness.**

6. PTTs that are called "complex" usually include a PTT coupled with

 A. A high-fidelity mannequin—NO, it is usually with VR.
 B. **Virtual reality—YES, this makes it more complex.**

C. A standardized participant—NO, it is usually with VR.

D. A standardized patient—NO, it is usually with VR.

7. PTTs are used for procedures to teach learners anatomical placements and

A. Landmarks—NO, this can be done with pictures.

B. Neurological responses—NO, this cannot be done with PTTs.

C. Correct pressure to apply—YES, this can be taught.

D. Patient sensitivity—NO, this can only be taught with humans.

8. When using PTTs that depict severe traumatic wounds or burns, it would be important to

A. Allow the students to orient to the PTT.—YES, the students should not be surprised, and they should see the severe injury so they can respond appropriately.

B. Make sure the student treats the PTT as if real.—NO, because it is only a PTT and this would be difficult.

C. Make sure the students do not act surprised when they view the PTT.—NO, this may happen and it is different than with a mannequin or human.

D. Cover the PTT until it is time to use it.—NO, this is for privacy when a real person is used.

9. Having students practice a procedure over and over on a PTT is subscribing to the concept of

A. Behaviorism—NO, this is a learning theory.

B. Surface learning—NO, this is a method of learning content.

C. Multitasking—NO, they can only do one skill at a time.

D. Deliberate practice—YES, PTTs are great tools for practicing.

10. Using the lowest fidelity equipment to facilitate learning outcomes effectively can be viewed as

A. Lack of equipment—NO, this is not always the case.

B. Cost-effective learning—YES, this is valuing resources.

C. Scaffolding—NO, this is increasing in complexity.

D. Leveled learning—NO, this is providing the appropriate learning activity for students.

CHAPTER 14 PRACTICE QUESTIONS

1. Which of the following best describes the World Health Organization (WHO) definition of interprofessional education (IPE)?

A. A form of testing in which different disciplines write questions for each other—NO, this is not the definition we need to embrace.

B. A form of didactic learning in which students learn about different professions—NO, this is not the definition we need to embrace.

C. A form of experiential learning in which students spend time observing other professions—NO, this is not the definition we need to embrace.

D. A form of experiential learning in which students from two or more professions learn about, from, and with each other—YES, this is the correct definition.

2. Which of the following are the four core competency domains identified for IPE?

   A. Values/ethics (VE), roles/responsibilities (RR), interprofessional communication (IC), and teams and teamwork (TT)—YES, these are the four core competencies that are important for all interprofessional healthcare teams.

   B. VE, individual scope of practice, team communication, and leadership—NO, it is VE, RR, IC, and TT.

   C. RR, evidence-based guidelines for care, IC, and TT—NO, it is VE, RR, IC, and TT.

   D. Professional ethics, team leadership, scope of practice, and teamwork—NO, it is VE, RR, IC, and TT.

3. Which of the following is an example of a simulation-based IPE program?

   A. Nurse practitioner students and undergraduate nursing students participating in rapid-response scenarios—NO, this only includes one healthcare discipline.

   B. Nurse practitioner students, medical residents, and respiratory therapy students participating in complex simulation scenarios—YES, this has multiple disciplines learning together.

   C. Undergraduate nursing students and medical students participating in individual SP scenarios—NO, although there are two healthcare disciplines in the laboratory, they are learning independently.

   D. Medical residents learning how to place central lines on a simulator—NO, this only includes one healthcare discipline.

4. Which of the following is a *primary goal* for the development of IPE competencies?

   A. For healthcare professions to understand each other's roles—NO, although this is a goal, it is not the primary driving force.

   B. To improve health outcomes in authentic patient care—YES, this is the goal.

   C. To increase the use of simulation to promote IPE—NO, simulation is just an excellent teaching strategy to reach the goal.

   D. To help the patient understand the healthcare team—NO, although patients should understand the roles of the members of the healthcare team, this is not the primary goal.

5. Which of the following has been identified as a barrier in developing and promoting simulation-based IPE?

   A. Persistent separation of healthcare disciplines—YES, learning in silos.

   B. Accreditation lagging behind practice—NO, this has not been identified as a major barrier.

   C. Students not interested in learning together—NO, students enjoy interprofessional learning.

   D. The reduction in tuition costs that would occur based on combining programs—NO, this would actually be an asset.

6. For an individual faculty member, which of the following activities would promote the development of simulation-based IPE experiences?

   A. Designing a simulation-based curriculum and then inviting students to participate—NO, the interprofessional team should be involved in the design, so their specialty is well represented.

B. **Inviting an interprofessional team of faculty to evaluate current curriculum and identify opportunities to design IPE experiences—YES, this will ensure all healthcare disciplines have a voice in the experience**.

C. Collaborating with one other discipline to design simulation-based IPE experiences to evaluate the two student groups at the end of their curriculum—NO, this is limited because learners are evaluated separately.

D. Publishing a review of IPE articles in your own profession only—NO, this does not assist in disseminating IPE.

7. The simulation educator overhears a particpant of the IPE experience barking orders at another member. The simulation educator understands that one of the main reasons this occurs is a violation of which of the following principles?

A. **VE—YES, this has to do with participants' values interposed in the situation.**

B. RR—NO, this has to do more with valuing others.

C. CC—NO, this has to do more with valuing others.

D. TT—NO, this has to do more with valuing others.

8. The simulation educator overhears a particpant of the IPE experience barking orders at another member. The simulation educator would best handle this situation initially by

A. Dealing with the behavior of the inappropriate participant at the end of the scenario—NO, detrimental behavior should be stopped as soon as recognized.

B. Developing a learning plan for the inappropriate participant—NO, detrimental behavior should be stopped as soon as recognized.

C. Asking the team to restart the scenario and provide additional patient background data—NO, this does not deal with the behavior.

D. **Stopping the scenario, discussing the actions with the team, and then restarting—YES, this will provide a venue to correct and establish better ground rules.**

9. The simulation educator overhears a particpant of the IPE experience continuously asking an ESL learner to speak up because he cannot be heard. The simulation educator understands that one of the main reasons this occurs is a violation of which of the following principles?

A. VE—NO, this has to do more with communication.

B. RR—NO, this has to do more with communication.

C. **CC—YES, this is a team communication issue.**

D. TT—NO, this has to do more with communication.

10. The simulation educator overhears a particpant of the IPE experience continuously asking an ESL learner to speak up because he cannot be heard. The simulation educator would best deal with this situation by

A. Dealing with the behavior at the end of the scenario—NO, this will alter the entire interprofessional process being sought.

B. Developing a learning plan for the inappropriate participant—NO, this can be done later but will not help "in the moment."

C. **Asking the team to restart the scenario and asking the person to speak up—YES, this is the best action to take and should not make the person feel disrespected.**

D. Stopping the scenario, discussing the actions with the team, and then restarting—NO, this is an individual, not a team issue; so just asking the participant to speak louder may correct the problem.

CHAPTER 15 PRACTICE QUESTIONS

1. The simulation educator requests a group of learners to gather in an auditorium-style room to debrief. In order to encourage active learning, the simulation educator may

   A. Request a spokesperson for the group—NO, this does not include all learners.
   B. Ask a question of each learner individually—NO, this is too time-consuming.
   C. **Bring in chairs, so half the learners can face the front row—YES, this will increase communication.**
   D. Use an audience response system to question about the scenario—NO, this works with pre-established questions or pre-established opinions, but is not good for reflection.

2. One of two debriefers for a group of learners states that the learner team was slow to respond to the simulated patient's deterioration. The second debriefer says that even though the learner team used time, they executed the resuscitation well. This type of debriefing can be described as

   A. **Good cop–bad cop—YES, this is a technique to present what went well and what needs improvement.**
   B. Advocacy–inquiry—NO, this is a different debriefing technique.
   C. Funneling—NO, this is a different debriefing technique.
   D. Plus–delta—NO, this is a different debriefing technique.

3. A novice simulation educator requires additional mentoring when he states

   A. "I will place the learners in a circle to debrief."—NO, this is correct.
   B. "I will provide adequate time for the learners to discuss the experience."—NO, this is correct.
   C. **"I will ask the learners to return tomorrow for the debriefing."—YES, debriefing should be done as soon as possible after the experience.**
   D. "I think the learners would benefit from high-intensity debriefing."—NO, this is correct.

4. The simulation educator asks the learners to take 5 minutes at the start of the debriefing session and write down what went well and what needs improvement in the performance of the team. This method of debriefing is known as

   A. Good cop–bad cop—NO, this is a different debriefing technique.
   B. Advocacy–inquiry—NO, this is a different debriefing technique.
   C. Funneling—NO, this is a different debriefing technique.
   D. **Plus–delta—YES, this compares the things that went well with the things that need improvement.**

5. The simulation educator understands that in the advocacy–inquiry debriefing technique, the goal of advocacy is
    A. Safe student learner space—NO, it is patient safety.
    B. Simulation educator's instruction—NO, it is patient safety.
    C. Patient safety—YES, the simulation educator is being an advocate for the patient.
    D. Teamwork development—NO, it is patient safety.

6. The simulation educator understands that when using the advocacy–inquiry technique, the goal is to
    A. Explain to the learners what needs improvement—NO, it is to have the student learn in a nonjudgmental environment.
    B. Understand the patient's perception—NO, it is to have the student learn in a nonjudgmental environment.
    C. Provide a nonjudgmental environment—YES, this provides the learner an opportunity for learning in a nonthreatening manner.
    D. Have the learner decide on the corrections—NO, it is to have the student learn in a nonjudgmental environment.

7. A useful tool when using case study analysis is to provide the learners with
    A. Past stories of the experience with other learners—NO, this is not appropriate.
    B. The patient outcome first, then the process—NO, this process should be discussed first.
    C. The actual written scenario that was used—NO, the scenario does not have to be reviewed.
    D. Objective data from observation or videotape—YES, this supports learning.

8. A novice simulation educator is asking questions during a debriefing that facilitate "yes" and "no" answers from the learners. This may be interpreted as a case in which the instructor is
    A. Overinstructing—YES, this is not letting the students express their perceptions.
    B. Using plus–delta—NO, this is overinstructing.
    C. Encouraging reflection—NO, this is overinstructing.
    D. Oversimplifying—NO, this is overinstructing.

9. Which of the following examples is a Socratic question?
    A. "Did you remember to turn the oxygen on when you placed the face mask on the patient?"—NO, this elicits a "yes" or "no" answer.
    B. "How did you feel about the family crying?"—NO, this promotes reflection.
    C. "Was patient safety your first thought?"—NO, this elicits a "yes" or "no" answer.
    D. "After the oxygen level was adequate, what was your next priority and why?"—YES, this assists the learner to think critically.

10. The simulation educator is viewing a scenario with a group of learners performing a sterile technique. The simulation educator observes two learners breaking the sterile technique and calls through the microphone to "freeze the action." This type of debriefing is known as

    A. Plus–delta—NO, this is done after the scenario is completed.
    B. Advocacy–inquiry—NO, this is done after the scenario is completed.
    C. In simulation—YES, the scenario is interrupted for learning.
    D. Spontaneous learning—NO, the simulation educator instructs during a scenario.

CHAPTER 16 PRACTICE QUESTIONS

1. One of the most beneficial uses of SPs is

    A. Summative evaluation—NO, this is final evaluation and should be done by an educator.
    B. Group enhancement—NO, this is not the purpose.
    C. Promotion of critical thinking—NO, this is not the purpose.
    D. Formative feedback—YES, to assist learners to improve and refine techniques.

2. Experiential learning is a learning methodology that combines

    A. Deep learning with hands-on experience—NO, this is not the best explanation.
    B. Personal experience with academic learning—YES, it allows students to construct knowledge.
    C. Academic learning and critical thinking—NO, it uses the students' experiences.
    D. Reflective learning and lecturing—NO, it incorporates students' experiences.

3. An experienced debriefer understands that the learner who is not ready to accept feedback may say

    A. "I understand that I was slow to react because I was overthinking the procedure."—NO, this is reflective.
    B. "I never thought that watching myself would be so revealing."—NO, this is reflective.
    C. "This is not like it is in the hospital, so I am not concerned about being slow."—YES, this is not reflective at all and does not take any responsibility for learning.
    D. "This experience made me look at things differently."—NO, this is reflective.

4. Adult learners may not respond to the debriefer's explanation about the simulation experience's

    A. Relevance—NO, they do respond to relevant learning.
    B. Use—NO, adult learners want to know how things can be used in the "real world."
    C. Theoretical background—YES, they are less concerned with theory.
    D. Applicability—NO, they like to learn things that are immediately applicable.

5. An SP is portraying symptoms of respiratory distress, and while the learners are doing lung assessments, continues to cough uncontrollably. This type of situation is referred to as

    A. A symptomatic SP—NO, this is not the term used to describe the situation.

    B. Overidentifying—YES, the SP is overidentifying with a patient role.

    C. Intentional obstruction—NO, this is not the term used to describe the situation.

    D. Overacting—NO, this is not the term used to describe the situation.

6. Foundational competencies for an SP include all of the following except

    A. Emotional intelligence—NO, this is needed.

    B. Reliability—NO, this is needed.

    C. Healthcare background—YES, this is not essential.

    D. Lifelong learning—NO, this is needed.

7. Advanced competencies for SPs include all of the following except

    A. The ability to understand the learning theory—YES, this is not essential.

    B. The ability to effectively communicate—NO, this is needed.

    C. Documentation skills—NO, this is needed.

    D. Evaluation skills—NO, this is needed.

8. It is important to carefully screen SPs because they should

    A. Be award-winning actors or actresses—NO, this is not essential.

    B. Be able to provide negative feedback—NO, this is not essential.

    C. Fit the physical role of the patient being portrayed—NO, this is not essential.

    D. Care about the learning process—YES, they are there to assist in the learning process.

9. During a group interview of four SPs, one actor keeps dominating the conversation by describing his many roles while name-dropping about famous people he has worked with. This may be a red flag because it can be interpreted as

    A. Narcissism—NO, this is not the description of the behavior.

    B. Emotional liability—NO, this is not the description of the behavior.

    C. Grandstanding—YES, this is bringing attention to oneself.

    D. Ineffective communication—NO, this is not the description of the behavior.

10. The following interaction describes sandwich-style feedback

    A. "I think you did a good job with the sterile technique initially, but then contaminated the field."—NO, this does not portray the technique.

    B. "I watched you contaminate the field and this concerns me. Can you tell me what you were thinking?"—NO, this does not portray the technique.

    C. "Contaminating the field is serious and can cause a patient to get infected; do you understand how necessary it is to be more careful?"—NO, this does not portray the technique.

    D. "You did a good job putting on sterile gloves, you reached over the corner of the field, but then you changed the contaminated sheet, which was good."—YES, this contains something they did well, something that needs improvement, and then finishes with something they did well.

CHAPTER 17 PRACTICE QUESTIONS

1. When choosing an avatar, the most important consideration is

   A. Design the avatar with as much humor as possible—NO, this is not the objective.

   B. Design the avatar as realistically as possible for the scenario—YES, in a professional virtual simulation, the avatar should represent the actual person participating in the virtual world (VW).

   C. The design doesn't matter and can be anything the participant chooses—NO, this is not the objective.

   D. To allow the learning platform to choose the avatar—NO, individual choice is important.

2. When designing a virtual learning (VL) platform using the constructivist theory, the designer bases the scenario on which principle of learning?

   A. Constructivist theory is experiential in nature—NO, it is not.

   B. Constructivist theory is based on adult learning principles—NO, it is based on pedagogy.

   C. Actions are based on building upon previously learned principles—YES, constructivist theory builds on previously learned knowledge

   D. Maslow's hierarchy of needs should be considered as part of the design—NO, this is inconsistent with a learning theory.

3. A major reason for choosing VL is which of the following?

   A. Self-learning is important when interacting in VWs—NO, it is really about learning new information and skills.

   B. VWs provide a safe environment for the learner to practice new skills—YES, participants can practice skills, make decisions, and implement actions without fear of harming a live person.

   C. Designers show off their creativity in designing a serious game—NO, this is not a valid reason.

   D. Outcomes of the activity are not important when interacting in VWs—NO, they are important for patient safety.

4. An avatar is best described as

   A. A three-dimensional (3-D) digitized person that best represents the participant—YES, the avatar is a 3-D representation of the person interacting in the VL environment.

   B. A passive figure created to mimic the nurse—NO, it could represent any healthcare provider or patient.

   C. A computer-generated representation of a person—NO, the computer does not have to generate it.

   D. A person who can only move in one direction based on input of the designer—NO, avatars are multidirectional action figures.

5. A major advantage or benefit of VL is that

   A. It does not require much work to complete the exercise—NO, this is not true.

   B. It is a cost-effective method of learning—NO, it can be costly.

C. It requires minimal preparation on the part of the designer—NO, it takes lots of preparation and design.

D. It allows interprofessional collaboration on best practices—YES, collaboration with members of other disciplines, as well as with professionals globally, is a key advantage to VL platforms.

6. When designing multiuser virtual environments (MUVEs), the briefing stage should be initiated. During this stage, which of the following occurs?

   A. Learners enter the VW to begin the simulation—NO, there needs to be an orientation.

   B. Learners make sense of the experience and build new knowledge—NO, there needs to be an orientation in order to do this.

   C. Faculty holds sessions with the learner to allow for reflection on the experience—NO, that is debriefing.

   D. Students watch videos before entering the VW as part of orientation— YES, the briefing stage is done before the experience begins in order to prepare the participant for the virtual simulation.

7. Instructional scaffolding means that the VL environment

   A. Can be applied to any level of the learner—NO, it is usually complex.

   B. Builds on previous knowledge and experiences of the participant— YES, instructional scaffolding is a part of the constructivist theory. VL simulations should be designed based on the level of the learner and become increasingly more difficult in nature.

   C. There is only one correct action or answer allowed in the scenario—NO, there may be many ways to accomplish an outcome.

   D. The scenario is linear in nature—NO, it is not.

8. Kolb's theory espouses which of the following principles?

   A. Reflections are assimilated into abstract concepts and applied to a new experience—YES, Kolb's theory is termed "experiential theory" in which the learner "experiences" the situation and makes meaning out of it, which can often lead to new learning experiences.

   B. Adults learn best when the material can be immediately applied—NO, this is not Kolb's theory.

   C. Andragogy is key to this theory—NO, this is not Kolb's theory.

   D. Learning is linear and is based on effective faculty teaching—NO, this is not Kolb's theory.

9. During the debriefing stage, which of the following occurs?

   A. Learners enter the VW using their avatar—NO, this occurs before the debriefing.

   B. Learners create an avatar for the virtual simulation—NO, this is done initially.

   C. Faculty develop outcomes for the VL experience—NO, this needs to be done initially.

D. **Educators facilitate learner reflection on the experience—YES, debriefing is an important stage in the VL environment. It allows the learners to reflect on their experience and provides opportunities for discussion and venting of feelings. The faculty role in debriefing is to allow learners to talk about their experience and facilitate further discussion on its meaning and ways to improve or change the experience.**

10. A limitation of incorporating MUVEs in the learning environment is

A. Participants view it as a game with no value in the learning process—NO, there is learning value.

B. VL does not provide opportunities for interaction with others—NO, it is interactive.

C. **The cost of developing an MUVE may be prohibitive—YES, this is a major disadvantage in VL. Cost may be reflected in many ways: amount of money needed to invest in the actual VW, time needed for faculty development of the modality, as well as technological support by the institution.**

D. It does not allow the transfer of knowledge to the real world—NO, it does teach things that can be implemented.

CHAPTER 18 PRACTICE QUESTIONS

1. A simulation educator is explaining to a novice the reason for completing a needs assessment prior to planning simulation activities. The best explanation is

A. "This allows the learner to choose what she really wants to learn."—NO, learners are not always in a position to understand their learning needs.

B. **"This is a starting point for assessing learner needs before the planning begins."—YES, having a clear understanding of learner needs helps to guide the goals and objectives for the simulation experience.**

C. "This is nice to do, but not always needed when planning for simulation."—NO, this should be done to ensure learners' needs are being met.

D. "This is a requirement for accreditation and must be done."—NO, this is not an accreditation requirement.

2. A simulation educator is teaching a class on planning for simulation activities. She determines that the instruction is effective when one of the learners states

A. "A goal should be short term and easily accomplished with simple activities."—NO, goals are usually longer term.

B. "Goals are very complex and may require several simulation activities to accomplish."—NO, goals can be the expected outcome at the end of any teaching–learning process.

C. **"Goals are broadly defined to identify the purpose and final outcomes of the simulation activity."—YES, the outcomes must relate back to the goals.**

D. "Goals and objectives are the same and the terms can be used interchangeably."—NO, these terms are erroneously used interchangeably, but have different meanings.

3. The simulation coordinator is assisting one of the hospital educators to develop objectives for a simulation experience for new nursing hires. The educator demonstrates understanding when she states

   A. "Objectives must be a measurable statement of a single behavior."—YES, this is a statement of what is to be accomplished after a teaching session.
   B. "Objectives are broad statements of what is to be attained."—NO, they need to be specific and measurable.
   C. "There is no need for objectives unless they are to be used for continuing education credit."—NO, objectives are used to describe what should be accomplished by the learner.
   D. "There should only be one objective per simulation activity."—NO, the number depends on the complexity of the simulation and what is to be accomplished.

4. Evaluating student learning during the simulation activity to facilitate further instruction and identify deficits is an example of

   A. Summative evaluation—NO, this is done at the conclusion of a learning activity.
   B. Debriefing—NO, this is done at the conclusion of a simulation activity and provides an opportunity for self-reflection.
   C. Outcome evaluation—NO, this is the same as summative evaluation.
   D. Formative evaluation—YES, this allows for assessment of learner progress toward achievement of learning objectives.

5. In discussing the debriefing process with a novice educator, the simulation coordinator's best explanation is that debriefing is

   A. "Ideally done after each simulation, but can be eliminated if time runs short."—NO, many experts agree that debriefing is the most important part of simulation.
   B. "An opportunity for learners to reflect and derive meaning from the experience."—YES, learners can process what they have learned.
   C. "The time to critique the learners' experience and point out all faults."—NO, although this is a time for constructive criticism, it should not be limited to what went wrong.
   D. "An activity that should be done on the following day after learners have had a time to reflect."—NO, debriefing is best done immediately after the simulation when the experience is fresh in everyone's mind.

6. In planning for a simulation activity, the simulation educator elects to use a simple pelvic model for learners to practice insertion of indwelling urinary catheters. This is an example of what type of simulation modality?

   A. High-fidelity simulator—NO, an example of this is a fully computerized mannequin.
   B. SP—NO, this involves live actors.
   C. Task trainer—YES, this is using a replica model to learn and practice simple procedures.
   D. VR—NO, this is a computer-generated environment.

7. The simulation coordinator is working with a graduate learner to plan a simulation activity. The learner correctly identifies that resources do not include

   A. Learners—YES, learners are the recipient of the simulation activity, not a resource.
   B. Location—NO, this is needed.
   C. Content experts—NO, this is needed.
   D. Laboratory technicians—NO, this is needed.

8. The clinical nurse educator and simulation coordinator are working together to organize a simulation team for a code II simulation activity. The first step is to

   A. Orient team members—NO, this cannot be done until all members are confirmed.
   B. Develop a training schedule—NO, this should not be done until the team is confirmed.
   C. Recruit content experts—YES, this must done first to confirm team members.
   D. Advertise the event—NO, this should be done after planning is complete.

9. While planning a simulation activity, a novice educator asks why an agenda needs to be prepared and sent out to learners ahead of time. The simulation coordinator's best response is

   A. "It is expected to always have an agenda for an educational event."—NO, although this is generally true, it is not the best response.
   B. "If there are any typos, we can correct them ahead of time."—NO, this is not a valid reason.
   C. "This is required for hospital employees to request time off to attend."—NO, this is not a valid reason.
   D. "This helps learners to know what to expect and identifies any preplanning needs."—YES, this often helps learners prepare for the simulation activity; it may identify equipment needs or preplanning assignments.

10. A content expert who has agreed to participate in a new simulation activity asks the coordinator why he needs to pilot the simulation ahead of time. The best response is

    A. "This is a good way to identify problems or issues before running a first-time simulation activity."—YES, this assists in the experience going smoothly.
    B. "This is something that should be done before every simulation activity."—NO, this is not necessarily required if the simulation has been used before and the team is experienced.
    C. "Piloting a simulation allows the planner to determine whether the content experts are appropriate for the simulation activity."—NO, the expertise of the content experts should be assessed before they are recruited.
    D. "This is the only way to make sure the equipment is all working."—NO, equipment can be checked in advance.

CHAPTER 19 PRACTICE QUESTIONS

1. A new faculty member wants to create and run a simulation "on the fly" to access the competency levels of the students for a pass/fail in clinical. The best response to this request is

   A. "We can try it, but I'm not sure this is the best way."—NO, there is no reason to try.
   B. "No, I don't think you should do that."—NO, you should explain why.
   C. "Best practices call for established objectives and learning outcomes."—NO, this is an evaluation.
   D. **"Summative evaluation requires a valid and reliable assessment."—YES, evaluating a student "on the fly" does not promote objectivity or fairness.**

2. A simulation activity involves the use of deliberate practice to learn and perfect a skill. Students are given immediate feedback as to the correct and incorrect steps taken throughout the simulation to enhance their learning. This is an example of a

   A. **Formative evaluation—YES, this type of feedback is considered formative evaluation.**
   B. Summative evaluation—NO, this assists the students to become more proficient.
   C. Self-evaluation—NO, this is done by the simulation educator.
   D. Peer evaluation—NO, this is done by the simulation educator.

3. The simulated patient has a terminal illness and is dying. The participant is evaluated on how professionally he communicates with the patient. This is an example of evaluating

   A. **Attitude—YES, professional behavior falls into this category.**
   B. Skill—NO, this is psychomotor ability.
   C. Psychomotor ability—NO, this is not what the scenario calls for.
   D. Emotion—NO, this is not part of a professional evaluation.

4. An evaluative instrument has criteria with possible scores from 0 to 5 in each category. This type of tool is best known as a

   A. Checklist—NO, this is done or not completed.
   B. Matrix—NO, this compares items in different categories.
   C. Rubric—NO, this describes behaviors at different levels of attainment.
   D. **Likert scale—YES, a Likert scale has ratings such as 0 to 5 and allows for measurement.**

5. Standardization of the evaluative process and evaluator training promotes which of the following?

   A. Increased reliability—NO, this is when the tool preforms well time after time.
   B. Improved validity—NO, this is when a tool is evaluated for eliciting the correct information.
   C. **Reduced bias potential—YES, standardization reduces the chance of bias from individual facilitator interpretations of the activity.**
   D. Evidence-based practice—NO, this is not evaluated in this process.

6. Following a simulation experience, students complete an anonymous online survey regarding their performance. This is an example of

   A. **Self-evaluation—YES, the students are reporting on their perceptions regarding what occurred during the simulation. This is the lowest level of evaluation.**
   B. Debriefing—NO, this is done with a simulation educator.
   C. Peer assessment—NO, this is done student to student.
   D. Formative assessment—NO, this is done by the simulation educator to increase performance.

7. A department head has mandated that faculty use a certain evaluation tool for summative evaluation with simulation. It is most important for faculty to

   A. Keep the evaluations hidden from the students.—NO, this is not the most important procedure needed.
   B. **Be educated in the appropriate use of the tool.—YES, it is essential that they all use the tool in the same way with the same processes.**
   C. Use the tool as much as possible.—NO, this is not necessary.
   D. Modify the tool as needed to meet the objectives of the course.—NO, this will change the statistics on the tool.

8. A hospital quality-assurance committee is analyzing patient satisfaction data related to communication between physicians and nurses following intensive team training with simulation. The results could support the achievement of which of the following?

   A. **Kirkpatrick's Level 4—YES, this would be a measurement and achievement of outcomes.**
   B. Translational Science Research (TSR) Phase 1—NO, this does not measure outcomes.
   C. Miller's pyramid base of "Knows"—NO, this does not measure outcomes.
   D. Kirkpatrick's Level 2—NO, this does not measure outcomes.

9. The hospital rapid-response team participates in simulation-based training (SBT). At the conclusion of the training, the teams' adherence to protocol is evaluated using a valid and reliable tool to determine the impact of the SBT on actual team performance. This evaluation is aimed at

   A. Miller's "Does" and Kirkpatrick's Level 4—NO, this speaks to translating into practice, which is described in Kirkpatrick's Level 3.
   B. Translating to practice and Kirkpatrick's Level 4—NO, this speaks to translating into practice, which is described in Kirkpatrick's Level 3.
   C. Miller's "Shows how" and Kirkpatrick's Level 3—NO, this speaks to translating into practice, which is described in Kirkpatrick's Level 3.
   D. **Translating to practice and Kirkpatrick's Level 3—YES, this is an example of an evaluation to determine whether the simulation training translates to practice. There is no evaluation of the patient outcomes or system needed to meet the criteria for the highest levels of evaluation.**

10. One of the most significant challenges in evaluating healthcare team performance is
    A. Understanding TeamSTEPPS as it relates to different types of healthcare teams—NO, these steps are clear.
    B. Recognizing individual team member roles, as the healthcare teams are not static—NO, this is explained also.
    C. Evaluating the impact of team members on the overall team performance—YES, if individual team members do not have the knowledge, skills, and attitudes needed to perform the tasks associated with their respective roles, the effectiveness of the team may be impacted.
    D. Evaluating communication strategies among team members—NO, this is also addressed.

CHAPTER 20 PRACTICE QUESTIONS

1. During a simulation, it is noted that some of the requested supplies and equipment are not in the room and available for learner use. What is the best initial step to take toward addressing this issue?
    A. Stop the simulation and ask the simulation technology specialist (STS) why the supplies are not available. Restart the simulation once the proper supplies have been obtained.—NO, focus on the simulation event first and then go back and resolve the issues related to why the supplies were not there. Maintain realism during a simulation for best learner outcomes.
    B. Continue the simulation with the STS introducing the supplies and equipment into the scenario, stating that these supplies have just arrived from central supply for this patient.—YES, using an "outside" lifesaver can help the scenario to progress and stay on target with the scenario objectives.
    C. Continue the simulation observing how the learners adapt to the lack of supplies and equipment.—NO, this would change the objectives; it is best to stay with the objectives.
    D. Stop the simulation and begin the debriefing, explaining to the participants that this is a common occurrence and that they are the unfortunate victims of a poorly managed center.—NO, marginalizing other team members is inappropriate. Items of this nature should be dealt with privately and not in front of the learners.

2. During a simulation, the wi-fi connection to the baby HPS is lost, and the baby becomes unresponsive. The learners believe that the baby has gone into cardiac arrest and begin cardiopulmonary resuscitation (CPR). As a facilitator, what is your best initial course of action?
    A. Stop the simulation and attempt to reestablish the wi-fi connection while you give the learners a break.—NO, valuable learner time may be wasted. Consider what you can influence inside and outside the scenario.
    B. Continue the simulation and modify the scenario on the fly as the learning outcomes are related to crew resource management and can be met within this evolving scenario.—YES, if the learning objectives can be met, then the evolving scenario is a good solution to this challenge.

    C. Stop the simulation and debrief the scenario based on the objectives the learners have met. Use the debriefing time for the STS to attempt to reestablish connection.—NO, the best response is to modify the scenario on the fly as long as the objectives can be met.

    D. Announce to the students that the wi-fi connection was lost and to please continue the simulation with modified objectives.—NO, maintain the original learning objectives.

3. The individual who schedules events (the scheduler) in your simulation center cancels a high-priority user and, in his place, schedules one of her friends' groups (a midpriority user) in the center. You are the director of the center, and you just received an e-mail complaint from your high-priority user. What is the most appropriate immediate action?

    A. Speak with the scheduler to find out why this action was taken.—YES, take time to find out why the decision was made to cancel the high-priority group before moving forward with other actions.

    B. Reschedule the event for the high-priority user and cancel the second group.—NO, speak with the scheduler first to determine the rationale for canceling the first group before moving forward with other actions.

    C. Do a resource assessment and, if able, negotiate so that both groups can use the center.—NO, speak with the scheduler first to determine the rationale before moving forward with other actions.

    D. Remove or severely restrict scheduling privileges until the scheduler undergoes retraining on scheduling policies and procedures.—NO, speak with the scheduler first to determine the rationale before moving forward with other actions.

4. An important tour is scheduled after normal working hours 2 months from now. Staffing this event has become a challenge because one of the employees in a leadership position has openly refused to modify her schedule to work for or support this event and has encouraged the other employees to refuse to work, as well. Alternate time off and compensation has been offered; their schedules are seldom modified. What resource can best help with this problem?

    A. Human resources personnel—YES, your human resources department can help you work through this problem and be there to provide guidance through challenging personnel issues.

    B. Resource allocation—NO, the human resources representative can help you work through this problem and guide you through the many legal issues related to challenges with personnel.

    C. Benefits specialist—NO, the human resources representative is best equipped to help guide you through the many legal issues related to challenges with personnel.

    D. Policies and procedures—NO, policies and procedures are a good reference, but your human resources representative is best equipped to help guide you through the many legal issues related to challenges with personnel.

5. During a scenario, the STS leaves the center, returning 30 minutes later. You are the instructor/facilitator and are upset because equipment malfunctioned and supplies were missing, creating a very difficult and stressful situation. You had

expected the STS to be there to help you if anything went wrong. You are upset and have only 5 minutes to do something about this situation. What is the best course of action?

A. Report this incident to the director and have her deal with the situation.—NO, try to resolve the issue with the individual first, before involving management.

B. Confront the STS, letting the STS know how upset you are at what happened.—NO, confrontation when individuals are upset can lead to breakdown in human relationships, and misunderstandings can result.

C. Ignore the situation; it just isn't worth the effort to try and resolve.—NO, this is avoidance and can lead to future problems.

D. Schedule a time in the near future to meet with the STS to discuss the incident.—YES, try to resolve the situation with the individual first, at a time when you are not upset and have adequate time to listen and understand.

6. Depreciation in relation to a simulation center's budget may be used for all of the following EXCEPT

A. To represent the loss in value of a piece of equipment—NO, this is considered part of depreciation.

B. In relation to capital equipment—NO, this is considered part of depreciation.

C. In calculated loss of value based on the projected lifetime—NO, this is considered part of depreciation.

D. To represent supply inventory—YES, depreciation is used for durable equipment, not consumable supplies.

7. While setting up for a simulation, you note that the HPS is not functioning normally. A few minutes later, it no longer responds to any input. What is the *best* initial course of action?

A. Shut down and then restart the HPS.—NO, this is a good step, but ensuring all connections are secure is the best initial step.

B. Call your sales rep.—NO, ensuring all connections are secure is the best initial step.

C. Consult the troubleshooting section of your user's manual.—NO, ensuring all connections are secure is the best initial step.

D. Check all cords and electrical plugs to ensure the connections are secure.—YES, this is the best initial step.

8. A recently purchased high-fidelity HPS does not function as intended for the third time this week. Each time this occurs, the HPS is turned off and then restarted, after which it begins to work properly. What action should be taken?

A. Review the troubleshooting section in the HPS manual.—NO, call your sales rep or tvhe manufacturer if the problem persists; simply documenting it will not bring the problem toward resolution.

B. Call the sales rep or manufacturer for customer service.—YES, report this problem and work with the company for resolution.

    C. Report your problems on Facebook.—NO, although you may feel justified, this will not resolve the issue with the HPS.

    D. Accept the fact that this is a normal challenge when working with this HPS.—NO, reporting the problem early can help to resolve this issue.

9. Recommended policies and procedures for a simulation center include all the following EXCEPT

    A. Center hours and scheduling guidelines—NO, these are recommended policies and procedures.

    B. Collections of prepackaged scenarios with debrief guide and checklist— YES, these are considered resources, not policies and procedures.

    C. Video retention, archiving, and access—NO, these are recommended policies and procedures.

    D. Course of action to resolve customer complaints—NO, these are recommended policies and procedures.

10. A mission statement is

    A. A statement of global plans and goals—NO, this is a vision. The mission statement is a statement that describes the purpose of the center.

    B. The road map of a simulation center—NO, this is a business plan. The mission statement is a statement that describes the purpose of the center.

    C. A statement that briefly describes the purpose for the existence of the center—YES, the mission statement is a statement that describes the purpose of the center.

    D. A comprehensive 3- to 5-year plan—NO, this is a strategic plan. The mission statement is a statement that describes the purpose of the center.

CHAPTER 21 PRACTICE QUESTIONS

1. A simulation educator is putting together a self-study report for accreditation. His coworker asks him why bother with accreditation. The simulation educator's best answer is

    A. "The provost will see what a good job I am doing."—NO, this is not a good reason.

    B. "The students deserve it."—NO, this is a good reason, but not the major one.

    C. "This is an excellent simulation laboratory and it should be no problem getting accreditation."—NO, this is not a good reason.

    D. "The goal is quality and safety in patient care."—YES, this is the ultimate goal.

2. A simulation educator is developing a self-study report for an accreditation process and is describing a simulation about a rapid-response team. This should be integrated in standard

    A. Professional integrity of the participant—NO, this addresses facilitation of leaning methods.

    B. Participant objectives—NO, this addresses facilitation of leaning methods.

    C. Facilitation methods—YES, this is the section that speaks about how learning is facilitated.

    D. The debriefing process—NO, this addresses facilitation of leaning methods.

3. Having a systematic plan of evaluation for ongoing excellence includes

   A. Aggregating data as evidence—NO, this is not the entire feedback process.
   B. Collecting data—NO, it needs to be aggregated, reported, and changes made if needed.
   C. **Making changes based on data—YES, this is using aggregate data to make decisions.**
   D. Developing a strategic plan—NO, this is not intricate to the systematic, continuous evaluative process.

4. A simulation educator is developing a self-study report for accreditation and includes a section on personnel qualification; this information should be included in

   A. Assessment—NO, this is part of teaching.
   B. Research—NO, this is part of teaching.
   C. **Teaching/education—YES, faculty provide the teaching and facilitate the education or learning.**
   D. Systems integration—NO, this is part of teaching.

5. The mission statement of a simulation laboratory should be

   A. General so that changes are not noticed—NO, this is not the purpose when devising a mission statement.
   B. **Congruent with the mission of the larger organization—YES, the missions need to be congruent in order for administration to work cooperatively.**
   C. Included in the literature about the laboratory—NO, this is a good idea, but not the best answer.
   D. Detailed so that specifics are understood by the public—NO, it should be fairly flexible.

6. Protection of learners in the laboratory against Family Educational Rights and Privacy Act (FERPA) violations would be best included in which section of a self-study?

   A. Mission and governance—NO, this should be included in the security section.
   B. Facilities, technology, simulation modalities, and human resources—NO, this should be included in the security section.
   C. Integrity—NO, this should be included in the security section.
   D. **Security—YES, students' rights are described in this section.**

7. An SP is doing a critical skills check-off evaluation of a learner. Which educational standard would this practice violate?

   A. Participant objectives—NO, this would be the evaluation of an expected outcome.
   B. Facilitation methods—NO, this would be the evaluation of an expected outcome.
   C. The debriefing process—NO, this would be the evaluation of an expected outcome.
   D. **Evaluation of expected outcomes—YES, qualified educators need to evaluate learners.**

8. A group of simulation educators are discussing the application for laboratory accreditation, and a member states that her new facility is state of the art and it should not have to prove that the facility is excellent. The best response is accreditation

   A. "Tells the world how good our facility is."—NO, this is not the best response.
   B. "Shows that we are experts, so everyone will know."—NO, this is not the best response.
   C. "Demonstrates expertise in teaching."—NO, this is not the best response.
   D. **"Validates more than just the excellence of the facility."—YES, the standards cover many areas of simulation education.**

9. When developing an accreditation self-study report, the simulation educator describes a student grievance incident and the due process that led to a resolution. This should be explained in which standard?

   A. Organization and management—NO, this is evaluation and improvement.
   B. **Evaluation and improvement—YES, this would speak to improvement in a process and how a process was handled.**
   C. Integrity—NO, this is evaluation and improvement.
   D. Security—NO, this is evaluation and improvement.

10. A key ingredient for a successful accreditation process is to have a

    A. Consultant—NO, this is helpful but not necessary.
    B. Simulation educator—NO, this is necessary for the functioning of the laboratory.
    C. **Project manager—YES, this person oversees the process.**
    D. Accreditation liaison—NO, this is not necessary.

CHAPTER 22 PRACTICE QUESTIONS

1. Professional development activities for simulation educators include all of the following EXCEPT

   A. Attendance at healthcare simulation conferences—NO, this is an excellent method to obtain state-of-the art information.
   B. Membership in professional healthcare simulation organizations—NO, this will provide the CHSE with up-to-date information.
   C. **Obtaining a higher degree—YES, this may not focus on simulation.**
   D. Reading journal articles on healthcare simulation—NO, this is encouraged.

2. The professional portfolio/dossier is used for the following:

   A. Appointments—NO, it can be used for new appointments to positions.
   B. Certifications—NO, the advanced certification is conducted by portfolio review.
   C. Promotions and tenure—NO, it is definitely used for promotion decisions as well as tenure.
   D. **All of the above—YES, all are applicable.**

3. Benner, Sutphen, Leonard, and Day support a three-pronged approach to health profession education, which includes all of the following EXCEPT

A. Knowledge acquisition—NO, this is included.
B. Career ladders—YES, this is not a personal attribute, but a method of career advancement.
C. Clinical integration—NO, this is included.
D. Ethical comportment—NO, this is included.

4. A portfolio or dossier is also a practical way to reflect on and document one's work with respect to

A. Teaching—NO, this is just one aspect of traditional scholarship.
B. Research—NO, this is just one aspect of traditional scholarship.
C. Clinical service—NO, this is just one aspect of traditional scholarship.
D. All of the above—YES, all need to be included.

5. The development of critical reasoning and professional development is best addressed via

A. Healthcare simulation—YES, this is an ideal method to develop knowledge, skill, and attitudes.
B. Didactic classroom sessions—NO, this basically addresses knowledge.
C. Role-playing—NO, this does not always include the ethical considerations.
D. Professional portfolio development—NO, this does not always demonstrate skill.

6. The process of professional development is best conducted in

A. The formative years of healthcare education—YES, this is the best time to develop knowledge, skill, and attitudes related to leadership.
B. Doctoral study—NO, this is focused on research.
C. Clinical environment—NO, this is focused on skill.
D. Continuing education—NO, this is helpful, but other avenues are also needed for a robust professional development.

7. Simulation is the most appropriate pedagogy for addressing

A. Crucial conversations—YES, this is an excellent method to teach crucial conversation technique.
B. Résumé building—NO, this can be done on an individual basis with a didactic method.
C. Career ladders—NO, this is done by documenting knowledge, attitude, and skill, not through deliberate practice.
D. Content deficits—NO, this is done through devising a coherent curriculum for whatever topic is needed.

8. Which of the following is considered one of the most powerful motivational predictors of success in one's career?

A. Education—NO, education alone may not suffice if the person lacks confidence.
B. Self-efficacy—YES, having the mindset that you can accomplish a task is important.

C. Advocacy—NO, the person must be able to advocate for self as well as others.

D. Occupation—NO, success can be obtained in all career paths.

9. The simulation expert has a responsibility to share expertise via a

A. Mentoring or consultant role—YES, this is a professional responsibility.

B. Clinical ladder—NO, this demonstrates individual accomplishments.

C. Advocacy role—NO, this is expected, but does not show one's own accomplishments.

D. Ethics training—NO, this is helpful, but does not demonstrate expertise.

10. The engagement in professional development by simulation educators is best evaluated by

A. Use of evidence-based simulation strategies—YES, this demonstrates professional engagement in the area of expertise.

B. Subscription to a professional journal—NO, this does not provide demonstration.

C. Attendance at health-related conferences—NO, this does not provide demonstration.

D. Attendance in a graduate program—NO, this does not provide demonstration.

CHAPTER 23 PRACTICE QUESTIONS

1. A new physician has heard about your simulation laboratory and is interested in scheduling a simulation. The physician would like to do a mock code. Based on simulation research and best practice, what should you have the physician do first prior to running the simulation?

A. Develop a scenario—NO, scenarios of mock codes have already been developed and are available on several websites.

B. Develop objectives—YES, developing objectives is a critical best practice in education.

C. Observe a mock code simulation—NO, although this may be helpful, it is not essential.

D. Notify participants as to date and time—NO, a mock code is usually not announced in advance.

2. An instructor who is new to simulation is pressed for time. In order to provide sufficient time for debriefing, the instructor skips the orientation. Why is orientation important? Orientation gives the learners

A. A chance to identify roles—NO, sometimes the faculty identifies student roles.

B. Time to plan their course of action—NO, students may want to do this, but because they don't know what's going to happen in the scenario, planning does not help.

C. Assistance in meeting objectives—YES, the orientation should include a brief overview of general objectives so that students know what is expected of them.

D. An opportunity to observe the environment—NO, students should receive a *focused* orientation to the environment prior to their first simulation.

3. Unless the simulation is for high-stakes testing, the main objective in simulation is
   A. Patient outcome—NO, students learn first prior to transferring to practice.
   B. Learner outcome—NO, formative assessment and feedback should precede summative.
   C. Task mastery—NO, this may be an objective when using task trainers, but simulations promote higher level thinking skills. Students should master procedures needed in simulation prior to the simulation.
   D. Learning—YES, simulation is all about learning in a safe environment. Students are free to make mistakes because they will learn more from errors than if they do everything perfectly.

4. A learner approaches you and confides that she has just had a death in her family. Her infant died after being in neonatal intensive care. She is not sure that she can handle participating in a simulation. The *best* course of action is to
   A. Send her for counseling.—NO, this is an option to offer, but not always necessary.
   B. Have her play a secondary role in the simulation.—NO, if the beeping of the monitor is the problem, playing a secondary role does not remove the trigger.
   C. Give her the opportunity to watch the simulation.—YES, because the literature shows that involved observers learn as much as participants, place the learner in the control room or debriefing room where she can observe the simulation.
   D. Tell her to come back another day.—NO, she will miss the experience with her peers.

5. Which of Kirkpatrick's levels of evaluation has been *most* heavily researched in simulation?
   A. Level 1, reaction—YES, satisfaction, learner perceptions, and self-confidence have been most heavily researched.
   B. Level 2, learning—NO, although some research has been done at this level, the rigor and design variance limits research.
   C. Level 3, behavior—NO, although some research has been done at this level, the rigor and design variance limits research.
   D. Level 4, results—NO, although some research has been done at this level, the rigor and design variance limits research.

6. The simulation researcher wants to study the live experience of the learner in a complex, interprofessional simulation. Which method should the researcher choose?
   A. Quantitative method—NO, quantitative methods are objective, not subjective.
   B. Survey method—NO, a survey is a quantitative method.
   C. Mixed method—NO, although mixed method may include the learner's experience, it is not the best choice.
   D. Qualitative method—YES, qualitative methods are used to study learners' live experience.

7. Which of these is *not* a credible source for up-to-date, simulation research information?

   A. International Nursing Association for Clinical Simulation & Learning (INACSL)—NO, this is a credible source.
   B. SSH—NO, this is a credible source.
   C. Association of Standardized Patient Educators (ASPE)—NO, this is a credible source.
   D. Simulator vendors—YES, simulator vendors may be biased.

8. Which debriefing method has *not* been found to be the *most* effective?

   A. Advocacy–inquiry—NO, advocacy–inquiry is a good debriefing method, one that stimulates conversation and deeper reflection.
   B. Critical judgment—YES, critical judgment occurs when the facilitator/instructor judges participant performance. Adult learning principles show that students learn more when they are actively engaged.
   C. Plus–delta—NO, plus–delta is a good debriefing method, one that stimulates conversation and deeper reflection.
   D. Debriefing for Meaningful Learning (DML)—NO, DML is a good debriefing method, one that stimulates conversation and deeper reflection.

9. What does the research on debriefing indicate?

   A. Effective debriefers should provide process feedback early.—YES, sometimes the unexpected happens in a simulation, which drives the learner to an invaluable lesson.
   B. Effective debriefers should initially focus on whether outcomes were met. —NO, this is critical judgment, an ineffective strategy. Research shows that once learners have expressed their feelings, the debriefing should focus on what participants did well.
   C. The debriefing should include a comprehensive review of all critical outcomes.—NO, debriefing should be limited to a few critical points focused on the learning objectives.
   D. An instructor who is a content expert will be an effective debriefer.—NO, an effective debriefer needs to be skilled in the process of debriefing.

10. Which norm will promote a quality simulation experience?

   A. A consistent template to develop scenarios—NO, although this may be important, it is not the best answer.
   B. Ensuring that all participants have the same knowledge base—NO, this is probably not feasible with all participants.
   C. Use of a confidentiality contract—YES, ensuring that what happens in simulation and debriefing stays in simulation and debriefing prevents other groups of participants from knowing what to expect, thus having an unfair advantage.
   D. An enforced time limit—NO, this restricts discussion.

Answers and Rationales

to Practice Test

1. One of the *most* important learning processes of simulation is
   A. High fidelity—NO, fidelity is not the most important learning aspect.
   B. **Debriefing—YES, much of the learning takes place during debriefing.**
   C. Teamwork—NO, sometimes individual simulation is needed.
   D. Suspending disbelief—NO, this is important, but not the most important aspect of the learning process.

2. Foundational to providing appropriate feedback is the concept that feedback
   A. Is provided by the instructor to the learner—NO, this is not always necessary; it can be peer feedback.
   B. Contains things done well and improvements needed—NO, this is not always the format.
   C. **Is a cycle of information and reaction—YES, it is cyclical and responsive.**
   D. Does not always respond with performance improvement—NO, it should lead to improvements.

3. A learning difference that is not attributed to adult learners includes
   A. **Flexibility in conceptualization—YES, many of the adult learner patterns are ingrained from previous experiences.**
   B. Ingrained personality traits—NO, this is an attribute.
   C. Previous experiences with learning—NO, this is an attribute.
   D. Relationship patterns—NO, this is an attribute.

4. When discussing contextual factors that influence feedback the simulation educator must think about
   A. The content to be discussed—NO, this is the information to be conveyed.
   B. **The place of the feedback session—YES, this may impact the effectiveness of the feedback.**
   C. The aim of the feedback—NO, this is the purpose of the feedback.
   D. The feedback recipient—No, this is the learner.

5. An attribute of traditional education includes
   A. Teamwork—NO, it is unidirectional from teacher to student.
   B. Experiential learning—NO, this is student centered.

C. Constructivism—NO, it is unidirectional, the teacher constructs the knowledge for the student.

D. **Unidirectional communication—YES, it is usually teacher centered.**

6. The novice simulation educator needs additional mentoring because he is providing weak feedback to the learners as demonstrated by the statement

A. "I was able to observe the entire procedure."—NO, this is necessary to provide accurate feedback.

B. "Let's review the learning objective before we begin."—NO, this is directing the feedback.

C. "I will reobserve you performing the procedure."—NO, this is reevaluating learning.

D. **"I heard from the simulation technician that it went well."—YES, this is using secondhand observations.**

7. Of the seven elements of debriefing defined by Lederman (1984), what or who produces the impact of the experience?

A. The debriefer—NO, this is the simulation educator.

B. The participants—NO, the participants are always the learners and it is assumed that they are there because they want to learn.

C. The recollection—NO, this is part of the post-process.

D. **The simulation scenario—YES, this creates the impact.**

8. The best method to objectively evaluate learner performance when doing a specialty examination would be

A. Reflective writing—NO, this is not objective.

B. Peer evaluation—NO, this does not include an expert.

C. Concept map—NO, this is used to plan care.

D. **Performance checklist—YES, this will record the important steps of the examination.**

9. When debriefing, the scenario may be interpreted differently from what happened if

A. **Excessive time has passed.—YES, time may alter perception.**

B. The learners are at varied stages.—NO, this would not necessarily alter the perception of the event.

C. The debriefer lacks experience.—NO, this would not necessarily alter the perception of the event.

D. The objectives were not met.—NO, this would not necessarily alter the perception of the event, just the outcome intended.

10. When evaluating learners' simulation performance, the evaluation tool should demonstrate interrater reliability, which is

A. Different learners score similarly on the evaluation tool.—NO, this is tool validity.

B. The evaluation tool works the same, group after group.—NO, this is tool reliability.

    C. **Different evaluators rate the same performance similarly.—YES, this is interrater reliability.**

    D. The items on the tool are deemed appropriate by experts.—NO, this is content validity.

11. The art of debriefing occurs when the debriefer moves the discussion from the personal accounts of the scenario to

    A. The "hot-seat" participant's account—NO, the debriefer wants to move the discussion away from the emotional components.

    B. A descriptive account of the event—NO, this is done initially, but then the discussion should move to a more global account.

    C. **An objective global perspective—YES, this facilitates the meaning of the event and promotes learning for future events.**

    D. A subjective descriptive account—NO, this is done in the initial phase.

12. A standardized (simulated) patient (SP) is used to demonstrate abnormal breath sounds. The SP has chronic obstructive pulmonary disease (COPD). This type of simulation is referred to as

    A. **A symptomatic SP—YES, this is an excellent learning opportunity.**

    B. An asymptomatic SP—NO, the patient actually has symptoms.

    C. Nonhealthcare provider instructor—NO, this is a trained SP to provide feedback.

    D. Confederate—NO, these are "other people" in the scenario that are not the patient.

13. A debriefing session should be tailored to the characteristics of the participants and

    A. The characteristics of the debriefer—NO, this is not relevant.

    B. The details of the experience—NO, this is not the global perspective of debriefing.

    C. **The learning objectives—YES, this is the important assessment during debriefing.**

    D. The feelings of the group—NO, this is dealt with initially, but it is not as important as discussing the learning objectives.

14. The three critical components found that influence learning in the simulation laboratory are

    A. Fidelity of the simulation, demeanor of the faculty, debriefing—NO, fidelity does not ensure success.

    B. Adequate preparation, skill of the faculty, and debriefing—NO, the faculty's skill is not as important as their demeanor in the learning situation.

    C. Fidelity of the simulation, demeanor of the faculty, and reflection—NO, these include adequate preparation, not just fidelity, demeanor, or reflection.

    D. **Adequate preparation, demeanor of the faculty, and debriefing—YES, these have been noted to be critical.**

15. The best teaching role for debriefers to assume is

    A. Authoritarian—NO, this will not facilitate learning in a debriefing session.

    B. Instructor—NO, the learning has to be from self-analysis of the learners

    C. **Facilitator—YES, the debriefer should be a colearner who guides and directs.**

    D. Observer—NO, the debriefer's is an active role.

16. The simulation situation that depicts a formative evaluation of learning is

    A. Specific body system examinations for a course grade—NO, this is at the end of the course, so it is summative.

    B. The objective structured clinical examinations (OSCEs) for medical students—NO, this is summative.

    C. **A midterm evaluation of a procedure—YES, this can be a learning experience because there is time left for improvement.**

    D. A scenario in which the simulation educator uses a final patient safety checklist—NO, this is summative.

17. The debriefer who takes a "back seat" during a debriefing session and only guides the group when absolutely necessary is said to be taking a(n)

    A. **High level of facilitation—YES, a high level of facilitation means low involvement.**

    B. Intermediate level of facilitation—NO, the team requires analysis at a deep level.

    C. Low level of facilitation—NO, the team needs active instructor involvement.

    D. Lassie-faire commitment—NO, this is not appropriate in any case.

18. The best simulation method for a summative evaluation of a sterile dressing change is to

    A. Observe the learners in a group format assisting each other.—NO, it is difficult to apply a grade to each individual learner.

    B. Videotape the procedure using a high-fidelity mannequin.—NO, high fidelity is not needed.

    C. Have an SP scenario.—NO, an SP would not be a good choice.

    D. **Observe them on a task trainer using an objective checklist.—YES, this will evaluate their technique.**

19. The novice debriefer is telling the team all about his impressions of the simulation event. The best response by the experienced debriefer would be

    A. "Thank you for the impressions, please continue."—NO, the debriefer is overinstructing.

    B. "The students need to tell their impressions."—NO, the novice debriefer should be acknowledged, then explain nicely that the students should speak.

    C. **"Thank you, let's hear from the students."—YES, this is the professional way to redirect the debriefing.**

    D. "Can you sum up the experience for us?"—NO, the novice debriefer needs to allow the students to contribute.

20. Scenario "lifesavers" are used primarily to

    A. Decrease the stress during a simulation scenario.—NO, this is not the reason.

    B. **Preserve the learning objectives of the scenario.—YES, this is done so students do not get too far off track.**

C. Keep the SP on track.—NO, this is not the main reason.

D. Change the content of the scenario as needed.—NO, this is not the main reason.

21. The debriefer of a simulation scenario develops a tool for the students that includes a column titled "What went well" and a second column titled "What can we change?" This type of facilitation is described as

A. Framing—NO, this is introducing the event to highlight its relevance.

B. Target focused—NO, this is when target behaviors are pointed out in the briefing to be discussed in debriefing.

C. Advocacy–inquiry—NO, this technique frames the experiences that need change by referring back to the way they were observed by the debriefer.

D. **Plus–delta—YES, this method looks at what went well and what aspects need improvement.**

22. The novice simulation educator needs better understanding of using a scenario "lifesaver" when the expert simulation educator asks him why he changed the scenario and he states

A. **"The learners did something wrong, but it was not life threatening."— YES, this is not a reason to change the scenario because it does not affect the objectives and can be discussed during debriefing.**

B. "The learners did not understand the scenario."—NO, this is a major flaw and needs to be addressed.

C. "The learners were having difficulty suspending disbelief."—NO, this will interfere with meeting objectives.

D. "The scenario was too complex for the learners' level."—NO, this is a major flaw and needs to be addressed.

23. The debriefer says to a learner, "I observed you checking the patient's identification band once before you administered the medication. That makes me uncomfortable because it is a double-check process. Can you tell me what you were thinking at the time?" This form of refection is known as

A. Framing—NO, this is introducing the event to highlight its relevance.

B. Target focused—NO, this is when target behaviors are pointed out in the briefing to be discussed in debriefing.

C. **Advocacy–inquiry—YES, this technique frames the experiences that need change by referring back to the way they were observed by the debriefer.**

D. Plus–delta—NO, this is listing what went well and what needs to be changed or improved during a scenario.

24. An example of a simulation scenario "lifesaver" from "within" would be

A. Stopping the scenario to get learners back on track—NO, this is a lifesaver from outside.

B. **Changing the patient's vital signs in order to demonstrate decomposition—YES, this is occurring within the scenario even though it may be controlled from outside the room.**

C. Telling the learners over the microphone that the IV is wide open—NO, this is a lifesaver from outside.

D. Coming into the simulation room and providing an instruction in intubation—NO, this is a lifesaver from outside.

25. When there is more than one debriefer, a technique that is effective to present opposing sides is

A. **Good cop–bad cop—YES, this promotes group cohesion.**

B. Target focused—NO, this is when target behaviors are pointed out in the briefing to be discussed in debriefing.

C. Advocacy–inquiry—NO, this technique frames the experiences that need change by referring back to the way they were observed by the debriefer.

D. Plus–delta—NO, this is listing what went well and what needs to be changed or improved during a scenario.

26. An example of a scenario "lifesaver" from "outside" would be

A. Changing the electrocardiogram (EKG) pattern on the monitor—NO, this is from within.

B. Telling the learners, through the mannequin, that he has a pain level of 8—NO, this is from within.

C. Having the SP demonstrate signs of an acute abdomen—NO, this is from within.

D. **Stopping the scenario to clarify the difference between respiratory wheezes and rhonchi—YES, this is a lifesaver and is needed to keep the students on track.**

27. An expert who brings specialized instruction postscenario to an experienced group of learners may be

A. An advanced student—NO, this person does not have the expertise.

B. A simulation technician—NO, this person also would not have the expertise.

C. A simulation educator—NO, this person may have the expertise, but do all debriefing levels.

D. **A content debriefer—YES, this person is an expert in this health-related area.**

28. One of the main learning strategies used in debriefing is

A. Information gathering—NO, this may be a part, but is not one of the main learning strategies.

B. **Reflective learning—YES, the student identifies what he or she did well and what could be done better through reflection.**

C. Discussion—NO, this may be a part, but is not one of the main learning strategies.

D. Socratic questioning—NO, this may be a part, but is not one of the main learning strategies.

29. The novice simulation educator needs further orientation when he stops a scenario for "in-scenario" debriefing, when he states

A. "Let's start that procedure over because the field is contaminated."—NO, if the aim is to teach a skill, it may be appropriate to stop the procedure.

B. "Stop the procedure; the mannequin is malfunctioning."—NO, it may be necessary if equipment is malfunctioning.

    C. **"Let's stop and talk about how you are feeling about the event."—YES, reflection should be done at the conclusion of the scenario.**

    D. "Stop the procedure to realign the catheter in order for it to work."—NO, if the aim is to teach a skill, it may be appropriate to stop the procedure.

30. During debriefing, the type of reflective learning that is used is

    A. Reflection in action—NO, this would be done during the scenario.

    B. **Reflection on action—YES, looking back on what took place.**

    C. Reflective consciousness—NO, this is not a valid term.

    D. Reflective reasoning—NO, this is not a valid term.

31. When debriefing a large group of participants, it may be more effective if the debriefer(s)

    A. Ask them to write their reflections.—NO, the discussion and perceptions are important for all.

    B. Break them into small groups and debrief one group after another.—NO, time is a factor that influences perceptions.

    C. Have them all sit in a classroom and pass around a microphone.—NO, this is traditional and authoritarian.

    D. **Break them into small groups with different debriefers.—YES, this would be most effective.**

32. A constructivist theory of learning includes

    A. Establishing baseline knowledge for the learner—NO, the learner links new knowledge to previous experiences.

    B. Group analysis that assists the learning process—NO, it is individually constructed through the reality of the individual.

    C. **Learning that is individually constructed—YES, it is learner centered.**

    D. New knowledge that is categorized simplistically—NO, new knowledge is linked to previous knowledge.

33. The following setup depicts the "fishbowl" method of debriefing (Steinwachs, 1992)

    A. **Arrange the learners in an inner and outer circle.—YES, the students who want to actively participate move voluntarily from the outer to inner circle.**

    B. Arrange the learners in large circle.—NO, this would be too large to be effective.

    C. Arrange the learners in three or more concentric circles.—NO, this would alienate some students in the outer circles.

    D. Arrange the learners in two semicircles facing each other.—NO, this would also be too large to be effective.

34. One of the main purposes of interprofessional simulation experiences is to foster

    A. **Communication—YES, this is to promote patient safety.**

    B. Procedural competence—NO, this is important, but does not have to occur interprofessionally.

    C. Role definition—NO, this is important, but does not have to occur interprofessionally.

    D. Scope of practice—NO, this is important, but does not have to occur interprofessionally.

35. During simulation debriefing, it is important to avoid creating "energy gaps." Therefore, simulation educators should try to (Steinwachs, 1992)

    A. Keep the group engaged.—NO, this is just facilitator or debriefer energy.

    B. Show enthusiasm.—NO, this is just facilitator or debriefer energy.

    C. **Seat learners next to each other. ——YES, so they feel as if they are part of a group.**

    D. Have learners make eye contact when speaking.—NO, this may still include excess space between learners.

36. Using simulation to identify "tacit team voice" with interprofessional teams that have been together for a time is helpful to accommodate

    A. Differences in culture—NO, the team has been functioning together.

    B. Differences in roles—NO, the team has been functioning together.

    C. Conflict—NO, the team has been functioning together.

    D. **Newcomers to the team—YES, assimilating a new member into an established team is difficult.**

37. One of the major ways that debriefing contributes to simulation education is that it

    A. Provides the debriefer's instructions to the group—NO, this is not just about correcting or instructing.

    B. Helps learners to increase procedural proficiency—NO, that is done with task trainers.

    C. **Brings closure to the experience—YES, this helps the student to process events and place them in perspective.**

    D. Develops individual self-efficacy—NO, debriefing is done in a group.

38. Kneebone (2005) describes simulation as a method of learning with which of these four key aspects for healthcare providers?

    A. **Assisted learning, psychomotor skills learning, situated learning, and affective learning—YES, these are the four learning components.**

    B. Assisted learning, psychomotor skills learning, cognitive learning, and professional role development—NO, role development is not included.

    C. Professional role development, skills learning, cognitive learning, and affective learning—NO, role development is not included.

    D. Psychomotor skills learning, affective learning, team learning, and situated learning—NO, team learning is not included.

39. The novice in simulation education needs further instructions about debriefing when she states that debriefing

    A. **"Tells the entire scenario all over again."—YES, this is not what debriefing does.**

    B. "Focuses on perceptions."—NO, this is a big part of debriefing.

    C. "Provides closure for the learners."—NO, this is a big part of debriefing.

    D. "Adds useful insights."—NO, this is a big part of debriefing.

40. Successful deliberate practice (DP) involves four components, which include

    A. Knowledge facilitation, skill assessment, feedback, and reflection—NO, knowledge facilitation is a prerequisite and not part of DP.

    B. **Repetitive performance, skill assessment, feedback, and increased skill performance—YES, these are key to deliberate practice.**

C. Knowledge facilitation, skill performance, reflection, and increased skill performance—NO, reflection is not a component of pure skill development.
D. Repetitive performance, reflection, feedback, and increased skill performance—NO, reflection is not a component.

41. After a simulation scenario, the learners rate their own performance and use the rating as a talking point in the debriefing session. This is referred to as
A. Pre-debriefing—NO, this is not the terminology used.
B. **Self-debriefing—YES, this has been studied as a means to debrief.**
C. Peer debriefing—NO, this is done by another student.
D. Reflection—NO, this is less about rating and more about discussing perspective.

42. When developing an evaluation instrument, *content validity* includes
A. Items that are equitable in difficulty—NO, this adds to total test reliability.
B. **Items that measure the elements of the construct being tested—YES, the items measure the correct content that was taught.**
C. Items that yield the same results over and over—NO, this is reliability.
D. Items that discriminate learners who do not know the content—NO, this is item discrimination.

43. A tool used to distribute roles and responsibilities among simulation learners during a scenario that can be used to promote active learning for all the participants, is a
A. Rubric—NO, this is used for evaluation.
B. Content module—NO, this is not a term.
C. Team description—NO, this is not a term.
D. **Collaborative script—YES, this describes people's roles.**

44. Evaluating instrument *reliability* offers simulation educators the knowledge that the instrument can
A. Test the construct it is meant to test.—NO, this is construct validity.
B. Test the content it is meant to test.—NO, this is content validity.
C. **Yield the same results in different groups.—YES, it is consistently effective or ineffective.**
D. Yield the same results in the same group at a later date.—NO, in different groups.

45. A simulation educator understands that to produce the best physical fidelity, the scenario about a motor vehicle accident trauma victim's arrival to the emergency department should be conducted
A. In a simulation laboratory set up as a trauma bay—NO, this would not produce the best physical fidelity.
B. In a simulation laboratory set up like an examination room—NO, this would not produce the best physical fidelity.
C. **In an emergency department—YES, this is the actual environment.**
D. On the road where the accident occurred—NO, the scenario starts in the emergency department.

46. Curriculum recommendations for using simulation learning experiences for healthcare professionals include

    A. Use of simulation in clinical courses—NO, simulation should be integrated for all courses.
    B. Simulation of interprofessional events to promote communication—NO, this is one great use, but there are other uses.
    C. **Use of simulation throughout the curriculum—YES, students will use it more effectively if it is familiar to them.**
    D. Simulation for key procedures needed by each profession—NO, it can help learners with many aspects, not just psychomotor.

47. The simulation educator is trying to increase the psychological fidelity for a scenario that deals with end-of-life issues. The best mechanism to do this would be to

    A. **Hire an actor who is educated as an SP.—YES, this will provide the best psychological fidelity for the situation.**
    B. Use a high-fidelity mannequin that can simulate tears.—NO, this will not produce the best psychological fidelity.
    C. Videotape the scenario to use in debriefing to evaluate emotions.—NO, this is completed after the needed fidelity.
    D. Have other learners act as family members around the bedside.—NO, this will not produce the best psychological fidelity because they may not have acting experience.

48. Virtual reality (VR) simulators are *most* effectively used for

    A. Common procedures—NO, task trainers are used for these.
    B. **Complex procedures—YES, such as invasive cardiology procedures.**
    C. Interpersonal skills—NO, it is usually an interface with a computer.
    D. Decision making—NO, although some have algorithms, most are used for procedures.

49. The simulation educator is worried about the feel of the granulated skin on a mannequin that is simulating a burn patient. The simulation educator is concerned about the

    A. Physical fidelity—NO, this is the place in which it is held.
    B. Environmental fidelity—No, this is what surrounds the room.
    C. **Equipment fidelity—YES, this may be a shortfall of the mannequin's plastic.**
    D. Psychological fidelity—NO, this is the affective domain of the summation experience.

50. The simulation educator is developing a scenario for healthcare learners to focus on health history taking. The best simulation method to develop would be

    A. A high-fidelity mannequin—NO, this may not interact with the learner the way a person would.
    B. A task trainer—NO, this is better used to learn procedures.
    C. VR—NO, this is better used to learn procedures and decision making.
    D. **An SP—YES, SPs make the scenario more "real."**

51. The simulation educator is setting up the simulation room to depict the room of a confused patient. The simulation educator is ensuring
    A. Physical fidelity—NO, this is the place of the simulation experience.
    B. **Environmental fidelity—YES, this is the space in which the scenario takes place.**
    C. Equipment fidelity—NO, this has to do with the actual equipment used during a simulation experience.
    D. Psychological fidelity—NO, this is the affective domain of the summation experience.

52. The best method of simulation to use to combine communication and procedural skills is
    A. High-fidelity and low-fidelity mannequins—NO, this is not best for communication.
    B. Task trainer and VR—NO, this is not best for communication.
    C. **Task trainer and SP—YES, the task is done on the part-task trainers and the SP is spoken to.**
    D. VR and high-fidelity mannequin—NO, this is not best for communication.

53. The simulation educator understands that the novice simulation educator needs additional mentoring when she states
    A. **"I think that student learning outcomes will be better if the mannequins look more real."—YES, fidelity does not assure learning outcomes are met.**
    B. "I think that this fidelity is adequate for the objectives of this simulation."—NO, the fidelity should be addressed according to the learning outcomes.
    C. "I believe that the method of simulation must be coherent with the learning objectives."—NO, the fidelity should be addressed according to the learning outcomes.
    D. "The student learning outcomes may be able to be met with different simulation methods."—NO, different simulation methods can address learning outcomes.

54. Scaffolding scenarios and feedback to learners provide the learners with
    A. Different perspectives—NO, this is not the purpose.
    B. **Progressive knowledge building—YES, this helps students understand increasingly complex issues.**
    C. More reflective time—NO, this is not the purpose.
    D. Self-pacing—NO, although this can be incorporated, it is not the purpose.

55. The learners describe the respirations of the SP in breaths per minute. This is describing the simulation "realism" in which mode?
    A. Fidelity—NO, this has to do with the overall realistic portrayal of the scenario.
    B. **Physical—YES, physical modes of realism are described in measurable terms.**
    C. Semantical—NO, this has to do with description of the events.
    D. Phenomenal—NO, this has to do with affective elements in a scenario.

56. Serious gaming can be described as

    A. **Designed learning experiences—YES, these are well-designed learning experiences.**
    B. Free-flow decisional experiences—NO, the learning is structured by design.
    C. Fun learning with self-developed objectives—NO, there are objectives established.
    D. Interactive fun activities—NO, there are learning objectives.

57. A scenario is set up so the learners find a patient who is unresponsive, and they need to react to the situation and start cardiopulmonary resuscitation. This scenario prompts a cognitive structure process for learners to understand that they need to acknowledge the situation. This would be a

    A. Secondary affective-promoting frame—NO, secondary frames are not described in simulation; they are referred to as modulations.
    B. Modulation of a skill—NO, the skill needed and thought process are direct in this situation.
    C. Social primary frame—NO, this does not call for interaction.
    D. **Natural primary frame—YES, this is a physical occurrence that needs attention.**

58. Creating an avatar to interact in a learning game is establishing a(n)

    A. Learning objective—NO, this is done prior to developing the game.
    B. Identity—NO, the person's identity is not specified.
    C. **Pseudonymity—YES, this is the term used for avatar identities.**
    D. Dual role—NO, this is not the term used.

59. Learners in the simulation lab are briefed on a scenario. The simulation educator asks them to sign a contract that states they will treat this scenario as a real situation. The simulation educator is asking them to

    A. Acknowledge an informed consent—NO, this is not the purpose.
    B. Regulate their behavior and not laugh—NO, this is not the purpose, but is part of the expectations.
    C. **Suspend disbelief—YES, learners must understand that the scenario should be treated as real.**
    D. Interact professionally—NO, this is not the purpose, but is part of the expectations.

60. In serious gaming, endogenous games include games that

    A. **Have context and game play linked—YES, there is a purpose to the game.**
    B. Have context outside the actual game play—NO, this describes exogenous games.
    C. Provide context before the game—NO, the context is linked.
    D. Contain "in situ" instructions during the game—NO, the content is linked to the game.

61. A simulation scenario calls for a patient with an allergic reaction to an antibiotic. The SP asks the healthcare learner to look at the rash on his chest, which is not actually present. The healthcare provider examines the chest of the SP. By doing so, the healthcare learner is supporting which of the following simulation concepts?

    A. Moulage—NO, this is when the SP or mannequin has simulated physical signs on them.
    B. DP—NO, this is repeating a skill.
    C. Realism—NO, this is one of the theoretical bases for simulation.
    D. **As if—YES, this is suspending disbelief in a situation.**

62. The SP is trained to demonstrate hyporeflexia for learners when they are checking deep tendon reflexes. The SP is considered

    A. **An asymptomatic SP—YES, the SP is just "pretending" the symptom.**
    B. A symptomatic SP—NO, these are SPs who actually have the symptom.
    C. A confederate—NO, these are other people in the scenario.
    D. A hybrid situation—NO, this is usually an SP with a task trainer.

63. A simulation educator asks the learners to sign a statement that they will treat the scenario as if it is a real patient situation. The document they sign is referred to as a

    A. **Fiction contract—YES, this alerts the student to the expectation.**
    B. Informed consent—NO, this is not the terminology used.
    C. Suspending disbelief contract—NO, this is not the terminology used.
    D. Promise document—NO, this is not the terminology used.

64. A healthcare learner needs to perform a summative physical assessment evaluation. The best simulation mode for this evaluation would be

    A. A high-fidelity mannequin—NO, this is difficult to position.
    B. A task trainer—NO, this is confined, usually, to only one body part.
    C. **An asymptomatic SP—YES, this is a real person portraying a patient.**
    D. A VR avatar—NO, this will not demonstrate actual technique.

65. One of the key learning elements of simulation is that it can provide learners with

    A. Historical patient scenarios—NO, this would be any patient scenario that was experienced in the past.
    B. Common patient problems—NO, these can be gained in clinical practice.
    C. **Uncommon patient problems—YES, these may be difficult to experience in clinical practice.**
    D. Futuristic healthcare ideas—NO, learners are provided with actual clinical scenarios.

66. Types of test validity can be drawn from all of the following analyses EXCEPT

    A. Testing the constructs—NO, this is construct validity.
    B. Test content—NO, this is content validity.
    C. Relationship of test scores to other instruments—NO, this is a valid method to check that an evaluation is assessing a concept similar to another instrument.
    D. **The relationship of test items to each other—YES, this is reliability.**

67. Nurse anesthesia learners need to practice how to do a spinal tap on a patient for a blood patch. The best type of simulation to teach this would be

   A. A high-fidelity mannequin—NO, this would not be easy to position.
   B. **A torso task trainer—YES, this is a great way to practice a procedure.**
   C. An SP—NO, this procedure should not be done on a human actor.
   D. VR—NO, this would not give the feel of the instruments.

68. A form of simulation in which a person spontaneously demonstrates a personality trait or a characteristic of a patient–provider interaction is called

   A. An asymptomatic SP—NO, the SP is trained.
   B. **Role-playing—YES, this can be done by an untrained person.**
   C. Hybrid simulation—NO, this is usually an SP and task trainer.
   D. A symptomatic SP—NO, the SP is trained.

69. The novice simulation educator needs further instruction about simulation when she states simulation is an asset because

   A. "There is no risk to actual patients."—NO, this is true.
   B. "Uncommon patient problems can be presented."—NO, this is true.
   C. "Simulation can be stopped for teaching purposes."—NO, this is true.
   D. **"Each simulation scenario cannot be standardized."—YES, they can be standardized.**

70. During an SP interaction, the simulation educator calls a "time-out" in order to have the

   A. SP describe what is happening—NO, this is not the reason for a "time-out."
   B. Learners reflect on what they are feeling—NO, this is not the reason for a "time-out."
   C. **Provide instruction by himself or herself—YES, this is done to provide the students with instructions.**
   D. Confederates redo their parts—NO, this is not the reason for a "time-out."

71. Nursing learners are learning how to insert a sterile urinary catheter. The best method of simulation to teach this procedure would be

   A. **Male and female torso task trainers—YES, this is the best way to learn an invasive procedure.**
   B. SPs—NO, this is invasive.
   C. High-fidelity mannequins—NO, this is cumbersome.
   D. VR—NO, actually doing the task will assist learning.

72. During a simulation "time-out," the SP

   A. Is removed from the room—NO, the SP is present for the instruction to the learner.
   B. Discusses the diagnosis—NO, the simulation educator instructs while the scenario is suspended.
   C. Remains in role and speaks—NO, the simulation educator instructs.
   D. **Goes into suspended animation—YES, the SP stops and then resumes the role.**

73. Combining a task trainer in a simulation environment with an SP, simulation educators can

    A. Deliver low-fidelity learning—NO, hybrid increases the fidelity.
    B. Simulate VR in a simulation room—NO, VR is computer based.
    C. **Change a low-fidelity simulator into a high-fidelity experience—YES, using a person changes the scenario to one that has procedure and interaction.**
    D. Provide a DP situation—NO, this is usually done with task trainers.

74. The design of the simulation scenario should be determined by

    A. The simulation educator—NO, the learning objectives need to dictate the design of the scenario.
    B. The level of the learners—NO, the learning objectives need to dictate the design of the scenario and they should consider the level of the learners.
    C. The fidelity of the mannequins—NO, the learning objectives need to dictate the design of the scenario.
    D. **The learning objectives—YES, meeting the learning objectives is the goal.**

75. The last phase of the Simulation Learning Pyramid (Doerr & Murray, 2008) is

    A. Debriefing—NO, it is (1) the simulation plan, (2) the simulation, (3) debriefing, (4) transference.
    B. Simulation plan—NO, it is (1) the simulation plan, (2) the simulation, (3) debriefing, (4) transference.
    C. **Transference—YES, transferring knowledge to actual practice.**
    D. The simulation—NO, it is (1) the simulation plan, (2) the simulation, (3) debriefing, (4) transference.

76. During a scenario, using a high-fidelity mannequin as a recovering alcoholic, a faculty member takes the role of the patient's belligerent spouse. The role being played by the faculty member is that of a

    A. Standardized patient—NO, this is a trained person who acts as a patient.
    B. Simulated patient—NO, this is a trained person who acts as a patient.
    C. **Confederate—YES, this is someone other than the patient.**
    D. Extra—NO, this is called a confederate or participant.

77. To develop a simulation plan, the simulation educator understands that the first step is to

    A. Decide on a case to develop—NO, first, you need learning objectives.
    B. Script the SPs—NO, objectives are needed first.
    C. **Develop the objectives—YES, these determine the purpose of the experience.**
    D. Establish time limits—NO, this is done after the objectives are established.

78. An important aspect of briefing learners is to

    A. Have them decide what they need to learn—NO, the objectives should be done first before other parts of the scenario.
    B. Develop the scenario—NO, this should be completed.

    C. Discuss debriefing expectations—NO, this will be done after the simulation scenario.

    D. **Orient them to the equipment—YES, this should decrease anxiety about simulation.**

79. "Confederates" used in simulation scenarios are actually

    A. **Other people in the scenario besides the learners and SPs—YES, they can be consultants, family, or ancillary healthcare providers.**

    B. SPs—NO, they are not in the patient role.

    C. Mannequins with moulage—NO, they are actors in a role other than the patient.

    D. The learners who have secondary roles in the simulation experience—NO, all learners learn in a simulation experience, even those who do not have a primary role.

80. A learner is able to perform a procedure with real patients after DP in the simulation laboratory. This demonstrates which step of Kilpatrick's (1998) four-level training evaluation model?

    A. Reaction—NO, this is how the learner perceives and reacts to the simulation experience.

    B. Learning—NO, this is the acquisition of knowledge from the simulation experience.

    C. **Behavior—YES, this is putting the knowledge into practice.**

    D. Results—NO, this is the outcome of patient care.

81. One excellent method used to enhance transference of knowledge is to

    A. Develop realistic moulage.—NO, this will help, but it is not the best method.

    B. Use SPs with symptoms.—NO, this will help, but it is not the best method.

    C. **Have the simulation experience "in situ."—YES, having the simulation experience in the actual place in which the healthcare learners would experience it, such as an emergency department or operating room, will help transference.**

    D. Have the simulation experience in a well-equipped laboratory.—NO, this will help, but it is not the best method.

82. Directive feedback provides the learner with

    A. Questions to reflect on—NO, reflection is not encouraged, direct knowledge for change is.

    B. **Items that require correction—YES, this is one of the main purposes.**

    C. Suggestions so learners can facilitate their own correction—NO, this is facilitative feedback.

    D. A grade for the experience—NO, it is usually formative feedback, not summative.

83. Simulation educators understand that a tenet of adult learning theory is that adults

    A. Do not need to know why they should learn something; they just need to know how to do it—NO, adult learners like to know why.

    B. They are interdependent learners—NO, they are independent learners.

C. **Like things that are immediately applicable—YES, adults learn for a direct purpose.**

D. Like subject-centered rather than life-centered learning—NO, they are life centered.

84. Facilitative feedback provides the learner with

   A. Questions to reflect on—NO, it provides suggestions to the learner.

   B. Items that require correction—NO, this is directive feedback.

   C. **Suggestions so learners can facilitate their own correction—YES, it helps them focus on what needs improvement.**

   D. A grade for the experience—NO, it is a formative evaluation.

85. According to Kolb's experiential learning theory (1984), learning is

   A. Sequential—NO, it is a continuous process.

   B. Newly found knowledge—NO, it is built on previous experiences.

   C. Involves transaction between people—NO, it is between a person and the environment.

   D. **A holistic process—YES, it has many aspects.**

86. A *fundamental attribution* error of a learner during a feedback session is

   A. **Blaming external factors—YES, this is not being accountable for actions.**

   B. Not understanding the objectives—NO, this is blaming external factors, and not taking accountability.

   C. Admitting to being unprepared—NO, this is blaming external factors, and not taking accountability.

   D. Discussing the scenario with peers—NO, this is blaming external factors, and not taking accountability.

87. According to Kolb's experiential learning theory (1984), four different abilities are needed by the learner. The ability to become involved in a simulation scenario fully without bias is which ability?

   A. **Concrete experience (CE)—YES, this allows the learner to focus on the scenario at hand.**

   B. Reflective observation (RO)—NO, this is considering other perspectives.

   C. Abstract conceptualization (AC)—NO, this is developing theories that logically fit into the knowledge scheme.

   D. Active experimentation (AE)—NO, this is decision making.

88. Using *interactional justice* during a feedback session means

   A. Describing what went right and then wrong—NO, this does not always consider the psychological needs of the learner.

   B. **Balancing the feedback with the psychological needs of the learner—YES, this provides a positive learning experience.**

   C. Providing negative feedback only when necessary—NO, this does not always consider the psychological needs of the learner.

   D. Providing positive feedback only—NO, this does not give them information for improvement.

89. A simulation learner gives concentrated glucose during a scenario that simulates a diabetic patient in severe hypoglycemia. The learner is demonstrating
which learning ability identified by Kolb (1984)?

   A. CEs—NO, this is immersion into a learning situation with an open mind.
   B. RO—NO, this is considering other perspectives.
   C. AC—NO, this is developing theories that logically fit into the knowledge
      scheme.
   D. **AE—YES, this is decision making and problem solving.**

90. Feedback provided to learners is more beneficial if it is

   A. **Specific—YES, this will assist them to improve.**
   B. General—NO, they need specific feedback to improve.
   C. Conceptual—NO, they need specific feedback to improve.
   D. Overarching—NO, they need specific feedback to improve.

91. The goal of DP is

   A. **Performance improvement—YES, practice increases proficiency.**
   B. Getting practice before clinical experience—NO, even practitioners in
      clinical practice need to keep up skills and can benefit from DP.
   C. Developing intricate skills—NO, it develops all types of skills.
   D. Pure repetition—NO, it is repetition with refinement.

92. The biggest disadvantage of using SPs is

   A. Preparation—NO, this is time-consuming, but beneficial.
   B. Differences in acting for different learners—NO, the scenarios can be
      standardized.
   C. **Cost—YES, actors may be expensive.**
   D. Recruitment—NO, this is usually not the main issue.

93. A primary goal of a simulation educator is to

   A. Develop a realistic simulation scenario—NO, realism does not guarantee
      effectiveness.
   B. Establish teacher–student boundaries—NO, this is not the purpose.
   C. **Create a safe environment—YES, this promotes risk-free learning.**
   D. Decrease mistakes during simulation experiences—NO, mistakes can be
      learning experiences.

94. Trained SPs are able to provide

   A. **Assessment feedback—YES, they can assist with providing valuable
      information to the learner.**
   B. Course grade—NO, this is the responsibility of the simulation educator
      or faculty.
   C. Learning objectives—NO, this is the responsibility of the simulation
      educator or faculty.
   D. Summative evaluations—NO, this is the responsibility of the simulation
      educator or faculty.

95. Kneebone (2005) believes that simulation educators should do all of the following EXCEPT

  A. Encourage DP—NO, this is correct.
  B. **Provide peer tutoring—YES, expert tutors should be provided.**
  C. Correlate simulation with real-life experiences—NO, this is correct.
  D. Maintain a learner-centered environment—NO, this is correct.

96. SPs have their roles and script provided by

  A. Simulation educators—NO, this could be possible, but usually this role is called patient instructor.
  B. **Patient instructors—YES, they specifically prep SPs.**
  C. Lead actors—NO, they are not used.
  D. Theater coaches—NO, these are usually not available.

97. The first level of Kirkpatrick's (1959) four-level learning theory is

  A. Learning—NO, this is Level 2.
  B. Results—NO, this is Level 4.
  C. **Reaction—YES, this is Level 1.**
  D. Behavior—NO, this is Level 3.

98. A simulation scenario is about delivering bad news to family members of a motor vehicle accident victim. The best simulation methodology would be

  A. A high-fidelity mannequin—NO, this would not provide the human interaction needed.
  B. A low-fidelity mannequin—NO, this would not provide the human interaction needed.
  C. VR—NO, this would not provide the human interaction needed.
  D. **An SP—YES, because this is in the affective realm.**

99. The last level of Kirkpatrick's (1959) four-level learning theory is

  A. Learning—NO, this is Level 2.
  B. **Results—YES, this is Level 4.**
  C. Reaction—NO, this is Level 1.
  D. Behavior—NO, this is Level 3.

100. Characteristics of an SP that need to be considered for realism include

  A. Height and weight—NO, although these could help the realism, patients come in all sizes.
  B. **Age and ethnicity—YES, demographics may be important to the realness of the scenario.**
  C. Hair and skin color—NO, this is not as important as age and ethnicity.
  D. Education and articulation—NO, this is not as important as age and ethnicity because patients are at all different educational levels.

101. The best simulation method to promote changes in learner behavior in the affective domain is

  A. High-fidelity mannequins—NO, these can be used, but lack interrelational realism.
  B. Task trainers—NO, these are impersonal.

    C. **SPs—YES, live actors may be important to the realness of the scenario.**
    D. VR—NO, this is also more impersonal.

102. The best simulation method to promote changes in learner behavior in the psychomotor domain is

    A. High-fidelity mannequins—NO, this can be used, but usually is done for more situational learning.
    B. **Task trainers—YES, because this promotes deliberate practice.**
    C. SPs—NO, a task trainer allows repeated procedures.
    D. VR—NO, this is usually a computer interface.

103. A learning method used during debriefing that leads learners to the higher order of critical thinking is

    A. Faculty instruction—NO, this is teacher centered.
    B. Peer discussion—NO, this may assist, but it depends on the group.
    C. Direct questioning—NO, this lends itself to "yes" and "no" answers.
    D. **Reflection—YES, reflection encourages learners to self-modulate behavior.**

104. The *best* role for a debriefer to assume is

    A. Instructor—NO, this does not promote learner reflection.
    B. Coach—NO, this may be a method, but is more like coaxing than guiding.
    C. Advisor—NO, this is authoritarian.
    D. **Facilitator—YES, the learners should discover knowledge.**

105. The choice of fidelity when planning a simulation-based learning (SBL) experience should depend on the

    A. Skill of the simulation educator—NO, this should not be the determining factor.
    B. **Learning outcomes—YES, the learning outcomes should be considered when choosing a method.**
    C. Equipment available—NO, this should not be the determining factor.
    D. Cost—NO, this should not be the determining factor.

106. The *best* simulation method to use to teach professional behavior and decision making for an ethical issue is

    A. Low-fidelity mannequins—NO, this is impersonal.
    B. Task trainers—NO, this is impersonal.
    C. **SPs—YES, human interaction is the best method.**
    D. VR—NO, this may be impersonal.

107. Clinical management of the simulation laboratory by the simulation educator includes all of the following aspects EXCEPT

    A. Scheduling—NO, this is part of clinical management.
    B. Management of equipment—NO, this is part of clinical management.
    C. **Content expertise—YES, the simulation educator does not have to be the content expert for all simulation learning experiences.**
    D. Budgeting—NO, this is part of clinical management.

108. Factors that influence the SBL experience include all of the following EXCEPT
    A. Active learning—NO, this affects the SBL experience.
    B. **Cost of equipment—YES, expensive equipment does not guarantee best practice.**
    C. Faculty–student interaction—NO, this affects the SBL experience.
    D. Realism—NO, this affects the SBL experience.

109. Psychological fidelity can best be ensured by using
    A. SPs—NO, this may not ensure it if it is a tense interpersonal situation.
    B. The learning outcomes to guide the simulation experience—NO, it depends on what the learning outcomes are.
    C. Experienced simulation educators—NO, this may not ensure it.
    D. **A learner-centered approach—YES, the learner becomes the focus.**

110. The *best* simulation method to teach tracheotomies to otolaryngology residents is to use
    A. Patients that need the procedure—NO, this may be difficult to find.
    B. **Task trainers—YES, this is procedural practice.**
    C. Intermediate-fidelity mannequins—NO, the entire mannequin is not needed.
    D. VR—NO, the skill should be manually practiced.

111. The *best* simulation method to use for a delicate open-heart surgical procedure is
    A. Patients who need the procedure—NO, this is not realistic.
    B. Task trainers—NO, these are better for gross anatomy procedures.
    C. Intermediate-fidelity mannequins—NO, it is best done as a complex procedure on VR.
    D. **VR—YES, this method is good for complex procedures.**

112. Positive outcomes of interprofessional simulation education include all of the following EXPECT
    A. It decreases anxiety in emergencies—NO, this is true.
    B. **It increases autonomy—YES, there is an increase in teamwork, not individual autonomy.**
    C. It promotes communication—NO, this is true.
    D. It promotes retention of skills—NO, this is true.

113. When using volunteers as SPs, the simulation educator must
    A. Offer some compensation—NO, this is not necessary; they volunteered.
    B. **Maintain confidentiality—YES, this is important in all patient situations.**
    C. Get institutional review board (IRB) approval—NO, this is not necessary unless it is being published.
    D. Have insurance to cover any health issues diagnosed—NO, this is not necessary if the SPs have insurance.

114. An interprofessional healthcare team is responding to an SP emergency. The team does not recognize the need for a critical airway on the patient and it fails to call the anesthetist. The simulation educator would best intervene by

    A. **Stopping the scenario—YES, this may be the best method to get the team back on track.**
    B. Giving instructions through the microphone—NO, this is not realistic and does not promote critical thinking.
    C. Giving the team a hint from the doorway—NO, this is not realistic and does not promote critical thinking.
    D. Providing a written note to a team member to check the airway—NO, this is not realistic and does not promote critical thinking.

115. The simulation educator develops environmental fidelity when he

    A. Adds moulage to the mannequin—NO, this does not ensure environmental fidelity.
    B. Uses a hybrid SP and a task trainer—NO, this is equipment fidelity.
    C. Uses a high-fidelity mannequin as the speaking patient—NO, this is equipment fidelity.
    D. **Sets up the room to resemble an emergency department bay—YES, this is realistic.**

Index